WITHDRAWN

A Short Textbook of
MEDICAL MICROBIOLOGY

University Medical Texts

General Editor
Selwyn Taylor D.M., M.CH. [OXON], F.R.C.S.

A Short Textbook of Medicine Fifth edition
J. C. Houston M.D., F.R.C.P.
C. L. Joiner M.D., F.R.C.P.
J. R. Trounce M.D., F.R.C.P.

A Short Textbook of Surgery Fourth edition
Selwyn Taylor D.M., M.CH., F.R.C.S.
L. T. Cotton M.CH., F.R.C.S.

A Short Textbook: Ear, Nose and Throat Second edition
R. Pracy M.B., F.R.C.S.
J. Siegler M.B., B.S., F.R.C.S., D.L.O.
P. M. Stell M.B., F.R.C.S.

A Short Textbook of Chemical Pathology Third edition
D. N. Baron M.D., D.SC., F.R.C.P., F.R.C.PATH.

A Short Textbook of Orthopaedics and Traumatology Second edition
J. N. Aston M.B., F.R.C.S.

A Short Textbook of Psychiatry Second edition
W. L. Linford Rees B.SC., M.D., F.R.C.P., D.C.M.

A Short Textbook of Venereology Second edition
R. D. Catterall F.R.C.P. (EDIN.)

A Short Textbook of Gynaecology and Obstetrics
G. D. Pinker M.D., F.R.C.S., F.R.C.O.G.
D. W. T. Roberts M.CHIR., F.R.C.S., F.R.C.O.G.

A Short Textbook of Paediatrics
P. Catzel M.D., B.CH., F.R.C.P., D.C.H.

A Short Textbook of Medical Statistics
Sir Austin Bradford Hill C.B.E., D.SC., PH.D., HON. D.SC. (OXON),
HON. M.D. (EDIN.) F.F.C.M. (HON.), F.R.C.P. (HON.), F.R.S.

A Short Textbook of Preventine Medicine for the Tropics
A. O. Lucas M.D., D.P.H., D.T.M. & H., F.R.C.P., S.M.HYG., F.M.C.P.H.
H. M. Gilles M.D., F.R.C.P., F.F.C.M., F.M.C.P.H., D.T.M. & H.

A SHORT TEXTBOOK OF
MEDICAL
MICROBIOLOGY

Fourth Edition

D. C. TURK DM, MRCP, FRCPath.

Consultant Microbiologist,
Regional Public Health Laboratory, Sheffield
Hon. Clinical Lecturer in Medical Microbiology,
University of Sheffield

I. A. PORTER MD, FRCPath.

Consultant Bacteriologist, City Hospital, Aberdeen
Hon. Clinical Senior Lecturer in Bacteriology, University of Aberdeen

HODDER AND STOUGHTON

LONDON   SYDNEY   AUCKLAND   TORONTO

British Cataloguing in Publication Data

Turk, David Charles
  A short textbook of medical microbiology.–4th ed.–
  (University medical texts).
  1. Medical microbiology
  I. Title II. Porter, Ian Alexander III. Series
  616.01   QR46

  ISBN 0–340–23256–0
  ISBN 0–340–23257–9 Pbk.

ISBN 0 340 23257 9 Unibook
    0 340 23256 0 Boards

First published 1965
Second edition 1969 Reprinted 1971, 1972
Third edition 1974 Reprinted 1975, 1976, 1977
Fourth edition 1978

Printed and bound in Great Britain
For Hodder & Stoughton Educational,
a division of Hodder & Stoughton Ltd,
Mill Road, Dunton Green, Sevenoaks, Kent
by Richard Clay (The Chaucer Press) Ltd,
Bungay, Suffolk

Editor's Foreword

The series of Short Textbooks which, in their green livery, have proved so popular over the years were originally conceived to provide an up-to-date and concise introduction for the student of medicine. I would like to pay a special tribute to the late John Maitland of Hodder and Stoughton who was indefatigable in launching what was then a new concept in medical publishing.

My wish then, as now, was that these books should be inexpensive and compact, should fit into the pocket of a white coat and become faithful friends. I hoped that they would be so well used that they would begin to fall apart when three or four years old and we could then provide a new edition. Most medical books if they are to keep pace with modern development need revising, and sometimes even rewriting, at intervals of about four years.

'Turk and Porter', as this volume is usually called has been one of the most popular books in the series since it first appeared. The authors knew quite clearly what the student must grasp, they knew exactly for whom they were writing and they wrote it. These are three of the basic requisites for a good book. But better than this they have continued through four editions to correct, rewrite and bring in new advances while always pruning anything which was no longer really necessary. It is surprising if one compares the first edition of 1965 with the present one how much change has taken place in microbiology.

True, some of it is due to a change in accent or fashion and some is due to more stress being placed on such subjects as virology and immunology. There has been a steady increase in information about infections rarely seen in the United Kingdom, but there are two good reasons for this. First the book finds increasing popularity overseas and second, the increase in the number of people travelling, especially by air, makes the occurrence of almost any disease in any country a real possibility.

I am certain this *Short Textbook of Medical Microbiology* will continue to attract new readers and for myself, I always keep a copy with the reference books on my desk.

Royal Postgraduate Medical School,   SELWYN TAYLOR
Hammersmith Hospital,
London W12 OHS
1978

Authors' Preface

Our aim as we have prepared each edition of this book has been to provide medical students with a concise, readable, up-to-date account of Medical Microbiology, which will help them to understand man's relationships with his microbial parasites and will prepare them for further reading in the subject and for an informed approach to the investigation of patients and to the prevention and treatment of microbial disease. We have repeatedly asked ourselves two questions: 'What is essential for this purpose?' and 'What can we safely leave out?'; and of course our answers to these have changed with the passage of time, and each new edition has involved substantial alterations. This Fourth Edition is no exception, as indicated in the next paragraph. We are happy that this book, as well as being popular with medical students in our own and various other countries, has been found helpful by many others—notably by paramedical workers and also by qualified doctors, even including trainee bacteriologists; but we continue to regard it as primarily a book for medical students.

The fact that this edition has about 10% more pages than the Third may suggest that we have relaxed our determination to keep the book short. The increase is in fact due to a change to larger and (in our opinion at least) more easily readable type. We have made space for new material by careful pruning out of all that seemed to be no longer relevant and accurate, and by shortening the section on Immunology; this has been largely rewritten and is now incorporated in a single chapter, in recognition of the availability of a number of excellent student textbooks on this subject written in recent years by professional immunologists. Other major changes include a new introduction to Chapter Nine (Bacteria), giving a more adequate explanation of the problems and systems of bacterial classification and nomenclature; expansion of the information given in Chapter Fourteen about choice and collection of specimens from patients; and extensive revision of Chapter Twenty-one (Antibacterial Drugs), with increased emphasis on the principles that should govern choice and administration of these drugs. A number of bacterial or virus pathogens not mentioned in previous editions have been recognized or have achieved notoriety since 1974 and have thus earned themselves places in this edition.

As before, we have given no details of laboratory methods, as we have assumed that our readers have opportunities to learn all that they need to know about these in practical classrooms or from other sources. Nor have we catered for readers who want practical instructions about the use of sterilizers, antiseptics, immunizing agents or antimicrobial drugs, though we trust that what they read here will enable them to understand the principles of the use of all these.

Suggestions for further reading are given at the ends of most chapters, but a few books that would qualify for mention in many places are mentioned here instead. Of the two volumes of *Medical Microbiology*, 12th edition, edited by R. Cruickshank and others (Churchill Livingstone, Edinburgh and London, vol. 1 1973, vol. 2 1975), the first is 'aimed at medical and science students and doctors', whereas the second contains more technical laboratory information. On the clinical side there are two excellent books entitled *Infectious Diseases*, one by A. B. Christie (Churchill Livingstone, Edinburgh and London, 2nd edition 1974) and the other by A. M. Ramsay and R. T. D. Emond (Heinemann, London, 2nd edition 1978).

We are indebted to Margaret A. J. Moffat, B.sc. (Hons. Bact.), Ph.D., Senior Lecturer in the Department of Bacteriology, University of Aberdeen, for valuable assistance in prevision of the chapter on viruses; to various other colleagues for suggestions and criticisms; and to Susan Devlin and Carol Shave of the publishers' staff for help in overcoming problems.

D.C.T.
I.A.P.
1978

Contents

PART I

INTRODUCTION

I

'Medical Microbiology'

Medical students of only a few years ago were taught 'Bacteriology'. That simple name was adequate. There was little to be taught about micro-organisms other than bacteria; and since bacteriology had grown up mainly as a para-medical subject there was no need to stress that they were studying *medical* bacteriology. The change of name from 'Bacteriology' to 'Medical Microbiology' reflects both the increase in knowledge of viruses and other non-bacterial micro-organisms of medical importance and the growth of microbiology as an independent science, no longer preoccuped with medical problems. It is an exciting science, with many fundamental biological advances to its credit; but it is not the subject of this book. However, to get our subject in perspective it may be helpful to think about some widely different approaches to the study of micro-organisms.

Naturally enough, the medical microbiologist has always been interested chiefly in micro-organisms that are parasites of man, especially those that are able to cause disease. He has tended to regard other organisms as unimportant, or as nuisances that contaminate his cultures or confuse him in other ways; but in general he has managed to keep clear of them by using cultural conditions more favourable to the growth of parasites. His culture media have mostly been made from meat broth, blood and other complex animal materials; their exact composition has not greatly concerned him provided that they have suited the requirements of the species which he has wanted to grow. In his attempts at classification he has been preoccupied with the problem of recognizing pathogens; and as ability to produce disease is not consistently linked with other microbial properties, he has used a different set of criteria for the subdivision of each group of organisms. Many of his tests have been, and still are, empirical and scientifically crude—for example he talks of bacteria producing 'acid' and 'gas' from a sugar or an alcohol without reference to the nature of the acid or gas or the mechanism of their production. Yet by such means he has gone a long way towards unravelling the problems of human microbial diseases and has provided clinicians with much valuable information. Similar empirical techniques have been successfully applied in other fields, such as veterinary medicine, agriculture and industry.

In sharp contrast to the view-point of the medical microbiologist is that of the academic microbiologist who is interested in micro-organisms for their own sake, and to whom the question whether they can cause disease is merely one aspect of their biology. He wants to know the minutiae of microbial structure, and his knowledge of these has increased greatly following the development of electron microscopy. He wants to know the details of microbial metabolism, and for this purpose he has to use media of defined chemical composition and apparatus that maintains continuous control of that composition even while metabolism is going on. He investigates mechanisms of microbial reproduction and genetics, and attempts to evolve classifications based upon the properties of the organisms themselves rather than upon what they do to other creatures. In all of these respects his discipline differs widely from the traditional approach of the medical microbiologist.

Paradoxical though it sounds, there are other students of micro-organisms who are not primarily interested in the organisms themselves or in the effects that they produce on other creatures. Many biologists, physiologists and biochemists use bacteria or fungi as relatively simple and manageable models in which to study processes that also occur in the cells of more complex organisms. Such workers have incidentally added much to our knowledge of micro-organisms. So have those biochemists who use them either as sources of interesting compounds or as tools with which to carry out chemical manipulations.

Although we have described them separately, these various disciplines overlap and learn from each other. Medical microbiology today owes an increasing amount to workers in other parts of the microbiological field. The medical microbiologist is well advised to keep an eye on what these colleagues are doing, and to make use of their discoveries in his own territory. The medical student and the clinician, however, have no need to keep abreast of microbiology as a whole, nor do they need to know more than a little of the technology of medical microbiology. What matters to them is the help that medical microbiology can give in the understanding, investigation, treatment and (best of all) prevention of microbial diseases of man. That is what this book is about.

Major Changes Impending

The traditional task of the routine medical microbiology department is to look for and to identify actual or potential disease-producing micro-organisms in material from patients, and then to determine, so far as laboratory tests permit, what antimicrobial drugs—if any—are likely to be effective against them when given to the patients. The usual approach to these problems is to examine some of the material, suitably stained, under the microscope for preliminary clues, to grow the organisms in culture, to purify them by further cultures if necessary, and then by still further cultures to test their sensitivities to various drugs. Such procedures may take several days to produce results that are useful in the management of patients, and they are carried out by hand because of the technical problems of designing machines that can handle large numbers of specimens without cross-contamination.

The last few years have seen exciting advances in the development of rapid methods and of automation in medical microbiology. There are new ways of identifying organisms precisely within a few minutes of the arrival of a specimen in the laboratory—for example, by detection of specific microbial components by countercurrent immunoelectro-phoresis (C.I.E.), or of specific microbial metabolic products by gas-liquid chromatography (G.L.C.). A sensitive turbimetric system can provide early evidence of bacterial multiplication in a suitable liquid, as can measurement of release of radio-active CO_2 from a culture medium containing ^{14}C-labelled glucose; and since such procedures can also give indications, within the first few hours, of failure of bacterial multiplica-tion in the presence of certain drugs, it may well be possible to recom-mend the appropriate treatment for an infection well before the offending organism is identified. The number of bacteria in a liquid (e.g. a urine specimen) can be rapidly determined by microcalorimetry (a very sensi-tive means of detecting their heat output), or by luminescence biometry, in which the amount of bacterial adenine triphosphate—and thus the number of bacteria—in a given amount of the liquid can be assessed by measuring the brightness of the flash of light emitted when that amount is mixed with a standard preparation of luciferin–luciferase (the 'lighting system' of fireflies); such methods make it possible to recognize many specimens as not requiring further bacteriological investigation because they do not contain bacteria in the numbers found when there is a true infection. Problems of automated processing of microbiological speci-mens are being overcome, and the consequent increase in the capacity of laboratories to process large numbers of specimens will doubtless lead to the development of more screening tests. These will make possible the rapid exclusion of some of the possible diagnoses in appropriate cases—a contribution which is often at least as useful to the clinician as the belated production of a positive report.

These developments have not yet revolutionized the practice of routine microbiological laboratories, and so for the present have not made necessary radical revision of such technical information as we give in this book. Any subsequent edition will certainly have to take account of major alterations, not only of technical practices but of outlook within the laboratories and of the ways in which they can most effectively provide help for the clinician and so for the patient.

2

Historical Perspective

Man has always lived in an environment that abounded with minute living organisms, and he has always carried them in countless billions around and within his person; but because of their tiny size they escaped his direct observation until recent times. However, from the beginning of history some of their effects—especially those that he did not like—have commanded his attention and interest. The science of microbiology can be said to be little more than a century old, having its origins in the work of Louis Pasteur in the 1850's, but that great breakthrough was preceded by many centuries of speculation and investigation.

The Concept of Contagion

From the most ancient writings we can learn that plagues and pestilences were already well-recognized features of human existence. Not being able to see their immediate causes, man attributed them to all sorts of real and hypothetical factors in his environment, such as divine anger, cosmic influences, witchcraft, the seasons of the year or bad air. It was appreciated at an early date that the introduction of a sick person into a community could result in the spread of disease to the local population. The book of Leviticus indicates that the methods of spread of certain skin and venereal diseases were known, and that their victims were accordingly excluded from contact with their fellow men. In his *De Contagione* published in 1546, Fracastorius struck a remarkably modern note with the statement that diseases could be spread by direct contact between individuals, by the agency of inanimate objects such as clothing and personal possessions (which he called 'fomites') or through the air. He suggested that this spread involved the passage of small infective particles, 'seminaria', from an affected person to others, but since he could not demonstrate the existence of these particles, his theory received little attention.

In the late eighteenth and early nineteenth centuries the theory of contagion was again propounded vigorously by certain medical men. In 1795 Gordon of Aberdeen showed that an epidemic of puerperal fever 'seized such women only as were visited or delivered by a practitioner or taken care of by nurses who had previously attended patients affected with the disease'. He recommended washing and the changing of clothes to prevent carriage of contagion from one puerperal woman to another. Almost 50 years later Semmelweiss showed that the spread of puerperal infection by students and practitioners who commonly went straight from the post-mortem room to the maternity wards could be reduced by cleanliness and the washing of their hands in a solution of chloride of lime. Both of these men believed that the carriage of 'something' from one patient to another was responsible for the development of puerperal fever.

Early Observers of Micro-Organisms

In 1671 Kircher reported the presence of little worms in the blood of patients with plague, and claimed that they were responsible for the disease. However, it is likely that what he saw were aggregations of red blood cells, and that the honour of being the first observer of micro-organisms belongs to Antony Leeuwenhoek, the linen-draper of Delft in Holland. His hobby was the making of simple but ingenious microscopes, and with these he was able, in 1674, to observe minute living creatures in rain, sea and pond water, and in various other fluids. He communicated his findings in a series of letters to the Royal Society in London, but neither he nor his contemporaries appear to have realized the significance of his observations. During the eighteenth century several workers suggested that small creatures such as he had described might be responsible for various diseases, but their ideas were not accepted for lack of any factual support.

By the early nineteenth century improvements in microscope design had made possible the beginning of systematic description of micro-organisms. In 1838 Ehrenberg, in his work on 'Infusoria' (the small creatures found in infusions), introduced such terms as *bacterium*, *vibrio*, *spirillum* and *spirochaete*. Meanwhile, in 1835, Agostino Bassi had described the fungus (later named *Botrytis bassiana*) which caused muscardine, a disease of silkworms, and he had suggested that this disease was transmitted by contact or by infection of food. This, the first reliable report of a disease caused by a transmissible parasitic micro-organism, was followed in 1839 by Schoenlein's description of the fungus that causes the human disease favus. In 1850 Rayer and Davaine reported the presence of rod-shaped organisms in the blood of animals that had died of anthrax, and Davaine later showed that this disease could be transmitted by inoculation of blood containing such rods but not of blood from which they were absent. During this era other claims to have found microbial causes of disease were put forward with inadequate experimental backing, and in 1840 Henle pointed out that a micro-organism causing a disease should be present in every case and should produce a similar disease in animals into which it was inoculated – criteria which were later expanded into 'Koch's postulates' (see p 49).

The Theory of Spontaneous Generation

Up to the seventeenth century philosophers and scientists had generally accepted that at least some animals could develop entirely from non-living materials. Thus putrefying meat was believed to give rise to maggots and the mud of the Nile to snakes, whereas corn and a linen cloth stored in a jar were considered suitable ingredients for the production of mice! However, in 1688 Redi showed that putrefying meat did not produce maggots if flies were kept away from it, and thereby convinced many that the theory of spontaneous generation was inaccurate, at least in relation to flies and larger creatures. It survived in relation to microscopic creatures for another 200 years, and in the latter half of the eighteenth century it was the subject of a fierce controversy, with the Italian abbot Spallanzani and the Irish priest Needham as the central figures. Needham's claim that micro-organisms reappeared in infusions which had previously been heated to kill all living creatures was countered by Spallanzani's demonstration that this did not occur if the heating was vigorous enough and if air was subsequently excluded from the container. According to Needham, this was because excessive heat destroyed a 'vegetative force' that was necessary for the generations of organisms. In 1854 Schroeder and Dusch showed that the growth of micro-organisms which took place in a previously heated infusion if air was allowed to enter the container could be prevented by first passing the air through a cotton-wool filter – in other words, that the important component of the air was particulate. However, their later findings were erratic and confusing because the amount of heat that they used was inadequate to sterilize all of the fluids tested.

Pasteur, Lister and Koch

To the French chemist Louis Pasteur belongs the credit both for terminating the dispute about spontaneous generation and for establishing beyond doubt the role of micro-organisms in transmissible diseases. He entered the field of microbiology at a point far removed from medicine – the study of fermentation. This phenomenon had been known to man from very early times but was without an explanation until 1837, when Schwann and Cagniard-Latour discovered independently that the yeasts always associated with alcoholic fermentation of sugar solutions were living organisms. Their belief that these organisms actually caused the fermentations was disputed by Liebig and others who upheld purely chemical explanations. In a series of brilliant experiments and papers between 1855 and 1860 Pasteur showed conclusively that lactic and butyric acid fermentations were the work of bacteria, and that the fermentations involved in the production of beer and wines were the work of yeasts. He also showed that there was a relationship between the type of micro-organism involved and the type of fermentation produced. He then proceeded to destroy the theory of spontaneous generation (though its supporters were slow to admit defeat) by showing that living micro-organisms were invariably derived from exactly similar living organisms. In the course of this work he learnt a great deal about the scrupulous care needed in dealing with bacteria and fungi, and about their differing nutritional requirements, and so he laid the foundations of modern microbiological technique. But he was far more than a careful technician. His brilliance lay in his ability to see the far-reaching significance of his discoveries. From problems of preparation and preservation of wine, beer and vinegar he went on to rescue the silkworm industry from the scourge of an infectious disease called pebrine, to show farmers how the spread of anthrax among their animals could be prevented, and then to discover how to immunize these animals against anthrax, fowls against chicken cholera and finally man against rabies.

Meanwhile, news of Pasteur's work on fermentation reached Joseph Lister, the Professor of Surgery in Glasgow. At that time virtually all wounds suppurated and the mortality following surgery was fearful. Failure of wounds to produce 'laudable pus' was in fact considered a bad sign – quite rightly, as we can see today, for all wounds were infected and lack of suppuration frequently meant absence of resistance to infection on the part of the patient. Lister concluded that if micro-organisms caused fermentation they might also cause suppuration of wounds, and that in their absence wounds might heal cleanly and without risk to the patients' lives. So he introduced his *antiseptic technique*, which he first described in 1867. By washing wounds with carbolic acid, spraying this substance into the air of the operating theatre and applying protective dressings to keep fresh organisms from entering the wounds, he achieved a striking reduction of post-operative sepsis and mortality. Because carbolic acid was toxic to patients and to their attendants, it was far from being the perfect answer to the surgeon's problems, and today more emphasis is placed upon preventing the introduction of organisms into wounds (*asepsis*) than upon their destruction, but Lister's procedure proved their importance and prepared the way for modern surgery.

In 1870 a young German general practitioner, Robert Koch, began to follow up the work of Davaine on anthrax. He was able to grow in artificial culture the rod-shaped organisms seen in the blood of animals suffering from this disease, and to reproduce the disease by injecting his cultures into animals. He also showed that the rods could turn into resistant spore forms and then back into rods. During the last quarter of the ninteenth century, Koch and his bacteriological pupils identified the causative organisms of tuberculosis, cholera, typhoid, diphtheria and many other major diseases of man and animals, and began to establish a systematic classification of bacteria. This work was made possible by technical advances for which Koch himself was largely responsible, including the use of aniline dyes for staining micro-organisms, of oil-immersed microscope objectives for examining them and of media solidified with agar for growing them.

The Beginnings of Immunology

Immunization against smallpox, by inoculation with material from a lesion of a patient (*variolation*), had been practised for centuries in the East before its introduction into Britain in 1721. It was a hazardous procedure, but smallpox was a widespread and terrible disease. In 1796 Jenner discovered that protection against smallpox could be achieved much more safely by inoculation with material from a lesion of cowpox, a natural disease of cattle. This process became known as *vaccination*, from the Latin *vacca*, a cow. We now know that its success was due to the close relationships between the viruses of cowpox and smallpox (variola).

Almost a century later Pasteur found that fowls inoculated with an old laboratory culture of the organism of chicken cholera developed only a mild illness and were subsequently resistant to infection with fresh cultures of the organism. Then he discovered that sheep could be protected against anthrax by inoculation with cultures of anthrax bacilli attenuated (i.e. rendered harmless) by growing them at 42 °C. This work provided a basis for a rational approach to the prevention of microbial diseases, and it was found possible to attenuate many other pathogenic organisms. Then in 1890, following the discovery by Roux and Yersin that the symptoms of diphtheria were mainly due to the release of a soluble poison (toxin) from the bacteria, von Behring showed that guinea-pigs could be protected against this disease by injections of diphtheria toxoid (toxin so treated that it became harmless). With Kitasato he similarly immunized animals against tetanus. The sera of such immunized animals were shown to neutralize the appropriate toxins specifically, and also to give protection against the appropriate diseases to other animals into which they were injected. Within a few years the treatment of human diphtheria was greatly advanced by the introduction of effective antitoxic sera (animal sera that neutralized diphtheria toxin) which could be injected into human beings with reasonable safety.

Thus the second half of the nineteenth century saw not only the establishment of the microbial origins of many diseases and the identification of many of the responsible organisms, but also the introduction of the first specific weapons for dealing with them. The pace of development in the present century precludes a brief historical summary, but two major advances in clinical microbiology deserve mention before we end this preliminary survey.

Antimicrobial Drugs
Naturally occurring compounds have been used with success in the treatment of infections for several centuries–at least since the first recorded use of an extract of cinchona bark (quinine) for malaria in 1619; but it was in the opening years of the present century that Paul Ehrlich began the search for synthetic substances specifically designed to attack harmful microbes (his 'magic bullets'). His arsenical compounds were effective against a limited number of such organisms, notably those causing syphilis and trypanosomiasis; but it was from 1935 onwards, with the introduction first of the sulphonamides and then of the antibiotics and sundry other antimicrobial drugs, that major advances were made, so that by now virtually all bacterial, fungal and protozoal infections and even a few due to viruses have come within the reach of effective drug treatment. Many diseases that were virtually untreatable and commonly fatal a mere 30 years ago can today be treated with almost invariable success. Medical bacteriology has been transformed by these developments, since its contributions have become far more relevant to patient care and are more urgently needed; but the transformation has included the whole of medical practice and indeed the way of life and life-expectation of us all. In almost any branch of medicine a doctor frequently has to decide whether to use an antimicrobial drug, and, if so, which to choose from the increasingly and confusingly wide selection available to him. A firm grasp of basic microbiological facts and principles provides the best foundation for his decisions.

Routine Diagnostic Virology
From the time of Koch the techniques of bacteriology could be applied, in almost any hospital laboratory, to the routine investigation of patients. Virology, however, although it began in the nineteenth century, remained a subject for research workers because of the difficulty and complexity of its techniques. The overcoming of these problems in the 1950's opened the way to the provision of a routine diagnostic virological service. Today this is generally available and is being steadily developed,

though as yet it lacks the stimulus which it will receive when more effective antiviral drugs are discovered.

Suggestions for Further Reading

The Life of Pasteur by R. Vallery-Radot (Constable, London, 1923).

Microbe Hunters by P. de Kruif (first published 1926, currently available as paper-back, Pocket Books Inc., New York).

Milestones in Microbiology trans. and ed. by T. D. Brock (Prentice-Hall London, 1961).

A History of Bacteriology by W. D. Foster (Heinemann, London, 1970)–for the period 1840–1940.

Changing Patterns: An Atypical Autobiography by Sir Macfarlane Burnet (Heinemann, Melbourne and London, 1968)–for developments in bacteriology, virology and immunology as seen and influenced by an eminent worker in these fields.

Microbes and Men by Robert Reid (British Broadcasting Corporation, 1974).

PART II

BIOLOGICAL BACKGROUND

3

'Concerning Little Animals'

(Leeuwenhoek, 1676)

Micro-organisms can be defined as living creatures so small that individuals cannot be seen without the aid of a microscope; and microbiology is the study of such organisms. The 'little animals' which Leeuwenhoek saw and described in various natural fluids (see p 8) doubtless included micro-organisms that we should today classify as bacteria, fungi, protozoa and algae, but we now know of other groups far too small to have been seen with his instruments.

Micro-organisms of medical importance can be classified in five large groups: (1) Bacteria; (2) Rickettsiae and Chlamydiae; (3) Viruses; (4) Fungi; (5) Protozoa. Whereas fungi and protozoa have cells essentially similar in structure to those of higher plants and animals, and are therefore know as *eukaryotic,* bacteria, rickettsiae and chlamydiae are known as *prokaryotic* because their cells have a much simpler nuclear structure, do not have nuclear or other internal dividing membranes and have in their walls a mucopeptide substance not found in eukaryotic cells (see below). Viruses are even simpler in structure and cannot be described as cells.

Bacteria

These are cellular (usually unicellular) organisms. A typical bacterial cell is able to carry out many different metabolic activities and to increase its size and reproduce itself by fission. Individual cells are of the order of $0.5-1$ μm broad by $0.5-8$ μm long (1 μm = a micrometre, a thousandth of a millimetre). The shape of a bacterial cell is determined by its rigid but permeable *cell wall*, which also prevents it from swelling up and bursting as the result of osmosis. The main structural component of this wall is *mucopeptide* (or peptidoglycan), which consists of chains of alternating molecules of N-acetylglucosamine and N-acetylmuramic acid cross-linked by peptide chains. Within the cell wall is the *protoplast*, which is mainly semi-solid *cytoplasm* surrounded by a thin elastic semi-permeable *cytoplasmic membrane*–a complex structure which is of great importance in determining what substances can enter or leave the cell and is the site of most of its enzymic activities. Among the structures to be found within the cytoplasm are many granular *ribosomes*, which contain much of the cell's ribonucleic acid (RNA) and a *chromosome* or *nucleus* (sometimes more than one), consisting of a long double-stranded deoxyribonucleic acid (DNA) molecule in the form of a much twisted and contorted ring; other DNA may be present in the form of small extra-chromosomal portions called *plasmids*. Some bacteria form *capsules*, usually composed of polysaccharide, outside their cell walls. Some have fine whip-like organs of locomotion called *flagella* (singular *flagellum*) protruding from their surfaces. Some have numerous shorter hair-like protrusions called *fimbriae* or *pili*; most of these are apparently organs of adhesion, enabling the bacteria to attach themselves to surfaces such as those of host cells, and are therefore possibly of importance in the production of disease, but some have a special role in bacterial conjugation (*sex-fimbriae*, see p 34). A few bacterial species form *spores*, thick-walled structures, originally intracellular, with greatly reduced metabolic activity and greatly increased resistance to adverse conditions. (For more detail about these and other morphological features of bacteria see pp 86–8).

Bacteria reproduce by *binary fission*, one cell enlarging and then dividing into two approximately equal parts; this division is preceded by simple replication of the nuclear ring, without the polarized mitosis that is part of the reproductive process of most other types of nucleated cell.

Bacterial cells are of various shapes. If they are spherical or nearly so, they are called *cocci*. These are commonly grouped together. If in pairs, they are often referred to as diplococci. Repeated division in the same plane produces chains; division in two or three planes at right angles produces regular packets of four, eight or more; and division without any definite orientation produces irregular clusters. The *bacilli* or rods are elongated cylindrical forms, straight or slightly curved, with ends that are rounded, square, pointed or sometimes swollen to form clubs. Certain bacteria which resemble bacilli but are more definitely curved are known as *vibrios* or comma bacilli. The *spirochaetes* are corkscrew-like spirals. Some of these (e.g. the leptospirae) are tightly coiled, whereas others (e.g. the borreliae) have large open coils. Some of the *higher bacteria*, so called because they are thought to represent a more advanced stage of evolution, resemble the fungi in forming branched filaments (e.g. the actino-mycetes).

Rickettsiae, Coxiella burnetii and Chlamydiae

These organisms resemble bacteria in that they contain both RNA and

DNA, have muramic acid in their outer coats, reproduce by binary fission and are susceptible to the action of antibacterial drugs that have no effect on viruses. On the other hand, with diameters of only 0·25–0·5 μm they are nearer in size to viruses than to bacteria, and they are also (with only one known exception) virus-like in being unable to reproduce except inside the cells of the host organisms.

Viruses

Though some viruses are similar in size to the organisms just described, most of them are smaller–some very much smaller–than any other known living organisms, and are too small to be seen with an ordinary light microscope ('ultra-microscopic') unless they aggregate to form inclusion bodies (see p 177). The virus particle is called a *virion*, not a cell. At its simplest, as in the viruses of poliomyelitis, this is a mere 25–30 nm in diameter (1 nm = a nanometre, a thousandth of a micrometre) and apparently consists only of a nucleic acid core, the *genome*, and a surrounding protein coat, the *capsid*. At the other end of the range, the virions of pox viruses measure about 200 × 300 nm and are chemically and structurally a good deal more complex, though they are still developments of the same basic plan. The nucleic acid found in a virus of any given type is either RNA or DNA, but not both as in bacteria and other cellular organisms. Viruses increase in number not by fission but by *replication* inside bacterial, plant or animal host cells which they have converted into virus-production units (see p 172).

Fungi

These are generally larger than bacteria, and are commonly multicellular. Their relatively thick cell walls owe their rigidity not to mucopeptide, as do those of bacteria, but to chitin or other components. The *moulds* grow as tubular branching filaments (hyphae) which become interwoven to form a network (mycelium). In some families the hyphae are divided into short lengths by cross-walls (septa). Such fungi reproduce by forming asexual or sexual spores of various kinds. The *yeasts* are oval or spherical cells which commonly reproduce by budding, but may also form sexual spores. (These reproductive spores differ in nature and function from bacterial spores.)

Protozoa

These are unicellular organisms, mostly much larger than bacteria, which show clear differentiation of their protoplasm into nucleus and cytoplasm. Their reproductive mechanisms vary from simple binary fission to complex life-cycles involving sexual and asexual phases and the formation of cysts.

THE MICROSCOPE–THE MICROBIOLOGIST'S BASIC TOOL

Leeuwenhoek's simple optical instruments opened the door to the microbial world. Our subsequent exploration of it has been largely dependent upon improvements in microscope design and in methods of preparing organisms for microscopic examination. The ordinary light microscope has been joined in recent years by other instruments which have given important additional information. Detailed theoretical descriptions of these different microscopes are to be found in larger textbooks, and the practical knowledge which is essential for their efficient use should be learned in the laboratory. Here we deal only with the general principles of microbial microscopy.

Ordinary Light Microscopy

Organisms to be examined with the light microscope may be:

1 *Unstained ('wet preparation').* A drop of fluid culture or of any other suspension of organisms is placed on a glass slide, covered with a cover-slip and examined with the high-power dry objective of the microscope, using a restricted amount of light. In this way it is possible to determine the size and shape of the organisms and whether they are motile. True spontaneous motility must be carefully distinguished from the Brownian movement to which all small particles in a fluid medium are subject, and from drifting due to currents in the fluid. Differentiation between organisms in such preparations cannot be carried very far, and some bacterial groups, notably the spirochaetes, are so feebly refractile that they cannot be seen at all in this way.

2 *Stained.* Bacteria are commonly examined by fixing them to a glass slide (usually by heating) and applying stains. They can then be examined with the oil-immersion objective of the microscope, using a bright light source. Even if only a simple stain such as methylene blue or carbol fuchsin is used, this procedure usually enables us to see more of the shape, arrangement and structure of the organisms than is visible in unstained preparations, though allowance has to be made for artefactual changes due to drying and staining. Additional valuable information can be obtained by using differential staining techniques. Gram's method (see p 91), the most widely used of these, divides bacteria into Gram-positive (staining blue) and Gram-negative (staining red), a distinction which is of true biological significance and also of considerable practical value. The Ziehl–Neelsen staining procedure (see p 145) makes it possible to recognize a relatively small but important group of bacteria which are 'acid-fast'–i.e. cannot be readily decolorized with acid after being stained with hot carbol fuchsin.

Dark Ground Microscopy

With ordinary light microscopy, objects that absorb or refract light are seen as dark against a bright background. Some bacteria too feebly refractile to be seen in this way can be seen by dark ground illumination, which also shows up fine details of their shape.

Dark ground illumination is obtained by focusing a hollow cone of light from below on to the top surface of the microscope slide in such a way that, unless deviated from its path, the light will diverge again and miss the front lens of the objective. Thus the only light to enter the objective and reach the eye of the observer is that which has been deflected by striking bacteria or other objects on the slide. These objects shine brightly against a dark background. The process is essentially the same as that by which one sees fine dust particles when looking from the side at a shaft of bright sunlight. Dark ground microscopy is usually applied to unstained wet preparations, with water or oil between the condenser and the slide to prevent total internal reflection of light within the condenser, and between the cover-slip and the objective to prevent scattering of light.

Fluorescence Microscopy

Certain dyes fluoresce when exposed to light of appropriate wave-length. Tubercle bacilli can be selectively stained with one such dye, auramine, by a Ziehl–Neelsen-like procedure in which the auramine replaces the carbol fuchsin. They can therefore be recognized in smears of sputum or other material stained in this way and examined microscopically by ultra-violet light.

The fluorescent-antibody technique (immunofluorescence) uses the fact that fluorescent dyes can be coupled with the serum proteins known as antibodies (see p 60). When such an antibody combines with its appropriate antigen, the antigen-antibody complex is fluorescent. Micro-organisms and other antigens can be located and identified in sections and smears by 'staining' these preparations with dye-conjugated specific antibodies. Two fluorescent dyes commonly used, fluorescein-isothiocyanate and lissamine-rhodamine, give green and orange fluorescence respectively. This technique is discussed further on p 72.

Electron Microscopy

This procedure has much greater resolving power than light microscopy, and permits much greater magnification ($\times$ 300 000 or more, as against $\times$ 1500). It has made possible the determination of the size, shape and structure of viruses, and has added greatly to our knowledge of the finer structure of bacteria and larger micro-organisms. A beam of electrons, derived from an 'electron gun', is passed through a series of electro-magnetic fields which correspond to the lenses in an optical microscope in that they bring about convergence of the beam. The material to be examined is mounted on a thin membrane of collodion, polyvinyl formal or carbon, which is supported on a metal grid, and the examination is carried out in a high vacuum which inevitably produces some distortion. Ultra-thin sections of tissue or of suitably embedded microbial or other cells can be examined, and so can films made from suspensions of very small particles, such as the smaller viruses. To be clearly visible these objects must differ from their surroundings in their opacity to the electron beam. This can be achieved by supplying a background of more electron-opaque material, such as sodium phosphotungstate ('negative staining'); or by 'positive staining' with some electron-opaque material that will selectively adhere to the particles (e.g. various heavy-metal compounds, or ferritin-labelled antibodies – see p 72); or by 'shadow casting' – i.e. projecting a shower of metal atoms over the film obliquely, so that a thin layer of metal is formed all over it except in the 'shadows' of particles. After the electron beam has passed through the material to be examined it is made to produce a visible image on a fluorescent screen or to produce photographs that can usually be much enlarged. Whereas ordinary electron microscopy can show outlines and structural details in a flat plane, the more sophisticated technique of scanning electron microscopy can produce clear 'aerial views' of particles such as microbial and other cells, showing the contours, irregularities and texture of their surfaces.

4

Ecology

Micro-organisms are virtually ubiquitous. The distribution of any particular species is limited by its growth requirements and by its compatibility with other species, but micro-organisms of some sort are to be found in almost any environment. They are present in soil, water and air and in most kinds of inorganic or organic non-living matter, as well as within and on the surfaces of living creatures.

An important part in the balance of nature is played by the many bacterial and fungal species which live by breaking down the bodies of dead animals and plants. 'If microscopic beings were to disappear from our globe, the surface of the earth would be encumbered with dead organic matter and corpses of all kinds, animal and vegetable. . . . Without them, life would become impossible because death would be incomplete' (Louis Pasteur, 1861). Such organisms that live on dead organic matter are described as *saprophytic*. Some normally saprophytic species can occasionally invade the tissues of living animals and humans, but this is rare. Some writers also use the term saprophytic for organisms that are superficial and harmless parasites (e.g. 'saprophytic neisseriae' in the human throat), but these are better described as commensals (see below).

A small minority of micro-organisms, including nearly all those of medical importance, are commonly or necessarily *parasitic*–i.e. they live inside or on the surfaces of other living organisms. Bacteria themselves harbour parasitic viruses called bacteriophages, and plants and animals act as hosts to large and varied microbial populations. Parasites may be *commensal, symbiotic* or *pathogenic*. A *commensal* (literally, one that shares the table) derives nourishment from its host but does nothing in return–a non-paying guest. Many examples are to be found in the secretions of human skin and mucous membranes. A *symbiont* lives in partnership with its host, receiving nourishment but rendering service in return–a paying guest. Such are the nitrogen-fixing bacteria of the root nodules of leguminous plants, and the vitamin-synthesizing bacteria of the human intestine. A *pathogen* does harm to its host. These terms refer to relationships between parasites and hosts, not simply to properties of micro-organisms; the same micro-organism may exhibit different forms of parasitism in different hosts, or even in the same host at different times or in different sites. Pathogenicity is as much an expression of the host's susceptibility as it is of the organism's intrinsic power to cause disease. To use a well-worn analogy, the soil is as important as the seed in determining the outcome of infection.

MAN'S NORMAL MICROBIAL POPULATION

There is evidence that in at least some species an apparently healthy young animal may be harbouring in its tissues viruses which it derived from its mother *in utero* and which may cause it to develop leukaemia later in life. We do not know whether such transmission involves only leukaemia viruses, or whether anything of the sort occurs in man. With this reservation it seems permissible to say that the healthy human foetus has no resident microbial population up to the time of its birth. While passing down the mother's birth canal it acquires on its surface or swallows or inhales an assortment of micro-organisms, and these are soon reinforced by contributions from various human and inanimate (and possibly also animal) sources in the newborn infant's immediate environment. Those organisms which find themselves in suitable environments, whether on the outer or inner body surfaces, begin to multiply and to enter into complex competitive relationships with other potential colonizers. Within hours of birth the infant is on the way to acquiring a resident microbial population—or rather, a number of different populations, since some organisms thrive on the skin, others do better in the mouth or throat or nose, others in the intestine and so on. By degrees—and at speeds that depend on many factors, such as frequency and method of washing, diet and living conditions—the combinations of organisms that have taken up residence in different areas of the growing child's external and internal surfaces begin to resemble those commonly found in such sites in adults (often described as the *normal flora*). Some idea of the nature of these combinations is given in Chapter Fourteen (pp 241–52), but two points need to be remembered: that the range of organisms detectable in any situation depends on the methods used in looking for them as well as on the actual population, and that throughout life there are fluctuations and marked personal differences in the 'normal' microbial populations of the body, dependent on general health, diet, hormonal activity, age, race and many other factors.

It is important to appreciate that the very large microbial populations that we have been discussing consist of micro-organisms that are in commensal or symbiotic relationships with man. The pathogenic relationship is of course highly important in medicine and will be dealt with at length in the chapters that follow, but it is the exception – indeed, the rare exception. Normal microbial populations should be treated with due respect. In many different spheres man has discovered by costly trial and error that problems and dangers as well as advantages may result when he applies his advancing knowledge to the alteration of complex established ecological systems – in popular language, to upsetting the balance of nature. When our modern anti-microbial weapons are used against pathogens, their powerful effect on normal microbial populations is too often forgotten, sometimes with disastrous results. Pathogens have had most of the limelight, and we know all too little about the ways in which man benefits from the activities of his normal microbial flora (though a few ways are mentioned in later chapters, notably on p 53); but it is increasingly clear that the doctor must not take as his motto words that we once saw in an insecticide advertisement: 'The only good bug is a dead bug'!

'GERM-FREE' ANIMALS

If an animal is born by Caesarian section with care to avoid microbial contamination, and is then maintained in a germ-free environment and fed on sterilized food, it does not develop a microbial population. If it is given a special diet that compensates for its lack of intestinal flora which would normally help in the breakdown of food and in vitamin synthesis, it grows and becomes an adult – though different in a number of ways from normal adults. The appropriateness of the name 'germ-free' for such animals is open to question because of uncertainty about intra-uterine transmission of viruses (see the beginning of the previous section). The term *gnotobiotic* has been coined instead, to indicate that these are animals in which it is possible to study known biological relationships – e.g. such an animal can be exposed to a given bacterium with the knowledge that it has never encountered it or anything like it before and that its response will not be complicated by the presence of an unknown range of other bacteria. Use of such animals promises to throw much light on the role of normal flora and on the mechanisms of pathogenicity and host resistance; but when interpreting data obtained in this way allowance must be made for the large gap between the experimental and the 'real life' situations.

Suggestion for Further Reading

'Bacteria indigenous to man' by T. Rosebury, in *Bacterial and Mycotic Infections of Man*, ed. R. J. Dubos and J. G. Hirsch, 4th edn. (Pitman, London, 1965), chapter 14.

Invisible Allies: Microbes and Man's Future, by Bernard Dixon (Temple Smith, London, 1976).

5

Physiology

Micro-organisms are of diverse sizes, shapes and structures, and live in widely varied environments. It is not surprising that they also differ widely in the details of their physiology, even though their biochemical mechanisms in general are similar to those of all living creatures, including man. This chapter deals mainly with bacteria. The physiology of rickettsiae, viruses and most medically important protozoa is less easily studied because it is inextricably intertwined with that of their host cells. Points of special importance in relation to individual groups of micro-organisms will be discussed in the appropriate places in Part IV.

METABOLIC NEEDS

We have seen that the bacterial cell is a complex structure. Within its minute confines are included a wide variety of proteins, nucleic acids, polysaccharides, lipids and their derivatives. Some bacteria are motile, some generate light, but the main activity of bacteria as a whole is reproduction—that is, the making of new bacteria. This process may go on at an amazing speed. Under optimal conditions some species divide as often as three times per hour, which means that a single bacterium, visible only if magnified several hundred times, may convert itself overnight into a colony several millimetres in diameter, with a population of many millions.

Such a formidable synthetic operation requires an adequate supply of energy and raw materials and appropriate environmental conditions. We shall now discuss in general terms the nature of these requirements and how they are met. The precise needs of a particular organism depend largely upon the equipment with which it is provided for carrying on its work—in other words, upon what *enzymes* it possesses. Some of these are *constitutive*, produced by the organisms in almost all circumstances, and others are *inducible*, produced (after some initial delay) in response to special circumstances, usually the presence of their specific substrates.

Sources of Energy

Some micro-organisms are *phototrophs*, able to derive their energy from sunlight. The majority, however, including all of those which are important in medicine, are *chemotrophs*, getting their energy from the oxidation of chemical compounds

Oxygen

Organisms that grow readily in the presence of air are described as *aerobes*. (The word 'grow' in relation to micro-organisms is generally used to mean 'increase in numbers'.) Some species are *obligate* (or *strict*) *aerobes*, unable to grow in the absence of free oxygen, but others are *facultative anaerobes*, able to grow in its absence, though often with decreased vigour. *Obligate anaerobes* (cannot grow if more than a trace of free oxygen is present; in at least some cases this may be because they poison themselves in such circumstances by making peroxides, which they cannot destroy since they do not possess the enzyme catalase. *Micro-aerophiles* grow best in the presence of a little oxygen.

The oxidations on which chemotrophs depend for their energy can be carried out in three different ways: *aerobic respiration*, with free oxygen as the final hydrogen-acceptor in a chain of oxidation-reduction reactions; *anaerobic respiration*, with inorganic compounds (nitrates, sulphates and carbonates) as final hydrogen-acceptors; and *fermentation* of a carbohydrate or other organic substance, the hydrogen-acceptor being another molecule of the energy source or some other organic molecule. Various organic acids and the gases CO_2 and H_2 may be formed as end-products of fermentation. (In medical microbiological writings the word fermentation is commonly used in a less precise sense–see p 90).

Carbon Dioxide

This is probably necessary in small amounts, such as are present in the atmosphere, for the growth of most micro-organisms. A higher concentration, 5–10%, improves the growth of many parasitic species, notably of *Neisseria gonorrhoeae*, and is usually necessary for the primary isolation of *Brucella abortus* from pathological materials. Free CO_2 can be the sole carbon source for autotrophs.

Raw Materials

Some chemotrophic bacteria (called *autotrophs*) can grow in simple inorganic salt solutions. At the other end of the scale are the leprosy bacillus and the spirochaete of syphilis, which cannot be cultivated in non-living media, and organisms of the rickettsia group and viruses, which depend upon their hosts for essential enzymes as well as for raw materials. Between these extremes are innumerable gradations. Among common parasites of man, *Escherichia coli* can grow in a solution containing glucose, ammonium sulphate and a small range of other inorganic salts. In contrast, *Haemophilius influenzae* has very exacting requirements; as well as glucose or other suitable carbohydrate, various minerals and an assortment of amino-acids, purines and vitamins, this species must be supplied with nicotinamide-adenine dinucleotide or its phosphate as a codehydrogenase, and with haemin or some closely related substance as a substrate for the synthesis of various respiratory enzymes. Such differences in the needs of organisms are of great importance to the medical microbiologist in his choice of culture media.

Temperature

Psychropiles grow best at low temperatures, some below 0°C. They are therefore important in connection with cold storage of food and blood, but otherwise are not relevant to medical microbiology. *Thermophiles*, found in such situations as hot springs and rotting vegetable matter, are of no medical importance except as sensitizing agents in 'farmer's lung', etc. (see p 76). The majority of bacteria, including all of those parasitic upon man, are *mesophiles*, with optimal growth temperatures somewhere between 20 and 40°C.; they vary considerably in the ranges of temperature over which they will grow. As might be expected, nearly all of man's parasites are best suited by temperatures around 37°C. Many of them will multiply at lower temperatures, down to 20°C or less, but few at more than 45°C. Some will grow only within a narrow temperature range–e.g. *Neisseria gonorrhoeae*, 30–39°C. Unusual among human pathogens is *Yersinia pestis*, the causative organism of bubonic plague. Its optimal growth temperature of about 27°C is probably related to the fact that multiplication in the proventriculus of the rat-flea is an important stage in its transmission (see p 132).

Hydrogen Ion Concentration

Micro-organisms differ widely in their preferences and tolerances concerning the pH of their environment. Most of those of medical importance grow best when it is slightly alkaline. Artificial culture media must be carefully buffered to prevent the rapid lowering of the pH value by acid metabolic products to a level at which organisms can no longer multiply. Lactabacilli are unusual among the bacterial flora of the human body in that they prefer an acid medium (pH 4·0). Indeed, members of this genus have a protective function in the adult vagina because they form lactic acid from the glycogen of the mucosa and thereby keep the vaginal secretion too acid for the growth of most other organisms. The medium which Sabouraud devised for the isolation of relatively slow-growing fungi makes use of their ability to multiply at a pH value of about 5·4; this is inhibitory to bacteria which would otherwise overgrow them. At the other end of the scale, *Vibrio cholerae* grows best around pH 8·5.

METABOLIC PRODUCTS

Obviously the most important end-result of bacterial metabolism is more bacteria. This section deals with some other results, which for convenience of discussion are somewhat arbitrarily classified under four headings – toxins, extracellular enzymes, pigments and other products. Antibiotics are considered later, on pp 40–2.

Toxins

One of the most powerful poisons known is the toxin produced by *Clostridium botulinum*, a soil bacterium that sometimes grows in human or animal foods and renders them highly lethal (see pp 117 and 304). This toxin, a protein that is fairly easily inactivated by heat, is called an *exotoxin* because it is liberated by living bacteria into their environment. Similar exotoxins are released by the causative organisms of tetanus, diphtheria and scarlet fever while they are growing in host tissues, and travel to other parts of the body where they produce clinical features characteristic of these diseases. The bacteria which cause cholera and some types of dysentery multiply in the lumen of the host's intestine and produce exotoxins that damage the intestinal mucosa and are consequently known as enterotoxins. Among other exotoxins named according to their effects are the haemolysins (red-cell-destroying toxins) and leucocidins (leucocyte-destroying toxins) of streptococci and staphylococci, and the lecithinase of *Clostridium welchii* (one of the gas-gangrene bactilli) which hydrolyses lecithin, a constituent of cell membranes. The most important of the exotoxins are discussed more fully in later chapters.

Gram-negative bacteria have, outside the mucopeptide structural layer of their cell walls (p 17), a thicker phospholipid-polysaccharide-protein layer. The name *endotoxin* is given to complex lipopolysaccharide-containing material derived from this layer. It is more heat-stable than exotoxins and, unlike them, is mostly liberated only on the death and disintegration of the bacteria. The endotoxins of different species differ somewhat in composition and effect, but all are weight-for-weight less potent than the more active of the exotoxins and much less specific in their effects. When released in sufficient amount into the blood-stream of a human or animal host they cause fever (and so are called *pyrogens*) and also, among other things, intravascular coagulation and the clinical condition known as shock—more specifically, in these circumstances, bacteraemic shock or even 'Gram-negative shock'. (This condition seems to be related to the as-yet mysterious Shwartzman reaction, induced by giving a rabbit a small intradermal injection of endotoxin and then 24 hours later a small intravenous injection. The first injection produces only a slight local inflammation, but following the second there is a vigorous haemorrhagic reaction at the site of the first. If the first injection is given intravenously, the second results in a severe systemic reaction which may be fatal.) A sensitive and clinically useful test for the presence of endotoxin in body or other fluids is provided by its ability to cause a lysate of amoebocytes from the horseshoe crab *Limulus polyphemus* to form a gel (the Limulus lysate test).

Extracellular Enzymes

Some of these enzymes have already been mentioned in their capacity as exotoxins. There are others which, although they are not truly toxic, still contribute to the pathogenicity of the organisms. The coagulase produced by most pathogenic staphylococci may give some protection against the defences of their hosts by coating the cocci with fibrin formed from plasma fibrinogen. The pathogenicity of these organisms may also be enhanced by the fact that clumps of cocci in fibrin clots become trapped in capillary blood vessels and multiply there, whereas isolated cocci are removed from circulation by the reticulo-endothelial cells (see p 55). Conversely, the streptokinase of haemolytic streptococci probably facilitates their passage through clots by activating plasminogen to the fibrinolytic enzymes plasmin. The hyaluronidases formed by various species are spreading factors that open up connective tissues to bacterial invasion by destroying hyaluronic acid in the cement substance.

Many micro-organisms depend for their survival on enzymes that destroy toxic substances. We have already mentioned catalase, which destroys hydrogen peroxide (p 27), and we shall refer repeatedly to another group of enzymes which have acquired great medical importance—penicillinases, by means of which many bacteria can destroy penicillins.

Other extracellular enzymes are concerned with the nutrition of their producers. Before an organism can use nutrients of high molecular weights, it must be able to break them down extracellularly into molecules small enough to pass through its cytoplasmic membrane. Such extracellular digestion by excreted enzymes is of particular importance to saprophytic organisms (see p 23).

Pigments
Phototrophic micro-organisms trap the energy of sunlight by means of their pigments, in much the same way as do the blue-green algae and higher plants. All chemotrophs also contain pigments–flavoproteins and cytochromes–which participate in their respiratory mechanisms. The pyocyanin of *Pseudomonas aeruginosa* (formerly *pyocyanea*), which gives a characteristic green colour to its cultures and also to pus from infected wounds, may have a respiratory function. Red, yellow, violet and other pigments are produced by some bacteria, most of them saprophytes of no medical importance, and also by many moulds. Growths of such organisms have been responsible for a number of curious episodes, such as 'bleeding' of statues and strange discolourations of foods. There is a legend that one famous bacteriologist amused his visitors by painting pictures, using bacteria as 'paints' and culture plates as 'canvas'. A more practical application of pigment production is that it gives help in the identification of organisms. For example, some of the ringworm fungi can be differentiated by the characteristic colours that they release into media on which they are growing.

Other Products
Some of man's essential vitamins are synthesized for him by his intestinal flora–a point which it is sometimes dangerous to forget. We have seen signs of severe deficiencies of vitamins B and K appear with startling speed in a patient with ulcerative colitis whose intestinal tract has been virtually sterilized by antibiotic treatment. It frequently happens in nature that the waste products of one species are the food supplies of another. A well-known laboratory illustration of the same principle is the satellite growth of *Haemophilus influenzae* around colonies of other bacteria which supply it with V factor (see p 137).

However, many products of microbial metabolism are probably of no use to any organisms, and indeed accumulated waste products are often fatal to their producers and to others. The precise nature of the end results of the metabolism of any particular organism depends in part upon the organism itself and in part upon the substrates available and the conditions of growth. If the substrates and conditions are standardized, the nature of the end products may give clues to the identity of the organism. This principle underlies many of the tests used in medical microbiology. We have mentioned the crude but informative procedure of testing an organism's ability to produce acid and gas from various sugars and alcohols (p 3). Such investigations provide a basis for the classification of Gram-negative bacilli and of several other groups of bacteria and fungi. Some other tests commonly used for similar purposes are mentioned on p 124. Gas-liquid chromatography (p 5) can be used to identify products of bacterial metabolism, and thus to indicate the nature of the organisms present in some clinical specimens (see p 242).

REPRODUCTION
Genetics

In general, micro-organisms reproduce themselves either by simple fission of one cell into two or by some form of sexual process in which genetic material from two or more cells is pooled and subsequently redistributed. Virus reproduction (or replication) does not conform to either of these patterns; it is discussed in Chapter Eleven. Some of the pathogenic protozoa, notably the malarial parasites, have complex life cycles with sexual and asexual phases (see Chapter Thirteen). Many fungi also show both types of reproduction, but most of those of medical importance have no known sexual phase; they form reproductive spores, but these are asexual.

A bacterium that reproduces by simple binary fission, as described on p 18, gives rise to two identical organisms, and consistent repetition of this process would produce a population of identical organisms. However, changes in the genetic composition (*genotypic variation*) of bacteria can happen in several ways. These include:

1 *Mutation.*   The bacterial nucleus or chromosome consists of double-stranded DNA, which in many bacteria at least is in the form of a loop. Each of the two intertwined spiral strands is a long sequence of nucleotide units; and each unit consists of a deoxyribose component which is part of the backbone of the strand and a projecting nitrogenous base component which is linked with that of a unit on the other strand. The base may be any one of four substances – the purines adenine and guanine and the pyrimidines cytosine and thymine. The sequence in which these four bases occur down the length of the strand constitutes a code or formula which determines the structure of the cellular enzymes and therefore the properties of the organism. The two strands are not identical but are complementary, in accordance with the rule that adenine on one strand is always matched by and linked with thymine on the other, whereas guanine is similarly paired with cytosine. When the cell is about to divide, the two strands separate and each acts as a template or guide for the construction of its new partner, so that if all goes well two new double-

stranded molecules are formed, each identical with the original molecule. On the great majority of occasions all does go well; but it is not suprising that so complex and delicate a process is occasionally disturbed by factors that break the strands or in other ways cause errors of copying and consequent changes in the code. The altered pattern is then faithfully handed on to later generations, provided that it is compatible with survival.

In fact, spontaneous mutations are rare. Any given 'mistake' is unlikely to arise in ordinary circumstances more than once in many millions of divisions, though its likelihood can be considerably increased by exposure of the dividing organisms to ultra-violet or X-irradiation or to one of various 'mutagenic' chemicals. The significance of mutation is greatly enhanced by circumstances that favour the mutants. For example, if 100 million bacteria, including one streptomycin-resistant mutant, are added to a suitable streptomycin-containing broth, the broth will soon be populated entirely by streptomycin-resistant descendants of the one mutant. (Environmental selective mechanisms are similarly important in determining the significance of any other form of genotypic variation.)

Note that mutation occurs within a single cell. Each of the other three processes described below involves movement of genetic material from one cell to another.

2 *Transformation.*   Pneumococci are capsulated bacteria and can be divided into a large number of types according to the chemical composition of their capsules. It used to be thought that each type would always breed true–e.g. that the descendants of a type 1 pneumococcus would always have type 1 capsules, unless they lost the ability to form capsules at all. However, the possibility of type-transformation was first demonstrated by Griffith in 1928 and its mechanism was elucidated in 1944 by Avery, McLeod and McCarty, whose experiments provided the first clear evidence for the central role of DNA in the mechanisms of inheritance. They found that if pneumococci of one type are grown under defined conditions in the presence of soluble DNA from pneumococci of another type, a minute proportion of the dividing organisms take up the 'foreign' DNA, incorporate it into their genetic make-up, and produce progeny which can make capsular material appropriate to the type from which the DNA came. Soluble-DNA-mediated transformation has been shown to be possible in many bacterial species other than pneumococci, but it occurs only when donor and recipient strains are of the same or closely related species.

3 *Transduction.*   Sometimes when a bacterial culture becomes infected by a virus (called a bacteriophage–see p 210) from another strain, a small minority of the recipient organisms acquire some property of the donor strain and transmit it as a stable genetic character to their descendants. This happens because the bacteriophage brings with it some of its previous host's DNA. Since as a rule any bacteriophage has only a narrow host range, transduction is usually between closely related strains. *Lysogenic conversion,* a different form of genotypic variation due to bacteriophage, is described on p 212.

4 *Conjugation.*   The genetic material of bacteria is not all located in the nuclear chromosome. In some bacteria at least, part of it is in the form of extra-chromosomal DNA units (or units which alternate between being free and being integrated into the chromosome) known as *plasmids* or *episomes.* Such free units are reproduced independently of the nucleus. They determine possession of properties that are 'optional' in the sense that they are not essential for the survival of the bacterium in a favourable environment. Individual bacterial cells of many different species contain special plasmids, *transfer factors,* which confer on them the ability to form *sex fimbriae* (see p 18) by which they attach themselves to and conjugate with other bacterial cells that do not already have transfer factor plasmids. In conjugation genetic material–the transfer factor and one or more other plasmids or part of the chromosome–is transferred from the initiating cell to its partner, which can then pass on some or all of the newly acquired genetic material (and therefore the associated properties) to its progeny. This form of genetic transfer is in fact a great deal more complex than our brief outline suggests, and there are a number of variants of it. It does not depend on close taxonomic relationship between donor and recipient organisms, and this fact has important medical implications; it means, for example, that antibiotic-resistant but harmless organisms in the human or animal intestine can confer antibiotic resistance, by plasmid transfer, on potentially pathogenic but previously antibiotic-sensitive bacteria of other genera which the host happens to ingest. The practical significance of such *transferable* or *infective drug resistance* is discussed in Chapter Twenty-one.

Phenotypic variations are changes of appearance or behaviour which depend on environmental factors and involve no alteration of genetic structure. The microscopic and colonial appearances of bacteria, their possession of flagella or of capsules, and many of their metabolic activities vary according to their circumstances. Particularly clear examples of phenotypic variation are provided by bacteria that show enzymic induction; these inherit a potential ability to make certain enzymes but only 'learn' to do so after being exposed for a while to appropriate substrates (see p 27).

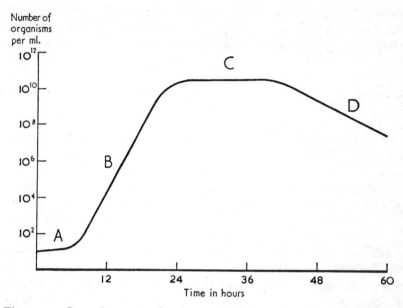

Figure 1   Growth curve of a bacterial culture in a liquid medium, showing lag phase (A), logarithmic phase (B), stationary phase (C) and phase of decline (D).

Phases of Growth

Many laboratory investigations of bacteria depend upon introducing them into or on to sterile culture media where they can multiply; and many experiments have been worthless because the experimenter failed to appreciate some of the factors determining their subsequent rate of multiplication. Each bacterial strain has its own maximal rate which it can achieve under optimal conditions; but it does not necessarily begin to reproduce at this rate straight away.

Fig. 1 shows a typical growth curve of a bacterial culture in broth. The logarithm of the count of living bacteria is plotted against the time after the inoculation of the broth. The exact shape of the curve depends on many factors, including the nature of the organism, the size of the inoculum, the age of the culture from which it was taken, the composition of the medium and the conditions of incubation; but four stages of activity can usually be discerned. In the first stage, called the *lag phase*, the inoculated bacterial cells adapt themselves to their new environment and prepare for division. They increase in size, but there is little increase in numbers. In due course division speeds up and is soon occurring at the maximal rate for the system. The increase in numbers is now exponential, the population doubling at regular intervals. Since such an increase takes the form of a straight line when plotted against a logarithmic scale, this stage is called the *logarithmic phase* of growth. The maximal rate of division continues until it is slowed by one or both of two factors—exhaustion of nutrients or accumulation of toxic metabolites. The population increase gradually comes to a standstill, the *stationary phase*, and this is succeeded by the *phase of decline*, in which the number of living bacteria slowly decreases. The speed and shape of this decline depends upon the susceptibility of the organisms to their own waste products; some delicate species are extinct within a few days, whereas cultures of others may continue to yield survivors for years. The total number of bacteria, living and dead, in a broth culture remains constant for a long period after the stationary phase, unless the organism is autolytic, producing enzymes that destroy its own cells.

One reason why it is important to know about these phases of growth is that the rapidly multiplying bacteria of the logarithmic phase are particularly susceptible to damage by antiseptics and antibiotics. They are also able to multiply at maximal speed immediately, without a lag phase, if transferred to suitable fresh medium. Therefore many *in vitro* comparisons between organisms are meaningless because the inocula are taken from cultures in different phases of growth.

A logarithmic rate of multiplication can be maintained indefinitely if the culture medium is repeatedly or continuously renewed. Such *continuous culture* has important industrial applications—e.g. in the manufacture of antibiotics—and also makes possible the study of bacterial metabolism under constant and controllable conditions.

SURVIVAL AND DEATH

Micro-organisms vary greatly in their resistance to adverse physical and chemical conditions. Some fail to survive minor environmental changes, whereas others are difficult to kill. Spore-forming species are the most durable. Spores have the physical protection of their thick coats, their metabolic needs are minimal and since they do not divide they avoid the increased susceptibility of dividing cells to various noxious agents. The tubercle bacillus and related organisms do not form spores, but having waxy hydrophobic surfaces and low rates of metabolism they are more resistant than most bacteria to drying and to chemical agents. They do not share the heat-resistance of the spore-formers.

In the sections and chapters that follow we use a number of technical terms relating to antimicrobial processes or substances. *Sterilization* means the killing or removal of *all* micro-organisms, including bacterial spores. *Disinfection* has a less precise meaning; it indicates the killing or removal of *potentially harmful* micro-organisms, other than resistant bacterial spores—and since potentially harmful bacteria have no particular susceptibility to such treatment, disinfection in practice means elimination of nearly all of the microbial population. The meanings of the terms *disinfectant*, *chemotherapeutic agent* and *antibiotic* are given on pp 38–40. We have abandoned the terms *antisepsis* and *antiseptic*, which were formerly used in much the same senses as disinfection and disinfectant. Applications of the processes of sterilization and disinfection are discussed in Chapter Seventeen.

Physical Agents

DRYING   Drying, as by exposure to ordinary atmospheric conditions, rapidly kills many bacteria and viruses, though some important non-sporing pathogens, such as *Mycobacterium tuberculosis*, *Staphylococcus aureus* and the smallpox virus, can survive in dust for long periods and sporing organisms can do so almost indefinitely.

FREEZING   Freezing kills some organisms, especially if they are in a liquid medium that is frozen slowly. However, even delicate organisms such as viruses and *Haemophilus influenzae* survive for many months at temperatures between − 20 and − 70°C if they are frozen rapidly.

A combination of drying and freezing known as *freeze-drying* or *lyophilization* is the most satisfactory method for long-term storage of bacteria. Broth cultures or bacterial suspensions are rapidly frozen and then evaporated to dryness in high vacuum. Alternatively, small volumes can be rapidly evaporated in the vacuum without preliminary freezing; they freeze in the early stages of this process as a result of loss of latent heat. Ampoules containing the lyophilized organisms are sealed while still attached to the vacuum pump, and can then be stored at room temperature.

HEAT   Heat is commonly used in sterilization. Most vegetative bacteria are killed in a few minutes at 60°C, but killing of spores by dry heat may take as much as 30 minutes at 160°C. Moisture increases their susceptibility, but even so they may survive prolonged boiling. With steam under pressure, as in the autoclave or in the domestic pressure cooker, sterilization can be achieved in 15 minutes at a pressure of 15 lb/sq. in.–i.e. at a temperature of 121°C.

RADIATION   Sunlight has an antimicrobial effect by virtue of its content of *ultraviolet light*, and artificial U.V. light is used in sterilization of air, of some forms of apparatus, and of materials such as plasma which would be rendered useless by heating or by chemical treatment. Although it has the merit of doing very little harm to the material treated, it has little power of penetration and can therefore sterilize only surfaces or thin layers of material. Its efficacy is greatly impaired by even a small amount of dust between the light source and the target. *X-rays*, *gamma-rays* and other penetrating radiations can kill micro-organisms, as can *sonic* or *ultra-sonic vibrations*.

Disinfectants

By this term we mean substances of useful antimicrobial activity which do not have serious general destructive effects such as are possessed by strong acids and alkalies, but which are too toxic for systemic use in the treatment of microbial infections. They are referred to as *bactericidal* when they kill bacteria (cf. fungicidal, germicidal) and as *bacteriostatic***** when they only prevent multiplication. It means nothing, however, to describe a substance as bactericidal or bacteriostatic without defining the concentration in which it is used, the identity and state of the organism and the conditions under which the two come into contact.

Some examples of well-known disinfectants are given in Table I. The useful applications of these varied compounds are determined by such properties as toxicity to human tissues, range of antimicrobial activity and degree of inactivation by organic matter. To give a few illustrations, cresols are too toxic to be applied to the skin, crystal violet is relatively ineffective against most Gram-negative organisms, and oxidizing agents are useless for the sterilization of faeces because they are reduced and inactivated by the large amounts of organic material present. But crystal violet is useful in the treatment of staphylococcal skin lesions, oxidizing agents can be used for the destruction of Gram-negative organisms so as to make water safe to drink, and cresols are suitable for sterilizing faeces. Other examples of the appropriate use of various disinfectants are given in later chapters, notably on pp 283–5.

Standardization of disinfectants presents serious problems. The Rideal-Walker coefficient was at one time widely used as a measure of the potency of a disinfectant. In fact it is only a measure of its superiority or inferiority to phenol for the single purpose of killing typhoid bacilli in the absence of organic matter. Even the Chick-Martin test, in which organic material is present in the form of sterilized faeces, tells us only what a disinfectant can do in those particular circumstances. Results obtained in a test-tube culture in a fluid medium may well be irrelevant to the choice of a disinfectant for the treatment of floors, furniture, or wounds. So far as practicable, such a choice should be based on 'in-use' tests specially designed to determine whether the disinfectant can do the job for which it is being used.

---

* The alternative spelling *bacteristatic* seems to be gaining support and is more consistent with *bactericidal*, but it is not yet generally accepted.

TABLE I
Some Properties of Some Commonly Used Disinfectants

Since the actions of disinfectants depend very largely on the conditions under which they are tested, entries in this table should be regarded as wide generalizations.

Class of compound	Examples and trade names	Vegetative bacteria killed[1]	Inactivation by organic matter	Toxicity to human tissues
Alcohols	Ethyl alcohol[2]	All	Moderate	Moderate
Aldehydes	Formaldehyde[3]	All	Moderate	Marked
Organic dyes	Crystal violet	Some	Moderate	Slight
	Proflavine	Some	Slight	Slight
Cationic detergents	Cetrimide ('Cetavlon')	Most	Marked	Slight
	Chlorhexidine ('Hibitane')	Most	Marked	Slight
Soaps, anionic detergents		Some	Slight	Slight
Phenols	Carbolic acid	All	Slight	Marked
Clear phenolics	'Hycolin', 'Stericol' 'Clearsol' }	All	Slight	Moderate
Cresols	'Lysol'	All	Slight	Marked
Chlorxylenols	'Dettol'	All	Moderate	Moderate
Hexachlorophane	'Phisohex'	Most	Slight	Slight
Oxidizing agents	Iodine, chlorine, iodoform, chloroform, sodium hypochlorite, potassium permanganate, hydrogen peroxide }	All	Marked	Slight to moderate
Salts of heavy metals	Mercuric chloride	All	Marked	Marked
Organic metal compounds	'Merthiolate'	All	Marked	Slight

[1] No available disinfectant is reliably effective against bacterial *spores*. The susceptibilities of rickettsiae, chlamydiae and viruses to disinfectants are considered on pp 161 and 181.
[2] Absolute alcohol is a relatively ineffective disinfectant; its activity is increased by dilution
[3] Formaldehyde can be used either as a gas or in aqueous solution; formalin is a 40% aqueous solution of formaldehyde.

Chemotherapeutic Agents

These are synthetic chemicals active against micro-organisms *in vitro* and of sufficiently low toxicity to be administered systemically. Scientific chermotherapy began in the first decade of this century (see p 12), when Ehrlich introduced the therapeutic use of the organic arsenical compounds, starting with atoxyl for trypanosomiasis and arsphenamine for syphilis. Then in 1935 Domagk showed that the newly-discovered prontosil (sulphonamidochrysoidin) could cure streptococcal infections in mice or human beings. Other therapeutically useful sulphonamides followed, differing from one another in solubility, toxicity and degree of absorption from the intestine but all acting in the same way upon bacteria. Being derivatives of *p*-aminobenzene sulphonamide, they all closely resemble *p*-aminobenzoic acid (PABA), an essential metabolite for many bacteria. If these organisms take up sulphonamide instead of PABA, their metabolism is arrested. Bacteriostasis depends upon there being a considerable excess of sulphonamide over PABA in the environment, and is reversible by the addition of more PABA. Sulphonamides are not bactericidal (see p 342 for the action of sulphonamide-trimethoprim mixtures). Their discovery was one of the great events of medical history because of the wide range of bacteria against which they are effective, and the great medical importance of some of these –e.g. haemolytic streptococci, pneumococci, meningococci, gonococci, dysentery bacilli and many of the Gram-negative bacilli causing urinary tract infections.

Many other chemotherapeutic agents are currently in clinical use, notably those mentioned on pp 341–3 and those used for leprosy (p 149), tuberculosis (pp 356–7), virus infections (pp 180–1) and protozoal infections (pp 223–30).

Antibiotics

This term, coined in 1942 by Waksman to describe a newly-discovered class of antimicrobial agents, is now a household word. According to Waksman's definition, an antibiotic is a substance, produced by micro-organisms, which can inhibit the growth of or even destroy other micro-organisms (the reverse of symbiotic activity). He also specified that dilute solutions of the substance must have these properties, thus excluding, for example, the lactic acid produced by lactobacilli (see p 28). The limits of Waksman's definition are now being stretched by man's activities in synthesizing compounds similar to or identical with those made by micro-organisms. It is hard to deny the name antibiotic to a substance such as chloramphenicol, which is man-made but is chemically identical with an antibiotic produced by a bacterium. The semisynthetic penicillins and other antimicrobial substances made in the laboratory by chemical alteration of microbial products are less easy to classify, and the dividing line between antibiotics and chemotherapeutic agents is now indefinite.

Very large numbers of antibiotics have been isolated from cultures of fungi or bacteria, notably from branching bacteria of the genus *Streptomyces*. Those with low toxicity to man coupled with high activity against his pathogens have been studied most fully. The first of these, *penicillin* (more strictly, benzyl penicillin), was isolated from the mould *Penicillin notatum* by Fleming in 1928 and made available for medical use by the work of Florey and Chain a decade later. It is remarkably non-toxic when pure; in concentrations which can easily be obtained in the body it is bactericidal to many important pathogens; and in the form of its sodium salt it is reasonably stable, except in acid conditions. It continues to be one of the most valuable antibiotics for clinical use, but falls short of the ideal in several important respects. It is ineffective against many pathogenic bacteria, including the tubercle bacillus and most Gram-negative bacilli, and against all non-bacterial pathogens; its use has resulted in the emergence of resistant (usually penicillinase-producing) strains of many species, notably *Staph. aureus*, and its effectiveness when given by mouth is limited by its acid-lability. Subsequent research has therefore been directed to finding other antibiotics free of these defects. Very large numbers of streptomycetes and other organisms have been screened for signs of antibacterial activity, and a number of useful compounds have been found by this empirical approach. Between them they have considerably expanded the range of pathogens susceptible to antibiotic treatment, so that this now includes the great majority of bacteria, the rickettsiae and the chlamydiae and some of the fungi. However, all of these compounds have at least some toxicity for man, and in concentrations that can be achieved in the body many are only bacteriostatic. Some of them can be given by mouth. Meanwhile it has been possible to produce variants of the penicillin molecule which are free from one or more of the defects of benzyl penicillin (see pp 344–5).

To be of clinical value an antibiotic must produce serious structural or metabolic lesions in the cells of the micro-organisms against which it is used, without at the same time doing significant damage to the cells of the human host. Hence the success of the penicillins and the related cephalosporins, which interfere with synthesis of cell-wall mucopeptide, a vital bacterial component not shared by human or other eukaryotic cells (see p 17); the consequences of such interference are, in some circumstances and with some organisms, inability of the bacteria to form cross-walls and so replicate themselves, and in other circumstances the formation of faulty cell wall which, like a damaged cycle-tyre outer tube, allows rupture of the unsupported cytoplasmic membrane (the 'inner tube') by osmotic pressure. Other antibiotics – the aminoglycosides, chloramphenicol, the tetracyclines, the macrolides and clindamycin – interfere at various points in the protein-synthesizing activities of bacterial ribosomes, and their clinical usefulness depends on differences between bacterial and mammalian ribosomes. Both these forms of interference with the processes of growth are effective only against multiplying bacteria, as is the inhibition of bacterial RNA synthesis by the rifamycins; but the damage that the polymyxins inflict on bacterial cytoplasmic membranes, leading to leakage of cell contents, is lethal even to resting cells.

Differences in antimicrobial drug sensitivities between bacterial species, or between strains within a species, are of great importance in medical microbiology and in the clinical management of bacterial infections. One species or strain may be more resistant than another to a particular drug for one or more of the following reasons: its internal biochemical processes may not be so dependent upon pathways susceptible to the action of the drug; its cell wall may be relatively impermeable to the drug; or, whatever its intrinsic susceptibility or permeability, it may be able to defend itself by producing a drug-destroying enzyme.

Further information about chemotherapeutic and antibiotic agents in common use in clinical medicine is to be found in Chapter Twenty-One.

Suggestions for Further Reading

Chemical Microbiology by A. H. Rose, 3rd edn. (Butterworth, Sevenoaks, 1976).

PART III

PATHOGENESIS OF MICROBIAL DISEASES

6

Transmission of Pathogens

The idea that diseases might be transmitted in the form of particulate matter rather than of abstract influences goes back at least to the sixteenth century. But, as we have seen (p 9), it was not until just over a century ago that Pasteur proved this to be true, showed that the transmissible particles are in fact minute living organisms, and finally destroyed the theory of heterogenesis or spontaneous generation, which postulated that micro-organisms in putrefying wounds and other lesions were formed on the spot from non-microbial materials. Today we know that the spread of microbial diseases depends upon the transmission of their causative organisms.

The term *infection* and related words occur frequently in most discussions of microbial diseases, but there is no general agreement as to their precise meaning–in particular, as to whether they imply actual invasion of host tissues or merely the presence of potential invaders. We think that infection is best defined as the arrival or presence of potentially pathogenic organisms on the surface or in the tissues of an appropriate host. We can then refer to an infected person, to an infected wound or part of the body, or to an infected animal or plant–even to a bacterium being infected with bacteriophage–but not to infected inanimate objects. For the latter, when they are carrying potential pathogens, and also when they should be sterile but have ceased to be so, we prefer the term *contaminated*. An infectious disease is one that is transmissible from patient to patient by transfer of the causative organism; and an infectious patient is one from whom such a disease can be acquired. Infection is called *clinical* when it is causing overt disease, or *sub-clinical* when there is little or no impairment of the patient's health. Persistent sub-clinical infection that may be converted into clinical infection by changing circumstances is described as *latent*.

Even these definitions do not eliminate all terminological

difficulties, since an aura of uncertainty surrounds the words 'potentially pathogenic'. For example, all human beings carry in their intestinal tracts *Escherichia coli* and related Gram-negative bacilli capable of producing disease in the urinary tract, in wounds and elsewhere. If we are to retain any useful meaning for the words that we are attempting to define, carriage of normal commensal or symbiotic organisms in normal sites must be excluded from their scope, even if those organisms are sometimes pathogenic elsewhere.

There is no ambiguity about the following terms commonly used in discussing microbial diseases; *epidemic*, a noun or an adjective, describing a temporary marked increase in frequency of a particular disease in a community; *pandemic*, referring to a world-wide epidemic; and *endemic*, used only as an adjective, describing a disease which is persistently present in a community. An endemic disease may from time to time flare up into an epidemic.

SOURCES OF PATHOGENS

Except when lowered local or general resistance makes a patient susceptible to the attacks of his resident parasites, pathogenic organisms are *exogenous*–that is, they come from outside the patient. With few exceptions (such as some fungi and possibly some clostridia), they come, directly or indirectly, from other human beings or from animals. These may themselves be clinically infected, or may be *carriers*, transmitting pathogens without showing any evidence of related disease. Carriers are important in the spread of epidemics, since they are hard to detect, mix freely with other people, and may disseminate large numbers of organisms over long periods; whereas victims of clinical disease are less 'successful' as distributors of the organisms because they are liable to be segregated, to some extent at least, and may even be permanently removed from circulation by death. Carriers may be *incubational* (or *precocious*) carriers, who will shortly develop the disease, or *convalescent* carriers, who have already had it. Often, however, they are *symptomless* carriers, whose infection is entirely sub-clinical. Typhoid is the classic example of a disease in which the carrier state may persist for many years, and may be very difficult to detect because excretion of the organism is intermittent. Hospital outbreaks of wound sepsis and other lesions due to *Staphylococcus aureus* are often traced to nasal or cutaneous carriage of the offending strains by members of the staff (see Chapter Eighteen).

TRANSFER OF PATHOGENS

Common routes for the spread of microbial diseases are indicated in Tables II and III. Only a few of the items listed there require further comment.

Droplets

'Coughs and sneezes spread diseases'. Even when talking or breathing quietly we constantly emit from our mouths and noses numerous droplets of moisture containing bacteria and viruses. The fate of these droplets depends on their size. The largest of them fall rapidly to the ground, where they dry and the organisms are added to the dust. Small droplets, however, evaporate to dryness in the air, leaving their solid contents as droplet-nuclei. These may remain airborne for long periods and travel considerable distances on air-currents, and they are readily inhaled by other people. Diseases spread largely by means of droplets include most bacterial infections of the respiratory tract, meningitis and many common virus infections.

TABLE II
Stages in the Transmission of Pathogens

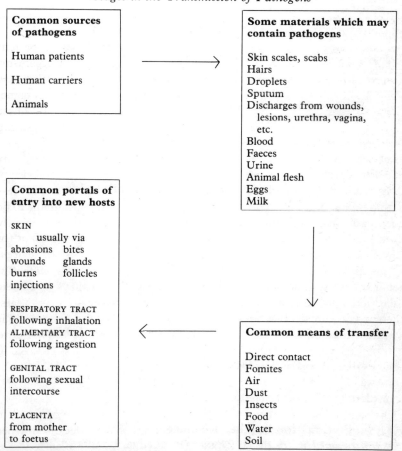

Direct Contact

Our ancestors used to talk of contagious diseases. There are certainly many which can be transmitted by direct contact, but only a few in which this is the principal means of spread. These few include the venereal diseases and probably leprosy.

TABLE III
Some Examples of Transmission of Pathogens

Disease	Type of organism	Source	Material containing pathogens	Common method of transfer	Common portal of entry
Syphilis	Bacterium	Human patient	Discharge from lesion	Direct contact	Abraded skin or genital tract
Tuberculosis	Bacterium	Human patient or Cow	Sputum Milk	Air, dust Food or drink	Respiratory tract Alimentary tract
Typhoid	Bacterium	Human patient or carrier	Faeces or urine	Food or water	Alimentary tract
Typhus	Rickettsia	Human patient	Blood	Louse	Bite
Smallpox	Virus	Human patient	Droplets or scabs	Air or dust	Respiratory tract
Influenza	Virus	Human patient	Droplets	Air	Respiratory tract
Ringworm	Fungus	Human patient or animal	Hair or scales	Contact, fomites	Intact skin
Malaria	Protozoon	Human patient	Blood	Mosquito	Bite

Fomites (p 7)

This is a useful comprehensive word for the patient's bedding, clothes, towels, books and other personal possessions and equipment. Sharing of such items may well transmit pathogens.

Soil

Contamination of wounds by soil is liable to result in gas-gangrene or tetanus. Both diseases are caused by sporing anaerobic bacilli of the genus *Clostridium,* which are commonly present in soil and also in the faeces of man and of animals. It is not certain whether their presence in soil is due to faecal contamination or whether this is their primary habitat.

PORTALS OF ENTRY

The way by which pathogens gain admission to the human body will be considered in the next chapter.

Suggestions for Further Reading

Rats, Lice and History by H. Zinsser (Routledge, London, 1942).

7

Pathogenicity and Host Defences

PATHOGENICITY

There is much in common between our uses of the words 'pathogen' and 'criminal'.

Some people are known to the police as specialists in particular forms of crime; others as more versatile wrong-doers; and others as generally law-abiding citizens who are liable to occasional lapses. To be a known criminal is not to be incapable of any other sort of existence; and to be unknown to the police is not necessarily the same as being innocent.

Similarly, some micro-organisms, such as *Corynebacterium diphtheriae* and *Clostridium tetani*, are known to be responsible for characteristic diseases; others, such as *Staphylococcus aureus* and *Streptococcus pyogenes*, can cause many different forms of disease; and others, such as *Str. viridans*, are usually harmless but in special circumstances may become pathogens. Most known pathogens are capable of existing as harmless commensals; and undoubtedly there are many species with as yet unsuspected pathogenic activities.

To establish beyond doubt that a given organism causes a given disease may be a difficult problem. It is not enough to show that it is constantly present in an appropriate distribution in each case of the disease, for its presence may be a result rather than the cause of the disease. According to the classical criteria of pathogenicity commonly known as Koch's postulates (though in fact Koch never formulated them so precisely) it should be possible to show that the organism is constantly present as already indicated, to grow it in artificial culture media, and to reproduce the disease in susceptible animals by administering such cultures to them. However, there are many diseases to which these criteria cannot be applied, but which can be confidently attributed to particular organisms. For example, *Treponema pallidum* cannot be grown in culture and does not produce in animals anything closely resembling syphilis, yet its association with that disease is so constant that nobody doubts its causative role.

Even when a particular microbial species is certainly pathogenic, this property is not necessarily, or even usually, shared by all strains of the species. It is common to find bacterial strains that are identical in all measurable characters except that one is pathogenic to certain hosts and the other is not. The term *virulence* is often used in an attempt to quantitate pathogenicity, but caution is needed here. It is sometimes convenient to be able to describe a strain as highly virulent, or of reduced virulence or avirulent; but we can give mathematical expression to virulence only if we define carefully the conditions under which it is measured. We can determine how many organisms of a particular strain constitute a lethal dose (LD) for a mouse, but this information is of little value because mice, like all other hosts, show wide variations of individual susceptibility. We have achieved rather more if we determine the number of organisms which, if administered to each of a large batch of closely similar mice, will kill 50% of them (the LD 50 for those mice); but even this information is only of value for comparison with the LD 50 of another strain grown under the same conditions in the same medium for the same length of time and administered in the same way to a batch of mice of the same strain which are strictly comparable with the first batch in regard to age, sex, size, nutrition, past experience of infection and any other features that may be relevant. Such a comparison will not necessarily tell us anything about the relative virulence of the two strains for another host species or even for mice of a different breed or age.

Implicit in what we have said about LD 50 measurements is an important concept – that the number ('dose') of organisms taking part in an infection has an important influence on its outcome. In an epidemic, or in an outbreak of common-source illness such as food-poisoning after a party, it is often found that some of those exposed have symptomless infections, some are mildly ill and some are more severely affected. In general such variations are likely to be determined, in part at least, by differences in the doses of pathogens reaching individuals, though other factors such as host immunity can also be important.

The impossibility of comparing virulence without specifying the host is well illustrated by the human and bovine tubercle bacilli (*Mycobacterium tuberculosis* and *Myco. bovis*). Both are pathogenic for man and for guinea-pigs, but cattle and rabbits are far less susceptible to human than to bovine strains. It is common practice to use guinea-pigs in testing the probable pathogenicity of tubercle bacillus strains for man; to use rabbits for this purpose would be grossly misleading.

The virulence of a microbial strain for a given host species may decrease progressively when the strain is maintained in laboratory culture or in an unrelated host species; such a strain is described as attenuated. Thus the *Bacille Calmette-Guerin* (*B.C.G.*) is a bovine tubercle bacillus strain attenuated by prolonged artificial culture. When injected into humans it causes only local lesions, but stimulates the development of immunity effective against natural tuberculosis (see p 310). Similarly, man can be protected against smallpox by inoculation with a strain of smallpox virus that has become adapted to living and multiplying in the skin of a calf, and has concurrently lost its ability to produce more than a local lesion in man (see p 206).

Characters of Pathogens

In some microbial species pathogenicity is closely associated with recognizable characters of the organisms, and strains without these characters are avirulent. Bacterial are sometimes isolated which have all the properties of the diphtheria bacillus except the ability to form exotoxin. Such strains are known as non-toxigenic *Corynebacterium diphtheriae*, and since it is the toxin which harms the host in diphtheria, it is not surprising that such strains are avirulent. Loss or reduction of virulence of *Streptococcus pneumoniae* occurs when it loses the ability to form a capsule. This too is understandable, since the capsule is known to protect the organism against ingestion by the host's phagocytic cells (see p 54), and may make other contributions to its pathogenicity. Other examples of such correlations could be given, but it is still true of a large proportion of pathogens that we have little or no idea what features make them pathogenic.

We can, however, make some generalizations about characters that pathogens must have:

1 Apart from a few special cases (e.g. botulism, which is due to the patient's ingestion of a ready-made bacterial toxin), a micro-organism *must be able to enter the host's body* in order to be able to produce disease. However, it may remain very near the surface, as do the ringworm fungi in the skin and *C. diphtheriae* and common cold viruses in the upper respiratory tract. Routes and methods of entry are discussed later in relation to the body's superficial defences.

The term *endogenous* is used to describe infections due to organisms that were previously present as commensals of the same host; and it appears to imply that they are exceptions to this rule. However, the organisms have of course come originally from outside the host; and their change to pathogenicity usually involves deeper penetration into his tissues or transfer to another part of his body.

2 *A pathogen must be able to multiply in the host's tissues.* Put the other way round, this means that the host's tissues must supply appropriate nutrients, atmospheric conditions and temperature for the pathogen's growth. Here we can see in broad outline the facts which determine the host ranges of all pathogens, and indeed of all parasites, but we can fill in very few of the details. Similar factors undoubtedly play a large part also in deciding the distribution of parasites within the body of the individual host, and the sites at which pathogens produce their characteristic lesions. For example, the fact that *Mycobacterium ulcerans* and *Myco.marinum* can multiply only in the temperature range 30–33 °C presumably accounts for their ability to produce lesions only in the skin of man and not in deeper tissues. (The distribution of leprosy lesions, due to the related *Myco.leprae*, suggests a similar temperature range for this organism, but confirmation of this awaits reliable means of growing it *in vitro*.) The restriction of the rhinovirus group of common cold viruses to the upper respiratory tract may be similarly determined (see p 188). Abnormal conditions in the tissues of a host may permit organisms to thrive which could not otherwise grow there. Hence diabetics are unduly susceptible to infections, probably as a result of the high glucose content and other chemical peculiarities of their tissues; and gas-gangrene, caused by anaerobic organisms of the genus *Clostridium*, occurs in tissues which have lost their blood supply and so their source of oxygen. The role of erythritol in localizing brucella infection in bovine abortion is considered on p 141. In the majority of cases, however, we do not know what determines the localization of organisms of microbial lesions.

3 It is self-evident that to be a pathogen an organism *must be able to damage the host's tissues*. This can happen in many different ways. As we mentioned on p 29, bacteria may produce local or more remote damage by releasing exotoxins as they multiply or endotoxins when they die and disintegrate. Viruses invade host cells and divert their synthetic processes to the production of more viruses – sometimes on a small scale, carrying on quietly for long periods without apparent damage to the host cells, but often on such a scale as to disorganize the cells' metabolism, impair their functional efficiency and even cause their rupture and destruction. Malarial parasites also multiply inside host cells, notably red blood cells, and rupture them, causing severe anaemia and other disorders.

4 In order to be able to do any of the things mentioned so far, a pathogen *must be able to resist and overcome the host's defence mechanisms*. These we will now consider, continuing to refer at appropriate points to some of the microbial 'answers' to them.

NON-SPECIFIC HOST DEFENCES

Defence mechanisms included under this heading are effective against wide ranges of micro-organisms. Some of them are somewhat dependent upon the body's previous experience of micro-organisms in general, but their effectiveness is not limited to organisms of the same kinds as it has met before.

Superficial Defences

Most of the outer surface of the body is covered by *skin*, which is both a mechanical barrier to micro-organisms and, by virtue of the fatty acid content of sweat and sebum, a death-bed for many of them. However, hair follicles and glands form comparatively weak points in the defences, and by multiplying in these *Staph. aureus* may give rise to pustules, boils and carbuncles. This same bacterial species, being resistant to the bactericidal action of the skin secretions, is commonly present on the surface and may be carried into the subcutaneous tissues by anything which pierces or lacerates the skin.

The *conjunctivae* are less of a mechanical obstruction, but they are constantly washed by tears and wiped by the movement of the eyelids. Tears contain an enzyme *lysozyme* (also present in most other body fluids and in polymorphonuclear leucocytes) which dissolves bacteria of many species.

Mucus, secreted by the membranes lining most of the internal surfaces of the body, prevents organisms from penetrating to the tissues over which it lies. Caught up in this secretion, microbial and other foreign particles are extruded from the body by various mechanisms; these include ciliary currents, coughing, sneezing and intestinal peristalsis.

Saliva is mildly bactericidal. A more effective barrier against entry of micro-organisms via the alimentary tract is provided by *gastric juice*, mainly by virtue of its acidity. However, some pathogens, of widely different sorts, can pass through the stomach unharmed.

The protective role of the *normal bacterial flora* has become increasingly apparent since the introduction of antibiotics. A number of diseases have greatly increased in frequency since we have had enhanced power to disturb the bacterial equilibrium of the body; these include infections of the mouth, respiratory or intestinal tracts and vagina by the fungus *Candida albicans* (candidiasis) and bronchopulmonary infection with intestinal Gram-negative bacilli (see p 125). Staphylococcal enteritis is a grave but fortunately rare consequence of the derangement of the bowel flora by antibiotics (see p 95). We have already mentioned the protective action of lactobacilli in the adult vagina (p 28); and the relative immunity of breast-fed infants to enteritis may be at least partly due to a similar action of acid-producing lactobacilli in their intestines. It is likely that organisms normally present in other parts of the body serve the same function of keeping abnormal and potentially pathogenic invaders at bay, but we know little about the mechanisms involved.

Cellular Defences

Organisms which get through the outer defences and begin to multiply within the tissues usually provoke inflammatory reactions. The vigour and pattern of these depend, among other things, on the nature of the organism and on the previous experience of the host. Full discussion of the mechanisms of inflammation is the province of the pathologist rather than the microbiologist. For our immediate purposes it is enough to say that part of the reaction, at least when the organisms are bacteria, is usually the emigration of polymorphonuclear leucocytes and larger mononuclear cells from the blood capillaries into the tissue spaces around the invaders. They are attracted there by a chemical signalling system (*chemotaxis*), and are able to engulf bacteria and other small particles (*phagocytosis*). Some bacteria, especially those equipped with capsules, are resistant to this process. It has been shown that phagocytes cannot grasp capsulate pneumococci when they are suspended in fluid, but can engulf them if they can first trap them against fibrin or other solid material. One simple explanation of these observations is that the capsulate forms are too slippery for the phagocytes to hold without the assistance of some relatively rough surface. Phagocytosis of these and other bacteria occurs more readily, in the host or *in vitro*, if specific antibodies called opsonins are present (see p 67).

Having been engulfed by phagocytes, bacteria vary greatly in their ability to survive the digestive activity of the cells; tubercle bacilli and typhoid bacilli are among the most resistant. Often it is the phagocytes which die first, either succumbing to the toxic action of bacterial leucocidins (see p 29) or being physically disrupted by the multiplication of the parasites within them. *Pus*, a frequent end-product of an encounter between pathogens and the host's defence cells, is a complex material that includes living or dead organisms and phagocytes (as a rule mainly polymorphs) and remnants of destroyed tissues. However, some bacteria—notably the brucellae and the tubercle and leprosy bacilli—survive for long periods, travel around the host's body and even multiply inside the long-lived large mononuclear cells (macrophages) which have engulfed them. In this situation they are protected against the body's humoral defences (though not against cell-mediated immunity—see p 73) and against antibiotics. Organisms of the rickettsia group and some viruses, fungi and protozoa make similar use of host macrophages.

Unless killed at the point of entry, invading bacteria usually find their way into the lymph capillaries, either in the free state or carried by phagocytes. On reaching the lymph nodes they may be taken up by the fixed phagocytic cells of the *reticulo-endothelial system:* but they may pass through the lymphatic system into the blood stream, from which they may be removed by other reticulo-endothelial cells in the spleen, liver or bone marrow. Mere presence of a few bacteria in the blood stream is a common state of affairs compatible with normal health, and is known as *bacteraemia.* It may follow every-day activities such as heavy chewing, which forces harmless mouth bacteria from the tooth sockets into the blood. When pathogenic organisms enter the blood stream in large numbers, or multiply there, and their presence makes the patient ill, the condition is described as *septicaemia.*

Human and other mammalian cells react to the presence of foreign double-stranded RNA by producing a protein called *interferon.* Replication of virus within a cell involves synthesis of virus RNA and is thus liable to be a potent stimulator of interferon production; some bacteria, rickettsiae and protozoa have the same effect. Interferon diffuses out from the infected cell into neighbouring cells, where it prevents replication of both the original virus strain and of other unrelated viruses that may be around. It is not toxic to animal cells, even when concentrated. Interferon production is not a property of special cells but has been demonstrated in many different tissues of various animals. So far it appears that the nature of the interferon produced by a given host is independent of the type of virus provoking it. There are, however, differences between interferons produced by different host species, so that interferon from the cells of one host gives effective protection only to cells of the same or related species. There can be no doubt that interferon plays an important part in the natural defences of the body against virus infections – particularly because, unlike specific immunity, it comes into play almost immediately after infection and is produced at the scene of the trouble. Great hopes have been aroused that it will also prove to be a valuable therapeutic weapon when it can be prepared in adequate quantities; but it cannot be synthesized, and the problems of large-scale *in vivo* production can easily be imagined. An alternative to administering it to a patient would be to give him some substance that stimulates his own production of interferon. So far substances that have been found to do this all have side-effects that make them unsuitable for clinical use. Moreover, not all viruses are equally sensitive to interferons, and it is in general true that the higher the virulence of a virus for a given tissue the less effective it is as a stimulus to interferon production in that tissue and the less sensitive it is to interferon produced by that tissue.

Humoral Defences

Cell-free serum and body fluids contain non-specific antimicrobial substances and mechanisms, but these are difficult to study; this is partly because they are of low potency and partly because all subjects except the newborn have many different specific humoral agents (*antibodies*–see below) in their body fluids as a result of their previous experiences of infection, and even newborn infants have antibodies derived from their mothers.

SPECIFIC IMMUNITY

Specific immunity, which is discussed more fully in the next chapter, is the resistance of an individual to a particular disease as a result of his ability to defend himself against its causative agent. It depends upon his genetic inheritance, his age, his general health and his past experience of micro-organisms. It may be classified as follows:

1 *Innate immunity.*   Each individual inherits certain susceptibilities and resistances peculiar to his species, his race and his family, and has his own personal combination of these. Presumably they depend upon his tissue chemistry, his superficial and cellular defence mechanisms, and possibly non-specific humoral agents. As he matures and ages, all of these factors vary through hormonal and other influences, so that immunity changes with age quite apart from the contributions mentioned in the next two paragraphs.

2 *Naturally acquired immunity.* Naturally occurring clinical or sub-clinical infection commonly provokes responses on the part of the host which enhance his ability to resist the causative organism when he meets it again. These responses involve production of agents that react specifically with the organism or its products–either special proteins called *antibodies* or special sensitized cells (the effect of which is described as *cell-mediated immunity*) or both. Immunity due to the host's own responses is called *active*, whereas immunity conferred by maternal antibodies that enter the infant's circulation via the placenta–or in some animal species via colostrum or milk–is called naturally acquired *passive* immunity because the infant itself has made no contribution to it.

3 *Artificially acquired immunity.*   Artificial stimulation of specific resistance to infection is called *immunization*, and is discussed more fully in Chapter Twenty. This also may be *active* or *passive*, in that the subject may be provoked to make his own antibodies or may be given some ready-made.

SOME POSSIBLE RESULTS OF INFECTION

A consideration of all possible outcomes of encounters between pathogens and host defences would be a review of the entire field of microbial diseases. The discussion would be further complicated by the need to take into consideration many different factors in the host's condition and circumstances which may affect the issue–e.g. injuries, anatomical abnormalities, presence of foreign bodies in wounds, nutritional state of the host and effects of treatment either with antimicrobial agents or with X-rays, steroid hormones or other agents that impair host resistance. However, it may be helpful to outline and illustrate a few of the situations which develop.

1 *Elimination of the pathogen without any clinical lesion.* This is undoubtedly the commonest outcome of infection by a pathogen, but for obvious reasons it is virtually never observed. If the elimination is not too rapid, it may be possible to demonstrate retrospectively that infection has occurred, because shortly afterwards specific antibodies appear in the host's blood or he develops a specific tissue hypersensitivity.

2 *Localization of the pathogen with production of a local lesion.* This is clearly illustrated by the common small staphylococcal pustule of the skin. There is no impairment of the patient's general health, tissue damage is confined to the immediate vicinity of the pathogen's point of entry, and as a rule the infection is soon eradicated.

3 *Localization of the pathogen with production of distant lesions.* C. *diphtheriae* is usually itself confined to the throat, but by means of its exotoxin it can produce distant lesions in the heart and nervous system. *Cl. tetani*, growing as a rule in subcutaneous tissue or muscle, also does serious distant damage by means of a neurotoxin.

4 *Extension of infection to surrounding tissues.* Because it produces hyaluronidase, *Str. pyogenes* is particularly liable to spread rapidly through connective tissue surrounding a primary lesion, causing the diffuse inflammation known as cellulitis. Such diseases as tuberculosis and actinomycosis spread in quite a different way, advancing slowly through the tissues and causing severe destruction as they go.

5 *General dissemination.* The majority of serious microbial illnesses involve entry of pathogens into the blood-stream at some stage. If they are present there in large numbers, they may kill the patient almost at once. If he survives this early septicaemic phase, multiple lesions in various organs may develop, their localization depending largely on the nature of the organism. Complete removal of the organisms from the

blood-stream by the reticulo-endothelial system, without the development of any secondary lesions, can occur spontaneously, but such an outcome is much more common now that the pathogens may be opposed by lethal or inhibitory concentrations of antimicrobial drugs.

HERD IMMUNITY

As we have seen, an individual's liability to become ill or to die as a result of exposure to a particular pathogen depends largely on his own immunity. His risk of being so exposed, however, depends largely on the level of immunity of those around him. This in turn depends on the community's experience of the pathogen and of artificial immunization.

The epidemiological story of poliomyelitis is particularly instructive. This virus infection occurs in all parts of the world, but does not take on epidemic form in communities with low standards of hygiene. Extensive studies of virus carriage and of antibody formation in such communities have explained the paradox of the greater susceptibility of more hygienic populations. The virus is excreted in the faeces, and in primitive communities everyone becomes infected in early life. Some infants get the disease, and a few die, but many first encounter the virus while they are still protected by maternal antibodies, and as this protection wears off continued exposure stimulates them to produce their own antibodies. Virtually all older children and adults are immune, though some continue to carry and excrete the virus, thus passing it on to succeeding generations. As hygienic standards improve, infants are less certain to be infected, until eventually a significant proportion of the population has no experience of the virus and therefore no immunity. In this situation an epidemic may occur, and the victims may include older children and adults. The better the standards of hygiene and the longer the interval since the last epidemic, the greater is the damage likely to be when the next outbreak does occur. This unsatisfactory situation can now be remedied by widespread immunization (see pp 315–6).

In other diseases also there is a danger that partial control may lead to low herd immunity. It is therefore a cardinal principle of preventive medicine that, when a potentially epidemic disease is being brought under control, herd immunity must be kept high by immunization.

Suggestions for Further Reading

The Pathogenesis of Infectious Disease by C. A. Mims (Academic Press, London, 1976).

Natural History of Infectious Diseases by Sir Macfarlane Burnet and D. O. White, 4th edn. (Cambridge University Press, 1972)–not specifically for medical readers, but an excellent account of matters relating to this chapter and many of the others.

8

The Host's Immunological Responses

Immunology began as the study of that specific resistance to further infection by a particular micro-organism which follows an initial natural or artificial encounter with that organism or with its products, and which we have already described as *acquired immunity* (p 56). This is now seen to be only part of a more general phenomenon – the initiation of processes in the body, as a result of meeting a foreign substance, which cause the body to react differently when it subsequently meets the same substance or one that closely resembles it. Immunology today concerns itself with all such processes and reactions, regardless of whether they have anything to do with immunity in the strict sense. The modified reactions may be either more or less vigorous than the original; they may be protective or harmful and in some cases they may be both at the same time. Organ transplantation, 'auto-immune' diseases and sundry other immunological topics are full of interest and excitement, but they are only indirectly related to microbiology. In this chapter we briefly review only those areas of immunology which seem most relevant to our subject. In places we present current beliefs and concepts with little or none of the supporting data and without the many qualifications and provisos that would make our account more accurate but longer, less readable and less intelligible. To fill out their knowledge of immunology our readers should go to such sources as those recommended at the end of the chapter.

ANTIGENS

An antigen is a substance capable of provoking some form of immunological response in a host. Its essential feature is that it is unfamiliar to those cells of the body that are capable of mounting an immunological response – the *immunologically competent cells* (see p 62). Foreign *proteins* with molecular weights above about 5000 are commonly antigenic to man and vertebrate animals, and in general their potency as antigens increases with their molecular weight. 'Foreign' in this context includes proteins from other species, some of those from members of the same species and even in certain circumstances some of the host's own proteins which have been altered or which are not normally permitted into the circulation. *Carbohydrates*, too, can be powerfully antigenic –notably the blood-group polysaccharides which constitute a major problem in blood transfusion, and in the microbiological sphere the capsular polysaccharides of *Streptococcus pneumoniae* and similar bacterial products. Some carbohydrates are complete antigens, but others are *haptens*–that is, they are antigenic only when combined with proteins, but in the uncombined state can usually react with antibodies formed in response to the combination. If, as often happens, the protein is supplied by the host, the situation is fairly straightforward, but it becomes more complicated if the hapten is combined with a protein that is itself antigenic. A wide range of small-molecule substances that cannot act as antigens on their own can provoke immunological responses by acting as haptens or by otherwise modifying host proteins. Examples are metal salts, azo-dyes, sulphonamides and various antibiotics.

Results of Antigenic Stimulation
The modes of encounter between the body and an antigen are innumerable. Among other variable factors, antigens may be soluble or particulate; they may be single substances or complex mixtures, such as whole organisms; they may be applied to the skin or a mucous surface, they may be ingested in food and absorbed from the gut, they may enter wounds or they may be injected–directly into the blood-stream in some cases. The body's response is affected by all of these variables, and different species may make widely different responses to comparable stimuli. But underlying this variety are two main classes of response, conventionally described as *humoral* and *cell-mediated* because in the first it is *antibodies*, present even in cell-free body fluids, that ultimately react with the antigen, whereas in the second it is host cells themselves that do so. However, as we shall see, host cells are the source of the humoral responses also.

THE NATURE OF ANTIBODIES
Antibodies are proteins, and in general they are most accessible to study when they are circulating as serum proteins. These can be fractionated in various ways, including the following:

(1) *Electrophoresis* separates them into albumin and α-, β- and γ-globulins. Antibodies are found mainly among the γ- and β-globulins.
(2) *Ultracentrifugation* separates proteins according to molecular

weight. Most human antibody globulins are 7S (i.e. have sedimentation constants of about 7 Svedberg units), corresponding to molecular weights around 160 000, or 19S, with molecular weights around 900 000.

(3) Being proteins, antibodies are themselves potential antigens to other species, and so antisera (sera containing specific antibodies) against them can be prepared in suitable animals. Such antisera detect similarities between antibodies which differ in some of their other properties. By such means human antibody molecules can be divided into 5 Ig classes. (Ig stands for *immunoglobulin*, another name for antibody globulin.) About 80% of the immunoglobulins in normal human serum are 7S globulins of the immuno-electrophoretic class IgG. Also present are other 7S immunoglobulins of class IgA; and 19S immunoglobulins (macroglobulins) of class IgM. In these three classes are to be found all of the 'classical' antibodies that give precipitation, agglutination and the other reactions, readily demonstrable *in vitro*, that are described later in this chapter; and they probably include all antibodies that are directly protective. Two other classes of human immunoglobulin are known; those of class IgD have not yet been shown to have any significance or function, but those of class IgE are the 'reaginic' antibodies whose formation gives rise to some of the hypersensitive states to be described on p 74.

Structure

A human IgG molecule can be visualized as a Y-shaped structure, with identical antigen-binding sites at the ends of its 2 arms; the distance between these 2 sites can be varied by alteration of the angle between the arms, up to 180°. The molecule is composed of 4 polypeptide chains – 2 identical long ones (the *heavy chains*) which run side-by-side up the vertical stroke of the Y and then diverge to go one along each arm, and 2 identical shorter ones (the *light chains*) lying outside and parallel to the arm portions of the heavy chains. Following early work on papain-cleavage of such a molecule the arm portions are called *Fab* (the antigen-binding fragments) and the remaining portion is called *Fc* (the crystallizable fragment). IgA, IgD and IgE molecules in serum are essentially similar 4-chain structures, but IgA found in mucous and other secretions – the situation in which its protective effects are mainly operative – has larger molecules consisting of 2 such 4-chain structures and an additional secretory component. An IgM molecule consists of 5 of the 4-chain units linked together by their Fc regions, so that each such molecule has 10 antigen-binding sites, of identical antigen-specificity, available on its surface. Within a class of immoglobulins are subclasses, differing in the composition of their constituent chains.

Before we can consider the actions of antibodies we need to know something of the cells that produce them and the circumstances in which they do so.

IMMUNOLOGICALLY COMPETENT CELLS

Immunological responses are initiated by cells which originate from bone marrow and are morphologically small lymphocytes. Some such cells have been prepared for immunological battle in such a way that they initiate the processes of humoral immunity. These are called *B-lymphocytes* because in the chicken their place of 'training' is the gut-associated lymphoid organ known as the bursa of Fabricius, but the location of the mammalian 'bursa equivalent' is uncertain; possibilities include the tonsils, the appendix and Peyer's patches. Other small lymphocytes are the initiators of cell-mediated immunity, and these are called *T-lymphocytes* because it is in the thymus that they acquire immunological competence.

Specificity and Diversity

Immunological competence means the ability to initiate, on encounter with a particular antigen, a response that relates precisely to the chemical configuration of some part of the antigen molecule–though the precision is not absolute, and reactions with substances presenting similar configurations may result. The mechanism of this specificity of response has been the subject of much speculation and research, but Burnet's *clonal selection* theory is now firmly established. Each B-lymphocyte or T-lymphocyte has on its surface antigen-binding sites specific for a particular antigenic configuration; in the case of B-lymphocytes these sites are in fact on immunoglobulins. Among the immunologically competent cells of the body there is such diversity of antigen-receptors that any of a wide range of foreign substances can find at least a few cells capable of binding it. Thus such a substance 'selects' its own lymphocytes, and they respond to contact with it by initiating clones of new cells, each clone producing a response that has the same antigen-specificity as the binding sites on the initiating lymphocyte. Because an antigen is bound most avidly by lymphocytes with receptors that give the best 'fit', a small amount of a new antigen will stimulate highly specific responses, but a larger amount will be more than enough for the most relevant lymphocytes and the excess will be available to bind with and stimulate others that are less appropriate. Thus the precision of response to a new antigen may be rather poor at first, but improves as clones of the most relevant lymphocyte types proliferate.

Although all lymphocytes stimulated by a given antigenic configuration will initiate responses of roughly or more precisely the same antigen-specificity, the nature of those responses may show great diversity in other respects. If both B- and T-lymphocytes are involved, both antibody production and cell-mediated responses will result. Furthermore, each *individual* B-lymphocyte that is stimulated initiates production of antibody of only one Ig class (indeed, of only one subclass within the class); but stimulation of a *population* of B-lymphocytes may well result in production of antibodies of various Ig classes and subclasses. Still further diversity of response to a given antigen molecule results if different areas of its surface can act separately as antigenic determinants.

Immunological Tolerance

The body's immunological mechanisms are usually debarred from operating against its own constituents, even though these may be antigenic to other animal species or even to other members of the same species. This obviously necessary state of affairs is thought to be achieved by destruction or long-term inactivation, during foetal development, of all lymphocyte clones with receptors for host components. This immunological tolerance of 'self' extends also to some 'non-self' potential antigens encountered *in utero* (or, in some animal species at least, shortly after birth). Tolerance of some antigens can also be induced experimentally in the adult, by means varying from giving repeated small doses ('low-zone tolerance') to giving very large doses ('high-zone tolerance'). These phenomena may occasionally have some relevance to the course of microbial infections.

Sometimes the ban on 'anti-self' responses is broken and *auto-immune diseases* result. Possible roles of micro-organisms in such diseases are indicated on pp 75–6.

B-LYMPHOCYTES AND HUMORAL IMMUNITY
Production of Antibodies

The encounter with antigen that stimulates an appropriate B-lymphocyte into immunological action usually takes place in a lymph node or in other lymphoid tissue. The antigen (or, in the case of a micro-organism, the consignment of different antigens) has probably first been taken up by a macrophage, which may have been responsible for transporting it to the site of encounter and may also have processed it in a way which enhances its antigenicity. Repeated division of stimulated B-lymphocytes and their progeny gives rise to a population of immature and then mature plasma cells, which are the main antibody producers. Mature plasma cells are thought to be 'end cells', which do not divide and have life spans of only a few days, spent at their sites of origin; but some of the immature cells travel via the lymphatic system and blood-stream to initiate centres of antibody production in lymphoid tissues elsewhere. The next histological change is the appearance of zones of lymphocyte proliferation (germinal centres) in the cortical areas of the stimulated lymph nodes. It is postulated that replicas of the original antigen-specific B-lymphocytes, persisting in these centres, are responsible for the phenomenon of 'memory', which enables the body to react months or years later in a way which indicates that it has not 'forgotten' the initial antigenic stimulus.

The full sequence of events just described does not follow initial transitory introduction of a new antigen into the body, but requires repeated or sustained exposure to it. No antibody response is simple, or easy to analyse and describe, but some idea of the general pattern of events following repeated stimulation with the same antigen can be obtained by studying a relatively simple example–the repeated intramuscular injection of appropriate doses of diphtheria toxoid (modified toxin–see p 11) into a healthy subject with no previous experience of this material or of the natural toxin.

1 *Primary response.*   After the first dose of toxoid, measurable antibody does not appear in the blood for 2 or 3 weeks, and indeed, may not do so at all. If it does, the amount is small.

2 *Secondary response.*   A second dose of toxoid given a few weeks after the first is followed within a day or two by a rapid and considerable rise of the antibody level. The size and duration of this response depends on the timing and amount of the second dose and on the toxoid preparation used. A third or even a fourth dose may be required in order to provoke the maximum antibody response of which the subject is capable. A few months after the final dose the antibody level begins to fall slowly, but measurable amounts may be present for years.

3 *Booster doses.*   When the antibody level has fallen, and even long after it has ceased to be measurable, it can be rapidly raised again by another dose of toxoid, which has an effect similar to the secondary response.

In this sequence of events the body behaves as though, on first meeting a new antigen, it has to set up a factory for the production of the appropriate antibody. This factory does at most only a 'trial run' until further contact with the antigen shows that the antibody is really required. It then goes into full production, but gradually slows down again when the need for its product appears to have ceased. However, once established the factory remains capable of renewed rapid output at short notice, and continues in this condition for many years, even possibly for life. The cellular basis for such a sequence of events has already been indicated.

In natural infection and in many forms of artificial immunization the story is more complex than that given in our example because the antigen is a living and multiplying organism. There is consequently no clear distinction between primary and secondary stimuli or responses. Stimulation is continuous, and at least for a time it increases in strength. The pattern of antibody production is modified accordingly. Similarly, non-living antigen can be injected into the tissues in a form in which it is only slowly dissolved or removed and so again provides a sustained stimulus. Substances such as alum, which are added to immunizing agents in order to delay their absorption and so to increase their effectiveness, are called *adjuvants*. This term is also used to describe substances that enhance the immunizing efficacy of antigens by quite different mechanisms. Thus Freund's adjuvant – a water-in-oil emulsion containing killed tubercle bacilli, commonly used in animal immunization experiments – achieves at least part of its effect by stimulating T-lymphocytes which themselves enhance the stimulating action of certain antigens upon their corresponding B-lymphocytes.

The first phase of the humoral response to microbial infection is commonly dominated by production of IgM antibodies, with IgG and IgA production gradually taking over later. In some diseases this pattern is so reliable that the presence of appropriate IgM antibodies in a patient's blood can be taken as evidence of continuing active infection. IgM is also virtually the only class of immunoglobulin made by the human infant before and in the first few weeks after birth. Therefore, since maternal IgM (unlike IgG) cannot cross the placenta, presence of IgM antibodies in an infant's blood cannot be a reflection of maternal infection but indicates that the infant itself has an active infection.

Before moving on in our discussion of antibodies to deal with their protective functions and laboratory behaviour we need an introduction to another important participant in many of the mechanisms of humoral immunity.

Complement

For many purposes complement can be considered as a single entity, a substance present in normal human and animal serum, which may be involved in almost any antigen-antibody combination and is essential for completion of some processes that result from such combinations – notably lysis of bacterial and other cells. One of its properties, important in certain *in vitro* tests, is that it is inactivated by heating at 56°C for 30 minutes, whereas most antibodies are not appreciably affected by such treatment. In fact, complement is by no means a single substance, nor even a mere collection of substances; rather, the name covers a complex system or 'cascade' of reactions, each one providing the stimulus for others that follow. The nine chief components of complement are designated C1, C2, etc. Reference to 'the amount of complement' in a serum sample is justifiable so long as it is understood that this means the amount of complement-activity, not the amount of a substance. Levels of complement-activity in serum vary somewhat from species to species, but are as a rule much the same in members of the same species and in any one subject at different times, except that they may be markedly reduced following certain massive antigen-antibody interactions, e.g. in glomerulonephritis.

The involvement of complement in certain specific manifestations of antigen-antibody interactions is mentioned below. Activation of the complement system has additional non-specific local effects – a chemotactic action which draws polymorphonuclear phagocytes to the scene and an inflammatory action which, by increasing local capillary permeability, allows more rapid access for reinforcements of antibodies and complement and other protective factors from the blood.

Antibodies and Protection against Micro-organisms

Antibodies that combine with and neutralize potent bacterial toxins have a protective value, recognized in the very early days of immunology (see p 11), which is relatively easy to understand and to study. The situation with regard to antibodies directed against components of micro-organisms themselves is very much more complex, partly because of the assortment of different components of one organism against which antibodies may be directed and partly because of the diversity of effects that can follow attachment of antibodies to surface components of organisms. Here are some examples of such effects:

(1) Many virus infections and some bacterial infections begin with the arrival of the organisms on one of the patient's mucous surfaces and their attachment to host cells there. If appropriate secretory IgA antibody is present in the mucous secretion it may coat the surface of the organisms in such a way as to prevent such attachment, and so abort the infection.

(2) Antibodies – particularly IgM antibodies with their multiplicity of antigen-binding sites – can act as *agglutinins*, holding micro-organisms together in clumps. This probably increases the efficiency of their removal from the blood-stream by the reticulo-endothelial system, and may put them at a disadvantage in other respects.

(3) In some circumstances antibodies are described as *bacteriolysins*, because their attachment to the surfaces of (Gram-negative) bacteria leads to cell-wall and cell-membrane damage and consequent disruption of the cells. This lysis is not, however, an activity of the

antibodies themselves but results from activation of the complement sequence. The antibody molecules are attached to the bacterial surfaces by their Fab regions, with their Fc regions directed outwards. Two suitable Fc regions (IgM or IgG) directed outwards can activate the complement sequence. Once again IgM antibodies, with their 5 Fc regions per molecule, are particularly effective. Human and animal cells are also susceptible to complement-mediated antibody lysis, and something similar happens to some viruses that have envelopes.

(4) Antibodies are called *opsonins* (from a Greek word relating to the preparation of food) when, by attaching themselves to the surfaces of micro-organisms, they make them more susceptible to phagocytosis (see p 54). This can be achieved by IgG antibodies alone or, more powerfully, by either IgG or IgM assisted by complement, since on the surfaces of polymorphonuclear leucocytes and of macrophages there are receptor sites both for IgG and for the C3 component of complement.

Although in these and other ways antibodies can contribute to the defence of the body against pathogens, mere presence of an antibody is evidence only that the body has been appropriately stimulated; it does not prove that the organism against which it is directed is a pathogen (a wrong assumption that is often made), and there are no grounds for assuming that the antibody is necessarily useful to the host. Indeed, there are some antibodies which seem to be far more useful to the clinician and the microbiologist, as the basis of diagnostic tests, than they are to the patients!

Antigen-Antibody Interactions in the Laboratory

Many experimental and diagnostic microbiological procedures make use of the fact that antibodies 'recognize' antigenic groupings with a precision that is often much finer than that of the most discerning chemical tests. Immunoglobulins made, say, by a horse differ considerably in *gross* chemical structure from those made by a rabbit or by a man, and as we have seen there are also major structural differences between immunoglobulins made by one species, or even by one individual; yet because of precise similarity in the *fine* structure of their antibody-binding sites, horse and rabbit and human antibodies to a particular antigen may agree in reacting with that antigen and in failing to react, or reacting much less strongly, with a compound that differs from it only in a small detail of molecular arrangement. This specificity of antigen-antibody interactions has a number of important practical applications, including the following:

(1) Two substances can be shown to be identical or closely similar by the fact that each reacts with antibodies produced in response to the other, and to some extent it is possible to estimate degrees of dissimilarity between substances by differences of reaction with the same antibodies.

(2) Consequently the identity of a micro-organism in culture can be established and its antigenic composition analysed by testing its reactions with antisera of known specificity – that is, sera containing antibodies against known antigens.

(3) Current infection with a particular micro-organism can sometimes be detected by demonstrating that the patient's body fluids contain antigens which react with antisera specific for products of such organisms – e.g. toxins or capsular polysaccharides.

(4) The presence, in human or animal serum, of antibodies specific for components or products of a particular micro-organism is presumptive evidence of infection at some time with that organism or with one that is antigenically related; and if the amount of such antibodies is still increasing, the infection was a recent one.

Techniques for demonstrating these and other interactions are outlined in this section, and many examples of their application to the problems of medical microbiology are mentioned in later chapters.

PRECIPITATION   A soluble antigen may combine with an appropriate antibody to form a precipitate. This happens maximally when the two meet in approximately *optimal proportions* and are both used up in the formation of large lattice complexes with alternating antigen and antibody layers. In the presence of substantial excess of either, there is a tendency to form much smaller complexes, each possibly consisting of just a single molecule of the scarcer component and enough molecules of the other to use up all of its binding sites; in antigen excess in particular such complexes are still soluble.

A precipitation reaction may be demonstrable by drawing up a small volume of antigen followed by a similar volume of antiserum into a capillary tube; the reaction then manifests itself as a layer of white precipitate near to the interface between the two fluids.

Alternatively, a *radial gel-diffusion* procedure may be used. Antigen solution and antiserum are placed in two suitably spaced holes cut in a layer of agar gel on a flat glass or plastic surface. Antigen and antibody diffuse out into the gel, and where they meet in optimal proportions a white line of precipitate is formed. Since the position of the line can be brought nearer to one hole by putting less of the relevant reactant into the hole in the first place, this procedure can be made quantitative. Multiple lines may appear if the two fluids contain several sets of antigens and corresponding antibodies. By using 3 holes it is possible to compare the reactions of, say, one serum and two antigen solutions, and so to arrange things that the lines formed by the two interacting systems meet at an angle. If the two antigens are the same, the two lines will merge into a curve—*the reaction of identity*; if the two are different, the lines will 'ignore' one another and cross.

In *immuno-electrophoresis* an electric current is used to separate out the components of an antigen mixture (or an antibody mixture) so that they are located at different points along a line in agar gel on a microscope slide or other suitable surface. Antiserum (or antigen solution) is then placed in a trough cut in the gel parallel to and at an appropriate distance from the electrophoresis line. Diffusion is then allowed to take place, and since the electrophoresed components set out from point sources on their line and meet a linear front of the reactant from the trough, precipitate lines are arc-shaped.

Cross-over or *countercurrent immuno-electrophoresis* (C.I.E.) is a rapid and very sensitive variant of radial gel-diffusion, in which an electric field is used to hasten the diffusion of the reactants towards one another.

AGGLUTINATION   Bacteria are commonly identified by preparing aqueous suspensions of them on glass slides or in tubes and seeing whether these are agglutinated into visible clumps on the addition of antisera specific for known bacterial surface antigens. Conversely, suspensions of known bacteria can be used to detect and quantitate antibodies in sera. Quantitation is achieved by testing a series of dilutions of the serum against a standard bacterial suspension and determining the highest dilution of the serum which still gives definite agglutination (the *titre* of the serum—see p 258). The *prozone* phenomenon (or *zoning*) sometimes encountered in such systems consists of absence of agglutination in the first few dilutions of a serum but its presence when the serum is further diluted.

For many purposes agglutination tests are easier and more satisfactory than precipitation tests. For *indirect* or *passive agglutination tests* soluble antigens are made particulate and therefore agglutinable. This is done by allowing or persuading the soluble antigens to adhere to the surfaces of particles that are themselves immunologically inert, at least so far as the test system is concerned. For example, many polysaccharides adhere readily and firmly to the surfaces of washed red blood cells; many protein antigens adhere similarly to red cells that have been treated with tannic acid or various other agents, or to particles of polystyrene latex; and antigens of many kinds adhere to particles of the mineral bentonite.

Co-agglutination depends on the high affinity of the cell-wall-associated protein A of *Staphylococcus aureus* for Fc regions of immunoglobulin molecules – IgG molecules only, in the case of human immunoglobulins. Staphylococci coated with immunoglobulins specific for antigens on the surfaces of bacteria or other particles co-agglutinate with these particles. Various other uses can be made of this immunoglobulin affinity of protein A.

CAPSULE SWELLING   This phenomenon, alternatively known by its German name 'quellung', consists of a change in appearance of the bacterial capsule when it is exposed to a serum containing antibodies specific for the capsular polysaccharide. The change in appearance is probably due in part to actual swelling of the capsule and in part to an increase in its refractility. The phenomenon is highly type-specific – i.e. it occurs only if the organism being tested shares a polysaccharide antigen with that against which the antibodies were formed. Accordingly, capsulate strains of *Str. pneumoniae* can be divided into a number of types, differing in their capsular antigens; and a similar process can be applied to the typing of other capsulate species, such as *Haemophilus influenzae* and *Klebsiella pneumoniae*.

COMPLEMENT FIXATION   It has been known since the end of the last century that certain antigen-antibody interactions which produce no visible result (such as a precipitate, agglutinates or changes in the appearance of organisms) can be detected by the fact that they use up or 'fix' complement so that it is no longer available to take part in other interactions. To demonstrate that such fixation has occurred in a tube which originally contained only a small known amount of complement, another antigen-antibody mixture can be added which will undergo a visible change only if complement is still present in adequate amounts. This is the basis of the *complement fixation test* (C.F.T.), which is most easily understood if considered in stages.

(i) Into a test tube are placed known amounts of antigen and of the serum to be tested for the presence of an antibody that will combine with the antigen and fix complement. This serum has previously been heated to inactivate the unknown amount of complement that it contained.

(ii) A known amount of complement is added to the mixture, usually in the form of guinea-pig serum. The amount is related to the known amount of antigen present, so that if the serum contains enough antibody all of the complement will be fixed.

(iii) After the antigen-serum-complement mixture has been given an adequate opportunity to combine, an indicator system is added. This commonly consists of sheep red cells and rabbit serum containing lytic antibodies for such cells. The serum must of course be heated to inactivate its own complement before it is added to the mixture in the test tube. If the original guinea-pig complement is still present in adequate amounts, the red cells will be lysed:

(i)   Antigen + serum containing no antibody   No COMPLEMENT FIXATION

(ii) Complement ⟶
(iii) Red cells + haemolytic serum ⟶ } LYSIS

whereas if the complement has been fixed in the first reaction, no lysis will occur:

(i)   Antigen + serum containing antibody ⟶ } COMPLEMENT
(ii) Complement ⟶ } FIXATION
(iii) Red cells + haemolytic serum ⟶ No LYSIS

It can be seen that there is a slight anomaly about the reading of this test, since the result is described as 'positive' if lysis fails to occur (indicating that antibody was present in the serum being tested) and as 'negative' if lysis does occur.

GLOBULIN DETECTION   The presence of non-agglutinating antibodies on the surfaces of particles can be demonstrated by the technique developed by Coombs and his associates. This depends upon the fact that the antibody is of necessity a globulin of a type peculiar to the animal species in question. Particles coated with it are therefore agglutinated by serum of an animal of another species which has received repeated injections of globulin derived from the first species. Thus, for example, the presence of human globulin on particles can be shown by exposing them to the action of the serum of a rabbit which has been stimulated to produce anti-human globulin (A.H.G.) antibodies. Furthermore, if the A.H.G. has been prepared by using purified immunoglobulin of one class only (e.g. IgM or IgG), it will agglutinate the particles only if they are carrying antibody molecules of that class. Originally devised for detection of blood-group antibodies, this technique has found various applications in microbiology–e.g. the exposure of a suspension of brucellae to the serum of a patient with possible brucellosis and then to A.H.G. to see whether they have picked up non-agglutinating antibodies.

LABELLING   This heading covers a wide and growing range of ingenious techniques, and brief outlines of a few illustrative examples must suffice here.

(1) The *fluorescent-antibody* technique (*immunofluorescence*) has already been outlined on p 21. This procedure is made even more useful by a modification (the *indirect* fluorescent-antibody technique) that is similar in its theory to the anti-globulin technique just described. As an example of this modification, a guinea-pig is given injections of rabbit gamma-globulin and the resulting anti-rabbit-gamma-globulin antibodies in its serum are conjugated with a fluorescent dye. This preparation can now be used to locate any rabbit gamma-globulin – e.g. in sections of tissue from a rabbit whose immunological responses are being investigated, or in material from a human patient which is suspected of containing certain micro-organisms and has therefore been treated with rabbit antiserum specific for those organisms. A similar technique can be used to locate human immunoglobulins, and like the anti-globulin technique described above it can be made specific for one Ig class. Antibody can also be located in tissue sections or other microscopy specimens by first treating the specimen with a solution of the antigen corresponding to the antibody, then washing off the unbound antigen, and finally locating the bound antigen by adding fluorescent antibodies specific for it (the *sandwich* technique).

(2) The iron-containing protein *ferritin* has various immunological uses because it takes up stains that have an affinity for iron, and so it is easily detected under the light microscope, or even naked-eye if enough of it is present; and because it is electron-dense, and so it is also recognizable under the electron microscope. When conjugated with antibody proteins it confers these same properties on them.

(3) *Enzyme-labelling* of antibodies allows them to be subsequently located, after they have attached themselves to corresponding antigens, by adding a substrate which undergoes a visible change under the influence of the enzyme. At microscopic level this technique permits detection and localization of antigens in tissues, but on a larger scale changes visible to the naked eye may be used. In the *enzyme-linked immunosorbent assay* (ELISA) procedure, for example, antigen which has been firmly attached to the inner surface of a tube or a well in a plastic tray is then exposed to the serum under test. The serum is then washed off, and anti-immunoglobulin of appropriate specificity, with enzyme linked to it, is given a chance to attach itself to any antibody bound by the original antigen. Finally, retention of the labelled anti-immunoglobulin by bound antibody is detected, after a further wash, by adding enzyme substrate to the tube or well and looking for the visible change (usually of colour).

Radio-active labelling has many applications in microbial immunology and the very sensitive procedure of *radio-immunoassay*, which is increasingly used in many other fields, can be used for precise quantitation of antigens or antibodies.

NEUTRALIZATION, BLOCKING, INHIBITION   Many antibodies can be detected and quantitated by means of their ability to interfere with the actions of micro-organisms or their products. Neutralization of toxin, as tested by comparing the action on susceptible animals of untreated toxin and of toxin mixed with the serum being investigated, is a simple example. Similarly, virus neutralization tests measure the ability of a serum to protect animals or tissue cultures against viruses. Other examples of this interference approach are metabolic inhibition tests, haemagglutination-inhibition tests and immobilization tests, which respectively test the ability of sera to prevent measurable metabolic activities of micro-organisms, to prevent the agglutination of red blood cells of various animal species which normally follows their exposure to certain viruses (see p 175) and to stop the spontaneous movement of flagellate or other motile organisms. Since such interference by antibodies is confined to particular species of organisms or even types within species, similar tests using antisera of known specificity can be used in identification of organisms.

T-LYMPHOCYTES AND CELL-MEDIATED IMMUNITY

Whereas B-lymphocytes mostly 'wait' in lymph-nodes for their antigens to be brought to them, many T-lymphocytes are in constant circulation in the blood-stream and even in extravascular fluids, 'looking for' their corresponding antigens. Encounter with its antigen provokes a T-lymphocyte to differentiate into a lymphoblast and then divide, thus initiating a clone of T-lymphocytes of the same antigen-specificity as their originator. This production of new T-lymphocytes occurs mainly in the paracortical areas of lymph-nodes. Returning to the sites where antigen is to be found, the stimulated T-lymphocytes release substances called lymphokines, the effects of which include attracting macrophages to the sites and provoking them to greater activity. This activity is not necessarily limited to organisms, cells of other structures carrying the original antigen, since macrophages are not antigen-specific. T-lymphocytes, in collaboration with macrophages, special lymphoreticular cells called K ('killer') cells and sometimes antibodies resulting from B-cell stimulation, attack and disrupt host cells which they have detected as carrying their particular antigens—an activity that makes them highly important in the body's defences against intra-cellular organisms such as viruses, the bacilli of tuberculosis and leprosy and brucellosis, and various protozoal pathogens. They are also largely responsible for graft rejection, since a graft of tissue from another body is a mass of cells containing foreign material; and for the Type IV hypersensitivity reactions described below, including many skin-tests that give information about possible microbial infections.

As with humoral immunity, cell-mediated immunity takes time to develop and requires repeated or persistent contact with the antigen. Its 'memory' mechanism is also similar.

Whereas microbiologists make frequent use of antigen-antibody reactions in the laboratory, the study of cell-mediated reactions is almost exclusively the province of the immunologist.

HYPERSENSITIVITY REACTIONS

Encounter with a foreign substance sometimes provokes immunological responses that lead to a state of *acquired hypersensitivity* to that substance. Such a state manifests itself in vigorous reactions that occur when the host again encounters the same substance, and such reactions cause damage to his tissues, varying in degree from minor local inflammation to severe illness or even death. Acquired hypersensitivity must be distinguished from *idiosyncrasy*, an abnormal sensitivity to a pharmacologically active compound (e.g. aspirin or morphine) which does not depend on previous experience of the compound and is often familial.

Harmful immunological reactions are classified according to their underlying mechanisms into four main types:

Type I   Antibodies attach themselves to host cells and sensitize them to react with antigen.

Type II   Circulating antibodies react with antigens that are components of, or are attached to, host cells.

Type III Free antigen and antibodies react in tissue spaces or in the bloodstream and are precipitated as antigen-antibody complexes in and around small blood vessels.

Type IV No demonstrable antibodies are involved; the reaction with antigen is cell-mediated.

Type I (Anaphylactic-Type) Reactions

These reactions depend on special antibodies, known as reagins or homocytotropic antibodies and belonging predominantly to class IgE, which become attached by their Fc regions to the host's mast cells. Binding of the sensitizing agent (antigen) by the antibody molecules leads to release of histamine and other pharmacologically active substances from the mast cells, and these substances are responsible for the local and systemic manifestations of this type of hypersensitivity.

If a small amount of the sensitizing agent is injected intradermally into an already sensitized subject, a local *immediate-type* reaction consisting of a wheal with surrounding erythema develops within a few minutes. Such a procedure is used in identifying the agent or agents to which a particular patient is sensitized, and also illustrates the course of events which follows natural exposure to such agents. Hypersensitivity of this type underlies the manifestations of the familial *atopic diseases* such as infantile eczema, hay-fever, asthma and urticaria, and these manifestations can sometimes be reduced or abolished by repeatedly injecting small amounts of the sensitizing agent. Such desensitization may depend on formation of IgG antibodies which bind the sensitizing agents more avidly than do the reagins. A much more serious form of type I reaction is *anaphylactic shock*. This can be induced experimentally in animals by repeated injections of foreign substances, usually proteins. Thus a guinea-pig, given a small intradermal dose of egg albumin followed by a larger intravenous dose of the same material 2 or 3 weeks later, will die in a few minutes. In this species the most striking feature of such anaphylactic shock is dyspnoea, with bronchial obstruction due to smooth muscle contraction and possibly also to interstitial oedema; other animals react differently, but with equally serious consequences. Anaphylaxis in man is fortunately rare, but it is a recognized hazard of repeated administration of heterologous serum (i.e. serum from another species, such as the horse) in passive immunization against tetanus toxin, for example. It also accounts for some of the very few deaths attributable to injections of penicillin, which can act as a sensitizing hapten. Atopic subjects may be more liable than others to develop anaphylaxis.

Type II (Cytotoxic) Reactions

By a complement-dependent mechanism similar to that of antibody lysis of bacteria (see p 66), or probably at times by collaboration with K cells (see p 73), IgG or IgM antibodies can destroy or severely damage host cells that contain or are coated with appropriate antigens.

'Auto-immune' diseases are mainly of this type, as are certain drug sensitivities which depend on reactions between antibodies and drugs that have become attached to cell-membranes. (Transfused incompatible red blood cells are attacked similarly, but they are not *host* cells.) Micro-organisms or their products can be involved in such reactions in the following ways:

(1) By stimulating formation of antibodies and also becoming attached to or incorporated into host cells, which are thus made the targets for antibody attack.

(2) By stimulating formation of specific antibodies which react with

components of host cells because these happen to resemble closely the original microbial antigens.

(3) By damaging host tissue components, turning them into 'foreign' and therefore antigenic substances.

(4) By disrupting host tissue organization, so that tissue components escape into the circulation which are not normally permitted to do so. Being 'unknown' to the antibody-forming cells, these components are antigenic, and the resultant antibodies may further damage the tissues from which they come.

Type III (Immune Complex) Reactions

When *soluble* antigen and corresponding IgG antibody meet in tissue spaces or in the blood-stream, they form complexes. This event activates the complement system and in other ways provokes an inflammatory reaction. Intradermal injection of such an antigen into a sensitized subject causes *local* erythema and oedema, with intense polymorpho-nuclear leucocyte infiltration and other features of acute inflammation, within a few hours (the *Arthus reaction*). This reaction differs both in appearance and in timing from the immediate-type skin reaction of Type I hypersensitivity and the delayed-type reaction of Type IV. Such a response depends upon excess of antibody over antigen, and deposition of small local complexes. Some reactions to antibiotics and other drugs are of this type. So are some of the forms of lung-damaging hypersensitivity reaction ('allergic alveolitis') that follow repeated inhalation of fine organic dusts–e.g. 'farmer's lung' caused by inhaling the spores of thermophilic actinomycetes that grow in mouldy hay; here the antigens are not injected but are absorbed through the alveolar lining. *Serum sickness*, on the other hand, is a *systemic* Type III reaction due to formation of large complexes in conditions of antigen excess. Typically it follows injection of a large dose of horse serum into a patient whose blood does not contain significant amounts of antibodies to the proteins in such serum. No reaction occurs in the first few days (unless as a result of existing IgE antibodies the patient develops a Type I response sometimes called 'immediate serum sickness'), but after about 10 days fever may develop, accompanied by joint pains, lymph-node enlargements and sundry other complaints. These result from the appearance in the circulation of IgG antibodies that react with one or more of the antigenic components of the horse serum. Such a reaction depends upon the dose of horse serum having been large enough and its elimination having been slow enough for a good supply of it to be still in the patient's circulation when antibodies begin to appear there. Many other antigens besides horse proteins can produce similar pictures.

Type IV (Cell-Mediated or Delayed-Type) Reactions

The mechanism of reactions of this type is that already outlined for cell-mediated immunity. The alternative name 'delayed-type' is derived from the fact that the reaction to intradermal injection of the sensitizing agent into a sensitized subject takes days rather than minutes (Type I) or hours (Type II) to develop; induration is its other important distinguishing feature, and is due to lymphocyte and macrophage infiltration of the dermis. The classic example of Type IV hypersensitivity is that to tuberculin which develops during tuberculosis. It can be demonstrated as follows:

If virulent tubercle bacilli are injected subcutaneously into a guinea-pig, it develops a local lesion during the next few weeks, with extension of the infection first to the local lymph nodes and then throughout the body. A second injection given a few days after the first produces similar results. But if more than 2 weeks elapse between the first and second injections, the latter provokes a vigorous local inflammatory response which begins within a day or two and often culminates in sloughing of the skin and subcutaneous tissues. This alteration of reactivity is called *Koch's phenomenon*, after its discoverer. He also found that for the second injection he could use dead bacilli, or even 'old tuberculin', a bacterium-free concentrate of broth in which tubercle bacilli had been grown. No local response follows the subcutaneous injection of either dead tubercle bacilli or old tuberculin into a guinea-pig which has no previous experience of tuberculosis.

These observations are the basis of the *tuberculin test*, in which tuberculin is injected into the skin of a human being or an animal. A local inflammatory reaction, including induration, which reaches its maximum after 2 or 3 days is evidence of past or present tuberculous infection. Similar specific hypersensitivities underlie a number of tests for past or present infection with bacteria (e.g. the brucellin test, p 142 and the lepromin test, p 148), with chlamydiae (e.g. the Frei test, p 167), with fungi (e.g. the trichophytin test, p 221) or even with larger parasites (e.g. the Casoni test for human infestation with the hydatid stage of the dog tape-worm, *Echinococcus granulosus*). In most of these infections, tests for humoral antibodies are far more useful than skin tests, and there is a risk that carrying out a skin test first may influence the results of antibody tests. (There is no useful test for humoral antibodies in tuberculosis.)

Contact dermatitis is a Type IV hypersensitivity to any of a wide range of chemicals that can interact with skin proteins – e.g. nickel from plated buckles and straps, detergents, hair dyes, and many forms of local medication including most antibiotics. Sensitization is usually a sequel to repeated or continuous application of the sensitizing agent to the skin, but it may follow oral administration or injection; penicillin injections, for example, can sensitize a patient so that dermatitis follows local application of any of the antibiotics in this group.

IMMUNODEFICIENCY AND IMMUNOSUPPRESSION

The immunological defence mechanisms that we have outlined are sometimes (but rarely) deficient from birth, or they may be impaired or suppressed later in life. Frequent and potentially overwhelming infections may result. When it is humoral immunity that is impaired, such infections may be due to any of a wide range of common bacterial pathogens, or to 'opportunist' pathogens from among the patient's normal flora – bacteria, yeasts or even the protozoon *Pneumocystis carinii*, which is normally harmless but can cause an unusual type of pneumonia in such circumstances. When the defect is in cell-mediated immunity, the patient is unable to deal adequately with many viruses, or with some bacteria of intra-cellular habitat, such as *Mycobacterium tuberculosis*; indeed, even vaccination with B.C.G., the tubercle bacillus variant used in immunization (see p 310), may result in serious systemic infection.

Congenital immunodeficiencies can be classified as follows:

(1) Deficiency of B-lymphocytes and so of immunoglobulins – hence the name hypogammaglobulinaemia.
(2) Thymic hypoplasia and consequent T-lymphocyte deficiency.
(3) Deficiency of the stem cells from which both B- and T-lymphocytes are derived, and thus deficiency of both of these cell-types.

The life expectation of patients with these conditions has been considerably increased by treatment with antibacterial drugs and injections of normal human gammaglobulin for (1), with grafts of normal thymus for (2) and with grafts of normal bone marrow for (3).

Some immunodeficiencies arising in adult life have no known cause, but some result from malnutrition and some from malignant proliferation of abnormal lymphocytes and related cells. Thus in multiple myeloma there is widespread proliferation of abnormal B-lymphocytes and their progeny, committed to the production of one particular type of immunoglobulin, with impairment of the body's ability to produce other and more useful B-lymphocytes and immunoglobulins. Similarly, in chronic lymphatic leukaemia there is a lack of normal B-lymphocytes. In Hodgkin's disease, on the other hand, there may be a serious shortage of T-lymphocytes.

An increasingly important cause of immunodeficiency is medical treatment. Radiotherapy can produce severe immunosuppression, as can cytotoxic drugs used against various malignant diseases. Furthermore, deliberate (as distinct from incidental) immunosuppression is now achieved in many patients, in order to prevent graft-rejection. All of these patients are exposed, in consequence of their treatment, to enhanced risks of microbial infection, and have to be protected accordingly. In special cases of extreme immunosuppression it may be necessary to reduce the patient's microbial population very substantially and to use strict protective isolation ('reversed barrier nursing' – see p 290) to protect him from all extraneous organisms. In less extreme cases it is usually wise to disturb the balance of the patient's normal microbial population as little as possible, and to use antimicrobial drugs for precise treatment of actual infections rather than for diffuse cover against a wide range of potential pathogens; a normal ecological balance may be the patient's best protection, in the absence of humoral and cell-mediated immunity, against external pathogens and even against 'opportunist' activity of normal residents.

Suggestions for Further Reading

Immunology: an outline for students of medicine and biology by D. M. Weir, 4th edn. (Churchill Livingstone, Edinburgh, New York and London, 1977).

Clinical Aspects of Immunology by P. G. H. Gell and R. R. A. Coombs, 3rd edn. (Blackwell, Oxford, 1975).

Essential Immunology by I. M. Roitt, 3rd edn. (Blackwell, Oxford, 1977).

PART IV

MICRO-ORGANISMS OF MEDICAL IMPORTANCE

9
Bacteria

BACTERIAL TAXONOMY

When a medical bacteriologist communicates with his bacteriological or clinical colleagues, or indeed with anyone, about a bacterium that he has isolated, he seldom wants to detail all of its observed properties; he usually needs a convenient short descriptive label. If he is fortunate he can use a simple term such as 'A typhoid bacillus'–short for 'A bacillus which we have shown, by tests generally accepted as conclusive, to have the properties of the well-known and clearly described organism that causes typhoid'. He can use this label because he has available: (a) an adequate description of an organism with which his isolate can be compared; (b) a widely used name for that organism–which in this case conveys to the informed recipient precise information about both the laboratory properties and the clinical significance of the isolate; and (c) generally accepted tests for demonstrating that in all important respects his isolate is the same as the named organism. (He also needs, of course, confidence that these tests are reliable when carried out in his laboratory!) Requirements (a) and (c) can now be met for most of the organisms that he isolates, but as regards (b) our example provided him with an exceptionally simple problem. In its early days much of the nomenclature of medical bacteriology was based on such organism-disease correlations (some true, some unfortunately false). This reflected the medical microbiologist's understandable preoccupation with the question whether his isolates could be equated with known pathogens (see pp 3 and 235). However, even among pathogens only a minority can be named in this way, and no provision is made for non-pathogens or for indicating degrees of similarity between organisms. Naming bacteria after their discoverers–Koch's bacillus, the Klebs-Loeffler bacillus, etc.–was an even less adequate system.

Clearly a comprehensive classification and nomenclature for bacteria was necessary, and an obvious choice was the system of orders, families, genera and species, with appropriate Latin (i.e. international) names, used so successfully in other branches of biology. However, vigorous efforts over many years to fit bacteria into such a system have met with limited success, for a number of reasons. Unlike most other biologists, bacteriologists are not dealing with individual organisms but, at best, with what are rather euphemistically described as *pure cultures*–i.e. populations of individuals all derived from the same single organism, but no longer necessarily identical in genotype or phenotype (see pp 32–4). The term *strain* is used for a group of pure cultures derived from a common source and thought to be the same–e.g. all apparently identical pure cultures derived from a single clinical specimen, or from different specimens from the same patient, or even from a number of victims of a common-source outbreak of infection. A group of closely similar strains can be said to constitute a *species*, but defining species boundaries among bacteria is a peculiarly difficult problem; cross-fertility, a valuable criterion for this purpose among higher organisms, has no relevance to predominantly asexual creatures that are capable of interchange of genetic material between manifestly 'unrelated' individuals (see p 34). Bacterial species have therefore to be defined according to other criteria, and there has been almost unlimited scope for disagreement as to what these should be. The larger the number of criteria applied, the greater the range of possible permutations becomes and the more apparent it is that the boundaries are in fact artificial. Grouping of species into *genera* also presents problems, and many bacterial taxonomists have given up trying to fit genera into families and families into orders.

An alternative to this approach of selecting *the important* criteria for classification into species and genera is the Adansonian or numerical approach of applying to each bacterial strain the same large range of criteria, all regarded as of *equal importance*; the strain is given a score of + 1 if the character sought by a given test is present, and − 1 if it is absent. This approach has its merits, particularly as a means of sorting large groups of basically similar organisms into clusters of strains of much closer similarity, or as a basis for computer-matching of the properties of an unidentified strain with those of a large number of reference strains; but it has not yet produced an overall system of classification which is of value to the clinical bacteriologist.

A different type of challenge to the older system has arisen from the introduction of a criterion of classification unlike any of those used previously–the ratio of guanine + cytosine to adenine + thymine base-pairs in the DNA of a bacterial strain; this is determined by procedures which are unsuitable for use in the routine diagnostic laboratory but have given interesting results in the hands of taxonomic specialists. These results do not provide any basis for positive classification, since similarity of base-pair ratios is not evidence of overall DNA similarity; but they can challenge the inclusion of a strain or species in a genus for which its base-pair ratio is anomalous, and can indicate a genus or genera more suitable for it.

Despite these problems and challenges, there is at present a useful level of international agreement about the classification into genera and species of most bacteria of medical importance, and about the standardization of Latin binomials for them. The International Committee on Systematic Bacteriology is making a major effort to tidy up outstanding problems in the next few years, to put an end to arguments about historical priority of names, and to regulate future changes of names. Scope must of course be left for discovery of new organisms or of new information invalidating the classification of known organisms, but not for the individual bacteriologist to revise names or introduce new ones according to his personal fancy.

Meanwhile the medical student needs a working knowledge of the language. He must reconcile himself to the fact that a Linnean binomial, while it tells the genus (first name, capital first letter) and species (second name, no capital) to which the organism is assigned, may for historical reasons suggest something which is no longer to be believed – e.g. that *Haemophilus influenzae* is the cause of or related to influenza. (Names of humans can be equally inappropriate!) History has created many other nomenclatural problems. For example, the word bacillus, without an initial capital, means any rod-shaped bacterium, and at one time most of these were given the generic name *Bacillus*; now, however, that generic name is confined to aerobic spore-bearing rods (see p 115), and other rod-shaped organisms (bacilli) are assigned to a large number of other genera. Many species have undergone several changes of name, and some still have alternative binomials in common use, as well as less formal names in many cases. Thus *Streptococcus pneumoniae* = *Diplococcus pneumoniae* = the pneumococcus. In this book we follow the general custom of using conventional abbreviations for generic names (e.g. *B.* for *Bacillus*, *Br.* for *Brucella*, *S.* for *Salmonella*, *Staph.* for *Staphylococcus*, *Str.* for *Streptococcus*) when the names are being frequently repeated or should have become familiar; and we sometimes employ widely used informal names instead of Linnaean names so that they also will become familiar to our readers. Alternative names are given in brackets following the headings of many sections dealing with individual species.

It is customary to print generic names in italics with a capital first letter when they are used in the singular – e.g. *Staphylococcus* or *Staph.* – but without italics and with a lower-case first letter when they are used as adjectives or in the plural as collective names for organisms belonging

to the genus – e.g. staphylococcus (or staphylococcal) strains and
staphylococci. Clearly the latter part of the convention cannot be applied
to the generic name *Bacillus*.

SPECIAL MORPHOLOGICAL FEATURES

We gave a brief account of bacterial morphology on pp 17–18, but
deferred until this chapter a fuller description of certain special features.

Capsules

A number of bacterial species – e.g. *Streptococcus pneumoniae*, *Klebsiella
pneumoniae*, *Bacillus anthracis* – characteristically form capsules which
surround their cell walls. In most cases these capsules consist of complex
polysaccharides, but that of *B. anthracis* is predominantly a polypeptide.
Capsules are not satisfactorily shown in preparations stained by ordinary
methods, but can be demonstrated by 'negative staining', in which the
bacterial bodies are stained and the spaces between the bacteria are filled
with some opaque material such as indian ink; the capsules then show up
as unstained haloes around the bacteria. Capsular development is
determined by environmental conditions, and is usually best when the
organism is growing in living tissues. The protective value of capsules is
discussed on p 51 and their immunological significance on pp 60 and 70.

Flagella

These are long, thin thread-like appendages, about 0·02 μm in diameter,
which project from the cells of certain bacteria. They have their origin in
basal granules in the bacterial protoplast and pass through the cell wall.
They are composed almost entirely of protein. The original Latin
meaning of *flagellum* is 'a whip', and it is to whip-like movements of these
appendages that flagellate bacteria owe their motility. Flagella cannot be
demonstrated under the light microscope unless they are first
considerably thickened by the deposition on their surfaces of special
stains. They can be studied more satisfactorily by electron microscopy.
Demonstration of motility due to flagella is mentioned on pp 20 and 123.

Spores

These are round or oval structures formed by bacteria of the genera
Bacillus and *Clostridium*. Sporulation appears to be in general a reaction
to conditions that are unfavourable for normal growth, in particular to
deficiency of essential nutrients. The spore has a low rate of metabolism,
and is surrounded by a thick protective coat which enables it to resist
heat, desiccation and other harmful agencies far better than do the
vegetative forms (see pp 36 and 39). Bacterial spores, unlike those of

fungi, are not reproductive; one vegetative cell usually produces one spore, which in turn germinates to form a single new vegetative cell. Certain trigger substances (e.g. L-alanine for some species) are needed to initiate the germination of spores.

A spore may be narrower than the bacillus in which it originates, or it may distend it (see Fig. 3, p 94). It may be at the end of the bacillus (terminal), near the end (subterminal) or in the middle (central). When mature it is freed from the bacillary cell, which then distintegrates.

Cell Walls, Protoplasts, Spheroplasts and L-Forms

The cell wall is a rigid structure which maintains the shape of the bacterium and prevents it from disrupting under the influence of high internal osmotic pressure. The component responsible for its rigidity is *mucopeptide* (see p 17). This constitutes 50–90% of the walls of Gram-positive bacteria but only 5–10% of those of Gram-negative bacteria, which have a thicker outer layer as described on p 29. Polymers of glycerol phosphate or ribitol phosphate known as *teichoic acids* are found in the cell walls of Gram-positive but not of Gram-negative bacteria. Gram's staining procedure (see pp 20 and 91) had been in use for about 75 years, as an empirical means of dividing bacteria into two major groups, before these differences in cell-wall composition of the groups were demonstrated; the cell wall of Gram-positive bacteria is relatively impermeable to the complex of dye and iodine. Some bacteria are particularly susceptible to the action of lysozymes (enzymes of human, animal or bacterial origin which attack mucopeptide—see p 53) and by such action they are converted into *protoplasts*. These are complete cells apart from the loss of their cell walls, or at least of important wall components, and consequent loss of rigidity, shape and osmotic resistance. They survive only if kept in suitably hypertonic environments. They are metabolically active and can grow but cannot multiply. Similar structures without cell walls can be produced from suitable organisms by the action of an antibiotic such as penicillin, which prevents mucopeptide synthesis (see p 41). But many bacteria, under the influence of penicillin or of any of a variety of other agents, *in vitro* or *in vivo*, produce either *spheroplasts* or *L-forms*. Spheroplasts have residual but damaged cell walls and assume bizarre shapes, but when transferred to suitable culture media free from the agent that caused them they may be able to produce orthodox colonies composed of normal individuals. L-forms, on the other hand, are not ordinary bacteria with damaged cell walls, but mutants that do not form cell walls and have been selected out by an environment unsuitable for those bacteria that do form them. As might be expected, these L-forms are delicate and friable, but they differ from protoplasts in being able to multiply. When grown on solid media they form characteristic small 'fried egg' colonies, with central smooth portions deeply embedded in the medium and consisting mainly of minute round forms, and more superficial peripheral zones in which much larger irregular forms are found. Attention has repeatedly been drawn in recent years to the possibility that many kinds of bacteria, when confronted with unfavourable conditions in the body, may persist there as relatively undetectable L-forms and in that state be in some way better able to resist the host's defences.

ISOLATION AND IDENTIFICATION OF BACTERIA

The hypothetical bacteriologist mentioned on p 83 had *isolated* his organism (i.e. obtained a pure growth of it, free from other bacteria) before he *identified* it with a described and named species. Isolation is usually a necessary preliminary to identification – though, as we shall see, a great deal of information about identity may be revealed during the process of isolation; but some bacteria can be identified, provisionally or even definitively, by direct examination of the original material. This may be achieved by microscopy of suitable preparations, looking for characteristic morphological features of staining reactions or for capsule swelling (see p 70) or for fluorescent-antibody attachment (see p 72); or by other methods: (e.g. C.I.E. or G.L.C., or p 5). Even so, it is still necessary in most cases to isolate the organism, so as to be able to confirm its provisional identification or to test its antibiotic sensitivities or to acquire other valuable information about it.

The common procedure for obtaining a pure culture of a bacterium is to spread a little of the original material over the surface of a solid culture medium in such a way that individual bacteria, or small clumps of attached and so presumably related individuals, are well separated from one another. On incubation of the culture a distinct pile or *colony* of bacteria is formed by each individual bacterium or clump of attached individuals (in technical language, each colony-forming unit or C.F.U.) that finds the conditions suitable for its multiplication. One of Robert Koch's valuable contributions to bacteriological technique was the use of *agar*, a seaweed derivative, as a means of solidifying media. Added in small amounts (1·5–2%) to a heated fluid culture medium, this substance causes it to set to a firm jelly when cooled to about 40°C. This low setting point allows heat-labile ingredients, such as red blood cells, to be added to a medium while it is still fluid. On the other hand, once set the medium will not melt until it is heated to nearly 100°C, and there is consequently no danger of its liquefying at ordinary incubation temperatures. Agar media are commonly used in circular, flat-bottomed glass or plastic *Petri dishes*, 9 cm or so in diameter, with close-fitting lids. Media and dishes must be sterilized before use (see Chapter Seventeen).

Isolation of pure cultures by using such plates is carried out as follows:

(1) The material to be investigated is spread over part of the surface of the medium.

(2) A wire loop, sterilized by heating in a flame and then allowed to cool, is passed several times through the inoculated area on to a fresh area of medium. The bacteria will thus be less thickly spread on this second area than on the first.

(3) Similar transfers are made from the second area to a third and so on until the whole surface of the plate has been used.

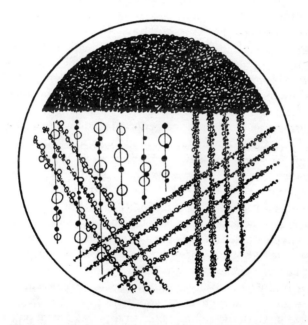

Figure 2   Diagram of plating out of a mixture of bacteria, as described in the text. Note that as the colonies become more widely separated, they increase in size and differences between them become obvious.

In this way, as illustrated diagrammatically in Fig. 2, there is usually at least one area of the plate on which the bacteria are deposited sufficiently far apart to form separate colonies after incubation. In medical bacteriology 37 °C is the usual incubation temperature and most organisms produce colonies large enough for identification within 18 hours. It is then possible to see whether the original material contained a mixture of bacteria, and to select single colonies for microscopic examination and subculture.

By this stage, we have already learned a lot about the bacterium that is being investigated. We know something about *conditions in which it will grow*, and if we have used several media and various conditions of incubation, we may also know something about conditions in which it will not grow. For example, it may have grown on *nutrient agar*–i.e. a simple broth solidified with agar–but failed to do so on *MacConkey's agar*, which contains bile salts and so is inhibitory to most non-intestinal organisms; or it may have grown on neither of these but on *blood agar*–i.e. nutrient agar to which has been added 5–10% of blood, commonly oxalated horse blood. It may have shown itself to be a strict anaerobe by growing only on plates incubated in an air-tight jar from which all oxygen has been removed; or it may have become clear that it is a strict aerobe or a facultative anaerobe. (Techniques for anaerobic culture are considered on pp 239–40).

Wherever the organism has grown, it will have revealed its characteristic *colonial appearances*. In the interpretation of these we have to make allowances for a diversity of factors, including the composition of the medium, the conditions and duration of incubation, recent exposure of the organism to antibiotics, and genotypic or phenotypic variations in the organism itself; so that a 'pure' culture may show two or more colonial variants on the same plate and widely different appearances on different media, and may undergo progressive changes of colonial morphology on repeated subculture. Despite all of this, it is possible to describe, for a given species grown under defined conditions on a specified medium, the size, shape, surface appearance, colour, opacity, consistency and other features of typical colonies and of common variants. Bacteriologists have built up a large vocabulary of descriptive terms for this purpose, but these need not concern us here.

We may also have observed *changes in the culture media* produced by the growing bacteria, such as the appearance of clear, colourless zones around and beneath the colonies of many species grown on blood agar; this is due to lysis of the red blood cells (haemolysis). Many culture media contain ingredients specifically intended to detect particular chemical activities of bacteria. For example, MacConkey's medium, mentioned above as containing bile salts, also contains lactose and neutral red, so that colonies of lactose-fermenting bacteria have a red colour on this medium due to acid-production. (From now on, we shall frequently use the term 'fermenting' as synonymous with 'producing acid from', rather than in the strict sense defined on p 27.)

It is likely that we already know something about the *microscopic appearance and staining properties* of our organism, having examined appropriate preparations of the original material. We can now confirm this morphological information by examining the pure culture. By far the most commonly used procedure for this purpose is to suspend a little of the growth in a drop of water on a microscope slide, dry it, fix the organisms to the slide by gentle heat, and then stain them by Gram's method. In this, methyl violet or gentian violet is applied first, followed by iodine as a mordant. After such treatment, some organisms, known as *Gram-positive*, resist decolorization by ethyl alcohol or acetone and remain violet or blue in colour. Others, known as *Gram-negative*, readily give up the violet dye and can then be stained red by a counterstain such as neutral red, dilute carbol fuchsin or safranin. This distinction is not absolute, in that faulty technique can give equivocal or wrong results and even in the most skilled hands some strains are difficult to classify. Very young or old cultures may give anomalous reactions. The procedure is open to criticism, in common with any similar staining method, on the grounds that the objects seen down the microscope are distorted artefacts, bearing little resemblance to the original live bacteria. Despite this, Gram's technique provides a division of bacteria, or at least of cocci and bacilli, which is of great practical value, depending as it does on a difference in cell-wall structure that has important effects on various properties of the bacteria.

In the great majority of cases we can now classify our bacterium as a Gram-positive or a Gram-negative coccus or bacillus. Distinction between cocci and bacilli is sometimes difficult if individual cells are studied, but is usually fairly easy if a large number of organisms from the same culture are examined together. Bacterial strains that are classified as cocci may show variation of individual shape from spherical to oval, but never to rod-shaped forms. Bacilli on the other hand may include many very short rods ('cocco-bacilli'), but indisputable rods are nearly always to be found and are usually predominant; filamentous forms also occur, and a culture which shows unusual diversity of size and shape is described as pleomorphic. When all organisms in a particular culture are of indeterminate cocco-bacillary shape, examination of a culture of the same strain grown on a different medium or incubated for a longer or shorter time will usually resolve the doubt.

Table IV shows the classification of the medically important genera of cocci and bacilli according to their Gram-staining reaction. Examination of a Gram-stained film may also enable us to place our organism in its appropriate genus or even species. For example, Gram-positive cocci in definite chains = *Streptococcus*; Gram-positive bacilli with spores = *Bacillus* or *Clostridium* (and the spores of the two genera are often distinguishable); lactobacilli and some members of the genus *Bacillus* are arranged in chains, whereas corynebacteria lie side-by-side or in bundles. These and other distinctive morphological features are illustrated in Fig. 3 (p 94). Among the Gram-negative bacilli, all the enterobacteria and members of the genus *Pseudomonas* look much the same in stained films, but are appreciably larger than most of the parvo-bacteria.

Having obtained our organism in pure culture, examined it by Gram's method and added up all of the evidence already available, we can

TABLE IV
Medically Important Genera of Cocci and Bacilli

Gram-positive	Gram-negative
COCCI	COCCI
Staphylococcus	*Neisseria*
Streptococcus	
	BACILLI
BACILLI	(a) Enterobacteria
Corynebacterium	*Escherichia*
Lactobacillus	*Klebsiella*
Bacillus	*Salmonella*
Clostridium	*Shigella*
(*Mycobacterium*)[1]	*Proteus*
	Yersinia
	(b) *Pseudomonas*
	(c) *Vibrio*
	(d) Parvobacteria
	Haemophilus
	Bordetella
	Brucella
	(e) *Bacteroides*

[1] Some mycobacteria, including *Myco. tuberculosis*, are stained only faintly or not at all by Gram's method.

proceed to further investigations appropriate to the group to which it seems likely to belong. These may include special staining procedures, subculture on other media or under different incubation conditions, tests of carbohydrate fermentation or other biochemical properties, or serological analysis of antigenic composition. Injection into animals may also be necessary, either in order to confirm the identity of the organism or to assess its virulence.

The rest of this chapter deals with groups of bacteria in the following order:

(1) Gram-positive cocci.
(2) Gram-negative cocci.
(3) Gram-positive bacilli.
(4) Gram-negative bacilli
    (*a*) Enterobacteria
    (*b*) *Pseudomonas*

(c) *Vibrio*
(d) Parvobacteria
(e) *Bacteroides.*
(5) Acid-fast bacteria.
(6) Branching bacteria.
(7) Spirochaetes.
(8) Mycoplasmas.

The properties of these organisms in laboratory cultures and also their recognition and isolation from clinical specimens are discussed here, but the collection and handling of clinical specimens is dealt with more fully in Chapter Fourteen. Treatment mentioned in the present chapter is purely antibacterial; no mention is made of the other aspects of the management of patients with bacterial infections.

GRAM-POSITIVE COCCI

The patterns of arrangement of cocci, as seen under the microscope, are a valuable guide to generic distinctions in this group (see p 18). The grape-like clusters from which the genus *Staphylococcus* gets its name are best seen in pus and other body fluids (Fig. 3(a), p 94). films made from cultures may show small clusters and short chains, but generally in such preparations the cocci are distributed at random throughout the microscopic field. Sets of 4 cocci in squares and larger geometrically-arranged packets are formed by members of the genus *Micrococcus*. Chain-formation is characteristic of the genus *Streptococcus* (Fig. 3(b), p. 94).

THE GENUS STAPHYLOCOCCUS

Staphylococci make a very large contribution to man's normal commensal flora and also account for a high proportion of his acute and chronic suppurative lesions. The majority of strains isolated from such lesions produce golden-yellow colonies on common culture media and so they have long been classified as *Staph. aureus*. However, pigment-production is a variable property, somewhat at the mercy of conditions of growth, and furthermore some strains which constantly fail to produce pigment are highly pathogenic. The capacity to produce *coagulase* (see below) appears to be a more stable character and is more closely correlated with pathogenicity. The name *Staph. aureus* is currently applied to all strains which are coagulase-positive (i.e. produce coagulase), including a minority which form white colonies. Strains belonging to this species are commonly found as commensals, as well as in lesions, but so far as our present knowledge goes they are all to be regarded as potential pathogens. On the other hand, many of the staphylococci found on the skin and in the upper respiratory tract are

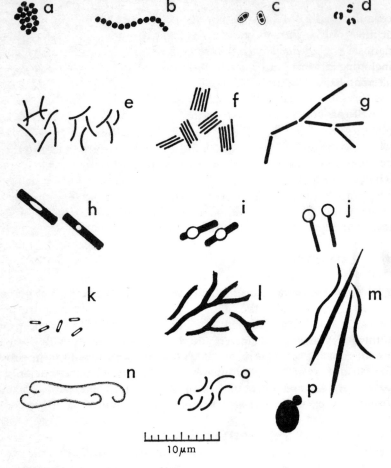

Figure 3 Morphological features of some bacteria.

(a) A cluster of staphylococci as seen in pus and tissues.
(b) A chain of streptococci.
(c) Pairs of encapsulated pneumococci as seen in sputum or pus.
(d) Pairs of kidney-shaped meningococci or gonococci as seen in pus (where as a rule most of them are inside pus cells).
(e) Diphtheria bacilli showing 'Chinese character' arrangement.
(f) Diphtheroid bacilli showing 'palisading'.
(g) Lactobacilli in branching chains (false branching).
(h) Members of the genus *Bacillus*, with spores narrower than the bacilli.
(i) Clostridia with central or subterminal spores wider than the bacilli.
(j) *Cl. tetani* with terminal drum-stick spores.
(k) Yersiniae showing polar staining.
(l) An actinomycete showing true branching and fragmentation.
(m) Vincent's organisms – *Borrelia vincenti* and *Fusiformis fusiformis*.
(n) Leptospires.
(o) Vibrios.
(p) A budding yeast for comparison of size.

coagulase-negative. These almost invariably form white colonies and are at most only low-grade pathogens. They are now classified by taxonomists as *Staph. epidermidis*, though the name *Staph. albus* (originally including all white-colonied staphylococci) is still in common use as an alternative.

Staphylococcus aureus

OCCURRENCE AND PATHOGENICITY   Organisms of this species are widely distributed, notably in air and dust and in human clothing and bedding. They reach such sites mainly from human patients and carriers. They are to be found as commensals on the anterior nasal mucosa of 40–50% of healthy adults, in the throats of many of them, in the faeces of about 20% and on the skins of 5–10%. As well as being carried in these situations they may also multiply profusely there, notably in the nose and on the perineal skin. New-born babies are rapidly colonized by this species, and 90% or more of those born in hospital carry it in their noses within 2 weeks of birth.

Staph. aureus is the commonest cause of pyogenic infections of man. The majority of such infections involve the skin or its appendages—e.g. pustules, furuncles, boils, impetigo, styes and infected surgical or accidental wounds. Abscesses of the subcutaneous and connective tissues are also commonly staphylococcal. Among the other diseases which this species can produce are osteomyelitis, bronchopneumonia and generalized septicaemia. It is also responsible for two forms of intestinal disorder. Staphylococcal food-poisoning, which is further discussed on p 302, is due to the eating of food in which staphylococci have multiplied and formed enterotoxin. Staphylococcal enteritis, on the other hand, is a rare result of serious derangement of the intestinal flora by antibiotic treatment (usually with a tetracycline or with penicillin and streptomycin). *Staph. aureus*, which does not multiply readily in the normal intestine, does so in these abnormal circumstances, causing severe enteritis which may be rapidly fatal unless treated with another antibiotic to which the offending strain is sensitive.

MICROSCOPY   Staphylococci are Gram-positive spherical organisms, 0·7–1 μm in diameter. Their arrangement has already been discussed. The species are not microscopically distinguishable from one another.

CULTIVATION   *Staph. aureus* grows well on nutrient agar and other common media under aerobic conditions, but less well anaerobically. Its optimal growth temperature is around 37°C, but it will grow within the range 10–44°C and pigment production is more marked at about 20°C. than at 37°C. On nutrient or blood agar, colonies are 2–4 mm in diameter after 18 hours incubation at 37°C, and are smooth, shiny, opaque, yellow or white domes resembling small drops of gloss paint. On horse blood agar, haemolysis is common but usually slight; it is more constant when sheep or rabbit blood is used. The ability of staphylococci to grow in concentrations of sodium chloride which are inhibitory to other genera (e.g. 7·5% in nutrient agar or 10% in nutrient broth) is useful for their isolation from faeces and other specimens likely to contain large numbers of other bacteria.

COAGULASE PRODUCTION   Coagulase is a thrombin-like enzyme that causes clotting of plasma from man and various animals. The probable relevance of this to the survival of *Staph. aureus* in the host's body has been discussed on p 30. It may well be that the walling off of staphylococcal lesions in the tissues is at least partly due to the deposition of fibrin by such means.

The ability of a staphylococcal strain to produce coagulase can be tested by the *tube coagulase test*. This can be carried out in various ways, but consists essentially of incubating together diluted plasma and a broth culture of the organism. Formation of a clot indicates that the organism is coagulase-positive. In routine practice the *slide 'coagulase' test* has the advantages of speed and simplicity, and its results agree with those of the tube test in the great majority of cases, but its mechanism is different. It is carried out by mixing part of a colony of staphylococci in a drop of water on a clean slide so as to make a homogenous suspension, and then adding a loopful of plasma. The test is positive if further mixing results in visible clumping of the bacteria, provided that spontaneous clumping (auto-agglutination) does not occur in a comparable suspension to which no plasma has been added.

STAPHYLOKINASE PRODUCTION   Most strains of *Staph. aureus* produce a substance which activates the plasminogen of blood, converting it into the proteolytic enzyme plasmin. This presumably facilitates the spread of staphylococci in tissues. Its importance in the laboratory is that the clot formed in the tube coagulase test may be subsequently lysed by the plasmin, so that undue delay in reading the results of the test may result in false negative readings.

TOXIN PRODUCTION   Many products of *Staph. aureus* have been shown to be toxic to animals, and some of them are undoubtedly relevant to human staphylococcal disease. These include the *alpha-toxin*, which causes constriction of small veins, and in the rabbit causes local necrosis if injected intradermally and death if injected intravenously; *leucocidins*, which destroy host white blood cells; and a heat-stable *enterotoxin* which is responsible for the manifestations of staphylococcal food-poisoning (see p 302).

PHAGE TYPING   Bacteriophages are virus parasites of bacteria (see p
210–12). Many *Staph. aureus* strains carry phages which, when spotted
on to plate cultures of other staphylococcal strains as described on p 211,
cause lysis of some of them. This phenomenon makes it possible to divide
the species *Staph. aureus* into phage-types–i.e. groups of strains having
the same or closely similar phage susceptibilities and resistances. For this
purpose a basic set of 2 dozen or so phage cultures is used. These are
numbered according to international agreement, and are divisible into 4
groups (I–IV) according to their antigenic composition. Any one strain of
Staph. aureus is likely to be susceptible to the lytic action of several
phages, which often belong to a single antigenic group. The phage type of
the strain is then designated by the numbers of the phages which can lyse
it under specified conditions. Thus strains of phage type 80/81, which
have received extensive publicity because of their exceptional ability to
cause outbreaks of sepsis in hospitals, are so called because they are lysed
by phages 80 and 81 (among others). Strains lysed only by a single phage
are rare. A minority of strains are not typable because they are resistant to
all of the phages used, but new phages are found from time to time which,
when added to the standard set, increase the number of strains that can be
typed. Some strains which are not lysed by phages in the dilution
routinely employed (Routine Test Dilution or R.T.D.) can be typed by
using more concentrated phage suspensions (1000 × R.T.D.).

We shall have more to say about applications of staphylococcal phage
typing in connection with hospital cross-infection (p 291) and food-
poisoning (p 303).

IMMUNOLOGY   Various antibodies are formed in response to staphylococcal infection, but their protective value is uncertain and their
measurement seldom gives much diagnostic help. Autogenous vaccines
(i.e. killed suspensions of the patients' own staphylococci) have been
widely used in the past in treatment of chronic skin infections.

ANTIBACTERIAL TREATMENT   Since antibiotics became available,
Staph. aureus has shown exceptional ability to produce variants which are
resistant to them. Consequently, infections acquired in a hospital are
likely to be due to strains resistant to antibiotics in common use in that
hospital. In such circumstances treatment should be guided by laboratory tests of the antibiotic sensitivity of the strain if time permits, or, if
the patient is seriously ill and there is no time for such tests, an antibiotic
known to be effective against all or virtually all of the prevalent
staphylococci should be employed (see p 352).

Other Staphylococci and Related Organisms

Staph. epidermidis, as already indicated, resembles *Staph. aureus* in most respects except that it is coagulase-negative, usually forms white colonies, and is almost non-pathogenic. It is found in large numbers all over human skin and on many mucous surfaces. It may play some part in the pathogenesis of acne and in other minor skin lesions, and has occasionally been incriminated as a cause of bacterial endocarditis (as have many other bacterial species which are otherwise virtually non-pathogenic). In recent years it has achieved greater medical importance as the organism most liable to colonize the fibrin overlying heart-valve and other prostheses, causing a low-grade but intractable infection which usually necessitates removal and replacement of the prosthesis.

Somewhere near to the disputed border between the genera *Staphylococcus* and *Micrococcus* are certain coagulase-negative non-pigmented strains, most easily distinguished in the laboratory from orthodox *Staph. albus* by their resistance to the antibiotic novobiocin, which quite commonly cause acute cystitis in young women, usually following sexual intercourse. These strains have been classified as *Micrococcus* type 3, but now seem likely to be reinstated as staphylococci—leaving the genus *Micrococcus* bereft of importance to the clinical bacteriologist.

THE GENUS STREPTOCOCCUS

Members of this genus are widely distributed in nature, largely as parasites of man and animals. They make a large contribution to the normal bacterial flora of the human respiratory, alimentary and female genital tracts. Certain types belonging to the species *Str. pyogenes* are highly pathogenic, though even these may occur as harmless commensals. *Str. pneumoniae* is an important pathogenic species but also a common commensal of the healthy respiratory tract. Some other commensal species are pathogenic in certain circumstances.

Streptococci are spherical or oval Gram-positive cocci, about 1 μm in diameter, non-motile, non-sporing, sometimes capsulate, and character-ized by their tendency to form chains (see p 18 and Fig. 3(*b*), p 94). Chain-formation is best seen in pathological materials or in fluid cultures—partly because chains are formed more readily in such si-tuations than on solid media and partly because the process of taking part of a colony from a solid medium and suspending it in water to make a microscopic film results in the breaking up of chains. Length of chains also depends upon the species involved. Some form chains containing scores of cocci, whereas at the other extreme *Str. pneumoniae* character-istically appears in tissues and exudates as pairs of cocci (diplococci—Fig. 3(*c*), p 94).

The genus can be divided into *aerobes* and *anaerobes,* most of the former being also facultative anaerobes. The *aerobes* (apart from certain intestinal streptococci, the *enterococci,* which will be discussed separately) can then be divided according to their *haemolytic* activities, as follows:

1 Beta-(or β-)haemolytic.   Beta-haemolysis consists of the production, around a colony of streptococci (e.g. of *Str. pyogenes*) on a blood agar plate, of a zone of clear, colourless medium, in which the red cells have been lysed and the haemoglobin decolorized. This activity may be shown in various degrees by the same strain grown on media containing bloods from different mammalian species and is often more pronounced when the plates are incubated anaerobically.

2 Alpha-(or α-)haemolytic.   Alpha-haemolysis consists of the production around the colonies of a zone in which the red cells are partly destroyed (so that the medium becomes somewhat less opaque) and haemoglobin is converted to a green pigment. Such a reaction is produced by streptococci of the viridans group and by *Str. pneumoniae.*

3 Non-haemolytic.   Many streptococci do not produce either of these forms of haemolysis. A few produce other changes, such as partial destruction of the red cells, with no green pigmentation or a brownish discoloration of the medium, but many have no visible effect on the medium and are described as non-haemolytic. They are as a rule harmless commensals.

Beta-haemolytic streptococci are divided into Lancefield groups A to T by means indicated below, in the discussion of the antigenic structure of *Str. pyogenes.* This species name is given to Lancefield group A streptococci, the predominant human pathogens of the genus. Strains of other groups (notably B, C, D and G) are occasionally pathogenic to man. In particular, group B strains have come into prominence in recent years, chiefly as causes of two distinct patterns of serious illness in newborn babies, due to strains of different types within the group: (1) infection acquired from the mother's genital tract during birth, leading to septicaemia (usually fatal) within the next 24 hours or so; (2) infection acquired from other sources, leading to meningitis 10 days or so after birth. Group D contains many of the enterococci (see below).

Streptococcus pyogenes (beta-haemolytic streptococci, group A)
OCCURRENCE AND PATHOGENICITY   Healthy human beings may carry in their throats, or less commonly in their noses, *Str. pyogenes*

strains which are potential pathogens; the skin and clothing of such carriers may become heavily contaminated. Strains of this species cause many different human diseases. To some extent the type of disease produced is determined by the portal of entry of the organism. The commonest picture is acute sore throat, often involving suppurative inflammation of the tonsils and cervical lymphadenitis. Such an infection may spread to the middle ears, mastoids and even meninges. Scarlet fever is a *Str. pyogenes* infection, usually of the throat, due to a strain which produces an erythrogenic toxin (see below). If the patient has no protective antibodies against this toxin, it causes the characteristic skin rash of scarlet fever. *Str. pyogenes* also causes infections of the skin (including impetigo and erysipelas), of the uterus following childbirth (puerperal sepsis) and of many other tissues. Spread into the lymphatic system (lymphangitis and lymphadenitis) and into the blood-stream (septicaemia) are common features of untreated *Str. pyogenes* infections. Immunological responses to *Str. pyogenes*, possibly involving one or more of the Type II mechanisms listed on pp 75–6, are thought to be responsible for acute rheumatism and acute glomerulonephritis, since onset of either of these diseases is commonly preceded by a streptococcal throat infection 2 or 3 weeks earlier. The strains associated with glomerulonephritis belong to a restricted number of Griffith types (see below, under 'Antigenic structure').

MICROSCOPY   Chain-formation is usually well marked. The cocci are spherical and conform to the general description given for the genus.

CULTIVATION   Growth is poor on ordinary nutrient media but better on those containing serum or blood. The species is aerobic, with rather less vigorous growth under anaerobic conditions. The optimal temperature for growth is 37°C, and no growth occurs below 18°C. Even under optimal conditions on blood agar, colonies are usually only 1 mm or so in diameter after 24 hours; they may be smooth and shiny, but are commonly dry and irregular in contour and outline, especially when they belong to virulent strains. They are greyish-white and opaque or semitransparent. The zone of beta-haemolysis around a well-developed colony may be up to 5 mm in diameter. In fluid cultures there is usually a granular deposit and a relatively clear supernatant, in contrast to the more uniform turbidity of broth cultures of staphylococci and of most other streptococci.

TOXIN AND ENZYME PRODUCTION   (1) *Streptolysin O* is a haemolysin which is oxygen-sensitive and is active only in the reduced state. It is a powerful antigen, and therefore anti-streptolysin O antibody (commonly referred to as A.S.O.) appears in the blood following a *Str. pyogenes* infection. This antibody can be measured by determining its power to block the haemolytic action of a standard preparation of streptolysin O. A raised level of this antibody is evidence of a recent *Str. pyogenes* infection (subject to the qualification that streptococci of groups C and G can also produce streptolysin O), and may therefore help to confirm a diagnosis of acute rheumatism or of acute glomerulo-nephritis. Streptolysin O is powerfully toxic to animals (and presumably to man), acting mainly on the heart.

(2) *Streptolysin S* is also a haemolysin. It is not inactivated by oxygen and is not demonstrably antigenic. It is responsible for the zones of beta-haemolysis seen on blood agar plates, and its action can be blocked by an inhibitor commonly present in human and animal sera.

(3) *Streptokinase*, when released by *Str. pyogenes* into blood or tissue fluid, plays a part in the activation of plasminogen to the proteolytic enzyme plasmin, which then breaks down fibrin. This process facilitates the spread of the steptococci through the fibrin barrier laid down as part of the host's defence mechanism.

(4) *Hyaluronidase* also facilitates the spread of *Str. pyogenes* by breaking down the hyaluronic acid of the connective tissue cement substance.

(5) *Streptodornase* depolymerizes DNA and deoxyribonucleoprotein. Since the latter material is largely responsible for the viscosity of purulent exudates, streptodornase makes them less viscous. Whatever the significance of this may be in relation to streptococcal infection, streptodornase has been used therapeutically as a means of liquefying pus and so hastening the cleaning up of wounds and abscess cavities. Streptokinase solutions have been used in a similar way.

(6) *Erythrogenic toxin* and its relationship to scarlet fever have been discussed above in connection with the pathogenicity of this species. The Dick test for the presence or absence of antibodies to this toxin is described on p 266:

(7) *Diphosphopyridine nucleotidase* is an enzyme produced by many *Str. pyogenes* strains. It splits off nicotinamide from diphosphopyridine nucleotides and is thought to be lethal to leucocytes.

ANTIGENIC STRUCTURE   Lancefield grouping depends on the cell-wall C polysaccharides possessed by most beta-haemolytic and some other streptococci. C polysaccharide can be removed from the organisms and obtained in solution by acid or formamide extraction or in other ways, and can then be identified by precipitation tests (see p 68), using antisera for the various Lancefield groups. Group A (*Str. pyogenes*) strains can be subdivided into about 55 Griffith types by study of their surface proteins, notably those designated M proteins which are important contributors to the virulence of the organisms. Such fine subdivision is sometimes useful in studies of the spread of infection, and certain types (notably type 12) are particularly associated with infections that precede the development of acute glomerulo-nephritis.

IMMUNOLOGY   Immunity following natural infection is highly type-specific, and immunization is impracticable because of the large number of types involved. Infection with a strain that produces erythrogenic toxin is followed by the development of immunity to such a toxin.

ANTIBACTERIAL TREATMENT   *Str. pyogenes* strains are sensitive to penicillin, which is therefore usually the agent of choice for the treatment of infections due to them. They are usually sensitive also to most other antibiotics except the aminoglycoside group, and to the sulphonamides. Tetracycline-resistant strains are now fairly common in many areas.

The Viridans Group of Streptococci (*Str. viridans*)

Alpha-haemolytic streptococci other than *Str. pneumoniae* (which is described below) have long been included in one species, *Str. viridans*. Such bacteria are almost invariably present in large numbers in the mouths and upper respiratory tracts of healthy people. As they have been studied more fully, it has become possible—and useful—to define a number of distinct species within the group. It now seems best to abandon the name *Str. viridans* and to refer to these organisms collectively as 'the viridans group' or 'viridans streptococci'—though in fact some of the new species incorporate non-haemolytic as well as alpha-haemolytic strains. Some members of the group are important in dental caries—notably *Str. mutans*, which turns sucrose into a sticky layer of dextran on surfaces of teeth. Apart from this the viridans streptococci are rarely pathogenic to man in their normal habitat, the mouth and pharynx, but they are liable to gain access to the blood-stream, particularly during dental filling or extraction. They are nearly always eliminated from the circulation without causing any trouble, but in patients with rheumatic endocarditis or congenital heart lesions they may invade the fibrinous vegetations attached to the valves or deformed structures, and they then cause subacute bacterial endocarditis. *Str. sanguis* is the species most likely to do this. Other named species in the group include *Str. salivarius*, *Str. mitior* and *Str. milleri*.

The microscopic appearances of members of this group are in general similar to those described for *Str. pyogenes*. So are their cultural characteristics, except that haemolysis, if present, is of the alpha type and usually not so extensive as the zones of beta-haemolysis around *Str. pyogenes*.

The use of antibiotics in prevention and treatment of bacterial endocarditis is discussed on pp 325, 328 and 353.

Streptococcus pneumoniae (*Diplococcus pneumoniae*, the *pneumococcus*)

OCCURRENCE AND PATHOGENICITY   This species is both a normal commensal and a common pathogen of the human respiratory tract, and it is therefore difficult at times to assess the significance of its isolation from sputum or other respiratory tract specimens. It takes its specific name from the fact that some types are the common causative organisms of lobar pneumonia and that many different types cause broncho-pneumonia, usually superimposed upon a virus infection of the respiratory tract or occurring in a bedridden or debilitated patient. Also in the respiratory tract pneumococci appear to play a part in the maintenance and aggravation of chronic diseases of the bronchi and paranasal sinuses. Infected pleural and pericardial effusions often accompany pneumococcal pneumonia. Other diseases caused by this species include otitis media, meningitis and peritonitis.

MICROSCOPY   The alternative generic name of *Diplococcus* for this species was derived from its characteristic diplococcal morphology in tissues, sputum and pus (Fig. 3(*c*), p 94). Typically, the cocci in such situations are somewhat elongated, and pointed at one end but rounded at the other (lanceolate), and the two members of a pair point away from each other. They are surrounded by a polysaccharide capsule. However, in artificial culture short chains are common and capsules tend to be formed poorly if at all, so that distinction from other streptococci is not possible on the basis of microscopic morphology. Furthermore, since a pair is the smallest possible cluster or chain, Gram-positive diplococcal forms may be seen in preparations containing staphylococci or streptococci of all varieties and are by no means peculiar to the species which we are discussing here.

CULTIVATION   *Str. pneumoniae* resembles the streptococci already described in its nutritional and environmental requirements except that it exhibits more definite enhancement of its growth by the addition of 5–10% CO_2 to the atmosphere in which it is incubated. Its colonies are surrounded by zones of alpha-haemolysis similar to those of the viridans group, but in general the colonies themselves are larger and more disk-shaped. Typically they have raised edges and concentric ridges on their surfaces which have earned for them the name of 'draughtsmen'. Some strains form moister, more mucoid colonies, whereas others have rough, granular surfaces.

OPTOCHIN SENSITIVITY Pneumococci differ from the viridans group in being inhibited by optochin (ethyl hydrocuprein hydrochloride), and indeed this is often the simplest way of distinguishing between the two in the routine diagnostic laboratory. Optochin sensitivity can be tested on blood agar by inoculating the organism on to the plate along a streak which leads right up to a filter-paper disk containing optochin, and seeing whether its growth is inhibited in the vicinity of the disk. Such inhibition of pneumococci may be detectable even in a mixed culture–e.g. a primary plate culture from a sputum specimen.

ANTIGENIC STRUCTURE Pneumococci form polysaccharide capsules which act as haptens (see p 60). Over 80 immunologically distinct pneumococcal capsular polysaccharides can be recognized, and all strains forming the same polysaccharide are assigned to the same type. Using type-specific antisera, strains can be identified by agglutination of capsule-swelling tests of the organisms themselves or by precipitation tests of solution of capsular polysaccharide. The possibility of immediate typing of strains in sputum by applying antisera to the sputum and looking for a capsule-swelling reaction was important in the past when antisera were the only effective treatment for pneumococcal infection, since it was essential to use antiserum of the right type-specificity. In Britain at that time, types 1 and 2 were responsible for more than half of the cases of pneumococcal lobar pneumonia and type 3, while less common, was responsible for a high proportion of deaths. Type 2 is now uncommon, and type 3 is the type most frequently implicated.

IMMUNOLOGY As already implied, immunity following infection is effective only against the capsular type involved. Active immunization was not used in the past but is now under consideration, especially in the U.S.A. This is because, in spite of the sensitivity of pneumococci to many antibacterial agents in vitro, pneumococcal infections still have a distressingly high mortality rate, mainly due to a number of pneumococcal types small enough for immunization to be praticable, and involving definable groups of specially susceptible people. Passive immunization is of historic interest only.

ANTIBACTERIAL TREATMENT Pneumococci are almost invariably sensitive to penicillin, and usually to the sulphonamides and to most antibiotics except those of the aminoglycoside group, though resistance to tetracyclines is now quite common. Strains relatively resistant to penicillin were first reported in 1967 from Australia, and constituted 12% of all pneumococcal strains isolated in a survey in New Guinea, but have fortunately remained very rare elsewhere.

Anaerobic Streptococci

There is no satisfactory classification of the strictly anaerobic and micro-aerophilic streptococci. Organisms of this sort are to be found as normal commensals of the adult vagina and also on other mucous surfaces. They may cause puerperal sepsis and septicaemia or chronic endometritis, and are also found in association with other pathogens in certain forms of gangrene of wounds and in chronic deep abscesses. Being markedly proteolytic and vigorous producers of hydrogen sulphide, they give an unpleasant smell to the pus from lesions in which they are involved. They are usually penicillin-sensitive.

The Enterococcus Group

This is a large and ill-defined group of streptococci which are normal intestinal organisms. As might be expected from this habitat, they differ from other streptococci in being able to grow in the presence of moderate concentrations of bile-salts, for example on MacConkey's medium. They tend to be oval cocci, and to form short chains. On blood agar their colonies are usually somewhat larger than those of *Str. pyogenes*. Some stains are beta-haemolytic, some are alpha-haemolytic, some are non-haemolytic, and some produce a brown discoloration of the medium. They mostly survive heating at 60°C for 30 minutes, treatment which is lethal to most other streptococci. Many of them belong to Lancefield group D; such strains are not necessarily beta-haemolytic. The specific name *Str. faecalis*, at one time applied to all group D enterococci, now strictly belongs to one of several species into which such organisms are divided.

Enterococci quite commonly cause urinary tract infections, either by themselves or in association with other common urinary tract pathogens such as *Esch. coli*. They are also important as invaders of wounds and ulcerative skin lesions and as low-grade pathogens in various other situations; and they may cause subacute bacterial endocarditis which follows gynaecological or genito-urinary instrumentation or surgery in much the same way as endocarditis due to viridans streptococci follows dental operations. It is particularly in this last context that their frequent resistance to penicillin and other antibiotics is important (see p 353).

GRAM-NEGATIVE COCCI
THE GENUS NEISSERIA

Member of this genus are non-motile and mostly non-capsulate. They include two important pathogens – *N. meningitidis* or the meningococcus and *N. gonorrhoeae* or the gonococcus–and a number of species that are common commensals of the human respiratory tract. In stained films made from cultures of any of the species, the cocci are usually arranged in pairs, each coccus being somewhat flattened or concave on the side facing its partner. In films of pathological material, such as cerebrospinal fluid or pus, the pathogenic species are characteristically found as pairs of kidney-shaped cocci (Fig. 3(*d*), p 94), many of which are inside pus cells. The pathogens are more exacting than the commensals in their nutritional, atmospheric and thermal requirements.

Neisseria meningitidis (the meningococcus)

OCCURRENCE AND PATHOGENICITY   This organism is an obligate human parasite. It is the cause of cerebrospinal (now more commonly referred to simply as meningococcal) meningitis, a disease of world-wide incidence occurring as sporadic cases or in epidemics. In temperate climates most epidemics have arisen in closely packed communities such as war-time barracks; but very large epidemics with high attack-rates sweep across extensive areas of Africa in dry weather. An outbreak in the city of Sao Paulo, Brazil, in 1974 produced more than 13 000 cases in 2 months. Septicaemia, with scattered petechial or larger haemorrhagic lesions of the skin, may accompany the meningitis or may occur without it. Such a septicaemia sometimes runs a prolonged sub-acute course, and sometimes is fulminating, with sudden death resulting from damage to the adrenal glands (the *Waterhouse-Friderichsen syndrome*).

CARRIERS   The meningococcus may be carried in the upper respiratory tracts of healthy people. During epidemics more than half of those at risk may become carriers, especially if they are living and sleeping in overcrowded conditions. During the First World War it was claimed that cases of meningitis were likely in barracks when the carrier-rate exceeded 20%, and that a rise to such a level could be prevented by adequate spacing of beds. Subsequent experience has not agreed very closely with these claims.

MICROSCOPY   See above, in the discussion of the genus. In stained films made from purulent cerebrospinal fluid the meningococcus can as a rule be rapidly identified and distinguished from other likely causes of meningitis by its characteristic shape, arrangement and predominantly intracellular situation.

CULTIVATION   *N. meningitidis* will grow on some of the richer varieties of nutrient agar, but does better on blood agar, and better still on a similar medium in which the blood has been heated and which is called *chocolate agar* because of its resultant brown colour. The species is aerobic; its growth is often enhanced by the presence of about 5% of CO_2 in its atmosphere (see p 240). The optimal growth temperature is about 37°C, but some growth will usually occur anywhere between 25 and 42°C. The colonies formed on a suitable medium are rather small (around 2 mm in diameter after 24 hours), smooth, greyish, semitransparent and devoid of striking positive features. Except on special storage media, cultures usually die within a few days.

The organism can be collected from the nasopharynx by using pernasal swabs (see p 244). These, and also blood and cerebrospinal fluid specimens when appropriate, are examined as described in Chapter Fourteen.

BIOCHEMICAL REACTIONS   In common with most other members of the genus, *N. meningitidis* produces an *oxidase* which can be detected by pouring a 1% solution of tetramethyl-*p*-phenylenediamine over the culture plate on which it is growing. Neisserial colonies become pink and then purple within a few minutes. This helps their detection in a mixed culture, but in order to survive they must be subcultured as soon as the colour change becomes apparent. A single colony can be tested by transferring part of it to a strip of filter paper that has been impregnated with the indicator; the colour then develops on the paper.

Carbohydrate oxidation by *N. meningitidis* and other neisseriae can be tested by growing them on a specially enriched nutrient agar to which have been added a sugar and an indicator. *N. meningitidis* produces acid from glucose and from maltose but not from sucrose, *N. gonorrhoeae* from glucose but not from the other two, and most of the commensal neisseriae from all three sugars or from none of them.

ANTIGENIC STRUCTURE   Seven or more serogroups of this species are currently recognized, but most epidemics of cerebrospinal meningitis are due to group A strains and most sporadic cases to those of group B or C.

IMMUNOLOGY   Natural active immunity follows asymptomatic carriage of meningococci, and there are encouraging reports about immunization with polysaccharides from group A and group C strains.

ANTIBACTERIAL TREATMENT   For many years sulphonamides were highly and uniformly effective and were the treatment of choice. They have also been of great value as cheap and acceptable prophylactics for use in control of the African epidemics. However, sulphonamide–resistant strains were reported in the U.S.A. in 1963 and now constitute a significant proportion of strains in many countries, including Britain; and they include some African group A strains. As yet, penicillin is effective against all such strains as a therapeutic agent, though it is less effective in prophylaxis.

Neisseria gonorrhoeae (the gonococcus)

OCCURRENCE AND PATHOGENICITY   This is also an obligate human parasite. Its transmission is nearly always by sexual intercourse, and the initial infection is then an acute suppurative urethritis, usually with involvement of the cervix uteri as well in the female. Infection may spread by direct extension to Bartholin's glands, the uterus and Fallopian tubes and the ovaries and peritoneal cavity in the female; and to the prostate, seminal vesicles, epididymis and testes in the male. Blood-stream spread may lead to suppurative arthritis and to tenosynovitis, and occasionally to endocarditis or other diseases. Non-venereal transmission is responsible for neonatal ophthalmia of babies born to infected mothers, and for vulvovaginitis of young female children; the latter may occur in epidemic form in institutions, being transmitted by towels and other fomites.

CARRIERS   The true carrier state probably does not exist, but patients with chronic infections, particularly prostitutes, play an important part in the maintenance and spread of the disease.

MICROSCOPY   The gonococcus is indistinguishable from the meningococcus by ordinary microscopy, but can be identified by the fluorescent-antibody technique (p 72). Characteristic intracellular Gram-negative diplococci are to be seen in urethral or cervical pus in the acute stages of gonorrhoea. In chronic infections microscopy often fails to reveal gonococci in material which gives positive results on culture.

CULTIVATION   The gonococcus behaves like the meningococcus in culture except that it will not grow on nutrient agar and has a narrower temperature range than the meningococcus, and that its colonies are usually slower to appear and smaller.

In the investigation of a patient, purulent material should whenever possible be transferred directly from the patient to culture plates, using a sterile wire loop. When this cannot be arranged, the material should be collected on swabs which are immediately placed in a special transport medium (e.g. *Stuart's*) for transmission to the laboratory. On ordinary dry swabs gonococci soon die. For their culture special media have been devised which contain mixtures of antibacterial agents to inhibit more robust bacteria commonly present in the relevant specimens.

BIOCHEMICAL REACTIONS   See under *N. meningitidis*.

IMMUNOLOGY   Immunity does not follow natural infection and cannot be produced artificially. The gonococcal complement-fixation test (G.C.F.T.) has been widely used, as an aid to the diagnosis of chronic infections, particularly the less accessible ones such as salpingitis and arthritis; but it has proved unreliable and even misleading, and its popularity has decreased.

ANTIBACTERIAL TREATMENT   Emergence of sulphonamide resistance was much more rapid and widespread among gonococci than among meningococci. The penicillins have remained effective far longer, and in a condition in which treatment failure is often the result of patient default they have had the advantage that adequate treatment could be achieved by a single injection of a long-acting preparation or by two oral doses accompanied by probenecid (see p 344) to delay excretion. However, over many years now it has been apparent in various parts of the world that the prevailing gonococcal strains were becoming somewhat less sensitive to penicillins, so that progressively higher doses have been necessary; and more recently strains have emerged which are penicillinase-producers and thus frankly penicillin-resistant. The subject of alternative treatment in such circumstances is too complex to be discussed here.

Neonatal opthalmia need never occur, as it can be prevented by the administration of silver nitrate drops to the eyes of all possibly infected babies as soon as they are born.

Commensal Neisseriae
Other species of this genus—e.g. *N. catarrhalis, N. sicca, N. pharyngis*—make a large contribution to the normal commensal flora of the human upper respiratory tract. They are virtually never pathogenic. They are distinguishable from the pathogenic species by their growth on simpler media and at lower temperatures and by their different sugar reactions.

GRAM-POSITIVE BACILLI
The four genera to be discussed differ in the following respects (among others):

Corynebacterium. Non-sporing; bacilli mostly in palisades or in 'Chinese characters' (see below); aerobic.

Lactobacillus. Non-sporing; bacilli commonly in chains; mostly microaerophilic or anaerobic.

Bacillus. Sporing, with spores usually not exceeding the bacilli in diameter; aerobic.

Clostridium. Sporing, with spores usually wider than the bacilli; anaerobic.

Their differences in microscopic morphology are illustrated in Fig. 3 (p 94).

THE GENUS CORYNEBACTERIUM

The genus owes its name to the club-shaped swellings often seen at the ends of the bacilli, especially in old cultures. It includes one important human pathogen, the diphtheria bacillus. Other species cause suppurative diseases of animals. Various non-pathogenic corynebacteria, known as *diphtheroid bacilli*, are normal commensals of human skin, upper respiratory tract, external ears and conjunctivae. Some of these have been given specific names – e.g. *C. hofmanni* and *C. xerosis*. Their properties will only be mentioned incidentally as part of our discussion of *C. diphtheriae*, but they are important to the clinical bacteriologist because they are present in a high proportion of the specimens that he receives.

Corynebacterium diphtheriae (the diphtheria bacillus, the Klebs-Loeffler bacillus)

OCCURRENCE AND PATHOGENICITY Diphtheria is now a rare disease in Britain, where widespread immunization against it was introduced in the early 1940s, and in other countries that have been able to afford comparable immunization programmes. Indeed, its near-elimination from such countries is one of the success stories of pro-phylactic immunization. However, it remains a common disease in other parts of the world; and rapid bacteriological confirmation of suspected cases is important in countries where it is rare. Its causative bacillus is an obligate parasite, with man as its only natural host. Typically, diphtheria is an infection of the upper respiratory tract, characterized by the formation of a thick adherent exudate or membrane; if this extends to the larynx it may cause respiratory obstruction. Exotoxin enters the patient's circulation and damages the heart, nervous system, liver, kidneys and adrenals. The severity of the resultant illness depends to some extent upon the variety of diphtheria bacillus involved. There are three of these – *gravis*, *intermedius* and *mitis* – which can be differentiated in the laboratory and in very general terms are associated respectively with severe, intermediate and mild illnesses.

Occasionally the primary infection is in the skin, a wound or the vagina. In such atypical cases systemic disturbance is usually not severe.

Non-toxigenic and consequently non-pathogenic strains of all three varieties occur (see below); they are most common in the *mitis* variety.

C. diphtheriae is not naturally pathogenic to animals, but guinea-pigs and rabbits are highly susceptible to injections of toxigenic strains or their toxins, and many other species are less markedly so.

CARRIERS   These play an important part in the spread of the disease. Some are convalescent, but many have had only subclinical infections. While the throat and nose are the common sites of carriage, the organism is sometimes carried in an ear or elsewhere.

MICROSCOPY   Corynebacteria divide like snapping sticks in which the bark fails to break on one side. In most diphtheroid bacilli the resulting arrangement tends to resemble a stake fence or palisade–rows of bacilli of rather irregular lengths lying side-by-side (Fig, 3(f), p 94). The rods of C. diphtheriae are slightly curved, and therefore form less tidy bundles, conventionally likened to Chinese characters (Fig. 3(e), p 94). An average diphtheria bacillus is of the order of 3 μm by 0·5 μm, and has terminal *volutin granules* which are clearly visible as dark dots at the ends of the bacilli in films stained by special procedures such as Albert's or Neisser's. Some of the diphtheroid bacilli also form such granules, but rarely in the characteristic bipolar distribution seen in C. diphtheriae.

The diagnosis of diphtheria cannot be reliably confirmed or excluded by microscopic examination of smears from pharyngeal or other lesions. In such situations the appearances of C. diphtheriae are not clearly distinguishable from those of commensal corynebacteria, and in any case diphtheria bacilli are often absent from smears made from undoubted cases of diphtheria.

CULTIVATION   C. diphtheriae grows on simple media, but better on those which contain serum or blood. On blood agar its inconspicuous small grey colonies are easily overlooked or mistaken for those of some of the diphtheroid bacilli. Many *mitis* and some *gravis* strains are more noticeable because they are haemolytic.

For the isolation of the diphtheria bacillus from clinical material, special media of two quite different types are commonly used. *Loeffler's serum* is an inspissated mixture of ox or horse serum and glucose broth. A wide variety of bacteria will grow on it, and colonial differentiation is very poor. However, the microscopic morphology and staining reactions of C. diphtheriae after 18 hours incubation on this medium are so characteristic that it can be recognized even in films containing many other organisms. Thus a presumptive diagnosis of diphtheria can often be made in about 18 hours or even less. Confirmation comes from the use of a selective *tellurite medium*, both for primary culture of the original material and for subculture of the Loeffler's serum. This medium is a blood or chocolate agar containing 0·04% of potassium tellurite, which suppresses the growth of most bacteria. It also slows even that of corynebacteria, so that they may take up to 48 hours to produce recognizable colonies. By naked-eye examination of these it is possible to distinguish *C. diphtheriae* from diphtheroid bacilli and from the few other species which are not inhibited by the tellurite. The three varieties of *C. diphtheriae* form colonies of somewhat different sizes and shapes, but all are predominantly dark slate-grey in colour, as a result of metabolism of the tellurite, whereas diphtheroid colonies are usually black, light grey or brown.

BIOCHEMICAL REACTIONS   Grown in a suitable medium *C. diph-theriae* ferments glucose and maltose but rarely sucrose, whereas most diphtheroid bacilli ferment all three or none of these. Only *gravis* varieties of *C. diphtheriae* ferment starch. *C. ulcerans*, an uncommon cause of diphtheria-like throat infection, gives the reactions of *C. diphtheriae gravis* in these tests but can be differentiated by other biochemical tests.

TOXIN PRODUCTION   This depends on a lysogenic relationship (see p 212) between *C. diphtheriae* and an appropriate bacteriophage; strains that lack the phage are non-toxigenic. Since pathogenicity of *C. diphtheriae* depends on toxin production, a strain isolated from a typical case of diphtheria can reasonably be assumed to be toxigenic. No such assumption can be made about a strain from a doubtful case or a carrier, and the matter may need to be investigated. The presence of diphtheria toxin in a broth culture can be demonstrated by showing that it produces typical lesions when injected into guinea-pigs, and that these can be prevented by prior administration of diphtheria antitoxin to the animals. An *in vitro* method of demonstrating antitoxin production is Elek's gel-diffusion procedure. A strip of filter paper soaked in diphtheria antitoxin is incorporated in a plate of a suitable serum agar, and known and suspected toxigenic *C. diphtheriae* cultures are streaked in single lines across the plate at right angles to the strip. The plates are incubated for 48 hours, during which time antitoxin diffuses out from the paper strip and toxin diffuses out from the growing toxigenic cultures. After incubation, fine white lines of toxin-antitoxin precipitate can be seen in the medium, radiating out from the points at which toxigenic cultures cross the strip. Lines due to antigens other than diphtheria toxin may occur; but a true positive reaction is shown by the fact that the line from the suspected culture, on meeting that from the known toxigenic strain, does not cross it but fuses with it to form an arch between the two cultures (the *reaction of identity*—see p 69).

IMMUNOLOGY   Immunity follows natural infection, often without any clinical illness, and can be detected by studying the patient's response to intradermal injection of a small dose of toxin (the Schick text, see p 265). Antitoxin can also be measured in serum. Active immunization (see p 312) has played a large part in reducing the incidence of diphtheria, as indicated above. Passive immunization–i.e. the administration of serum containing antitoxin–is the only effective treatment for an established infection, and must be given at once to any patient suspected of having diphtheria, without waiting for laboratory confirmation of the diagnosis.

ANTIBACTERIAL TREATMENT *In vitro* the diphtheria bacillus is sensitive to most antibiotics, but these are of little value in treatment because they cannot deal with toxin already in the patient's body. However, penicillin and other antibiotics can be used to prevent infection and to stop cases from becoming carriers, and are occasionally effective in dealing with established carriers.

LISTERIA MONOCYTOGENES AND ERYSIPELOTHRIX RHUSIOPATHIAE

These two species, which have many properties in common with one another and with the corynebacteria, are both animal pathogens that occasionally cause disease of man. Both are sensitive to most of the common antibiotics.

Listeria monocytogenes

This aerobic non-sporing Gram-positive bacillus differs from the corynebacteria in being flagellate and feebly motile (see p 123), in being agglutinable by known anti-listerial sera and in causing monocytosis in rabbits. In humans it may cause meningitis or a severe generalized septicaemic illness, usually during the first few weeks of life but sometimes in adults, and in particular in those on immunosuppressive treatment following renal or other transplants. It is said also to cause low-grade fever in pregnant women, sometimes leading to abortion or still-birth or to the neonatal infections already mentioned.

Erysipelothrix rhusiopathiae

This organism closely resembles *Listeria monocytogenes* but is non-motile and is usually micro-aerophilic. It is widely distributed in nature, causing swine erysipelas and other animal diseases, and it is present on the skin and scales of many kinds of fish. *Erysipeloid*, the human condition for which it is responsible, occurs mainly among those who handle meat, poultry or fish. The organism enters a skin abrasion, commonly on a finger, and causes a painful purplish local swelling that increases in area by peripheral extension but tends to heal centrally.

THE GENUS LACTOBACILLUS

This genus of long and slender Gram-positive bacilli, commonly occurring in chains (Fig. 3(*g*), p 94), deserves to be ranked as important in medical bacteriology because its members make a substantial contribution to man's normal flora. They are to be found in the mouth, the stomach, the intestines and the vagina, and are particularly abundant in the faeces of milk-fed babies. However, they are mostly anaerobic or micro-aerophilic, some of them will multiply only in an acid environment and they have unusual nutritional requirements. Consequently the average clinical bacteriologist does not grow many of them, and he has little incentive to try to do so, since they are generally regarded as non-pathogens. In the early days of bacteriology the *Boas–Oppler bacillus* was under suspicion as a possible cause of gastric carcinoma, because its long threads are frequently to be seen in the gastric juice of patients with that disease; but this was a classical example of confusion between cause and effect, since in fact they are also present there in many other conditions in which gastric acidity is reduced to a level that suits their growth. Similarly, the presence of abnormal numbers of lactobacilli in the stools in some forms of diarrhoea is probably a consequence rather than the cause of the intestinal upset. Indeed, ingestion of cultures of *L. acidophilus* and of *L. bulgaricus* (found in Yoghurt) has in the past been recommended as a treatment for some alimentary derangements. The most serious claim for the pathogenicity of at least some members of this genus relates to the production of dental caries. Decalcification of enamel, which is a stage in the pathogenesis of this condition, may be due to acid produced in the mouth by lactobacillary breakdown of food residues. However, it now seems likely that even in caries lactobacilli are innocent bystanders and that the damage is done by oral streptococci (see p 102).

On the credit side, we have already had several occasions to mention the protective activity of lactobacilli in the adult vagina (see p 28).

THE GENUS BACILLUS

The sporing aerobic bacilli include one highly pathogenic species, *B. anthracis*, and a large assortment of other species that are almost always saprophytic.

Bacillus anthracis (the anthrax bacillus)

OCCURRENCE AND PATHOGENICITY   Mainly a pathogen of herbivorous animals, in which it produces a disease varying from a fulminating haemorrhagic septicaemia to a chronic fever with pustules, *B. anthracis* is an occasional cause of human disease. This may take either of two forms. *Cutaneous anthrax* may occur in farm workers and others in contact with infected animals. In countries such as Britain animal infection is rare and human victims are mostly dockers or factory workers who handle imported hides, bristles, wool or bone meal. A papule at the site of inoculation develops into a blister, then becomes purulent (the 'malignant pustule'), and then becomes a dark-centred necrotic lesion surrounded by oedema, induration and a ring of vesicles. In the absence of effective treatment a severe and commonly fatal septicaemia may follow. The other form of human anthrax, 'wool-sorter's disease', is a severe haemorrhagic infection of the bronchi and lungs, often accompanied by pleural and pericardial effusions and by septicaemia. It affects only a small proportion of workers who are exposed to the hazard of inhaling anthrax spores in wool or hide factories.

Whereas man does not acquire anthrax readily, cattle and sheep are highly susceptible to natural infection. It also occurs in other herbivorous mammals, including goats, horses and camels. All of these are infected by ingesting spores. The organisms then pass from the intestine into the blood-stream. Laboratory infections can be produced in mice, guinea-pigs and rabbits by injecting cultures of B. anthracis, which cause fatal septicaemia.

MICROSCOPY   Anthrax bacilli are large–4–8 μm long and 1 μm or more wide. Their spores, situated near the centres of the bacilli, are not large enough to distend them (Fig. 3(h), p 94); they can be seen as non-staining areas in Gram-stained films and can be demonstrated even more clearly by special spore stains. The rods are non-flagellate and, in culture, non-capsulate. They are square-ended and are often arranged in chains.

In smears of vesicle fluid or other pathological material the presence of chains of large Gram-positive rods is strong evidence of anthrax, but not conclusive, since some of the other members of the genus can present similar appearances. In the body of its host B. anthracis does not form spores, but usually does have a capsule. Unlike most other bacterial capsules, which are composed of polysaccharides, that of B. anthracis contains a polypeptide. It gives a characteristic purple staining reaction with polychrome methylene blue (McFadyean's reaction).

CULTIVATION   B. anthracis grows well aerobically and anaerobically on most common media, but forms spores only in aerobic conditions. Its opaque, greyish-white, rough-surfaced colonies resemble tangles of fine hairs, often with loose curls protruding at the edges.

ANIMAL INOCULATION   The identity of the cultured organism is confirmed by inoculation into mice or guinea-pigs.

IMMUNOLOGY   Pasteur's conclusive and dramatic demonstration, at

Pouilly-le-Fort in 1881, of the possibility of immunizing animals against anthrax is one of the milestones of bacteriology. The story is well told in Vallery-Radot's biography. Pasteur used a vaccine of *B. anthracis* attenuated by prolonged growth at 42°C or higher. It has not been possible to produce in this way vaccines that are consistently effective and safe enough to be given to man, but dockers, factory workers and others whose work exposes them to special anthrax hazards can now be safely immunized by using a non-living protein antigen which can be precipitated from bacterium-free filtrates of broth cultures of *B. anthracis*.

ANTIBACTERIAL TREATMENT   Passive immunization, using serum of immunized animals, has been superseded by antibiotic treatment. The organism is usually sensitive to penicillin and to several other antibiotics, which are effective if not given too late, though the slow response of the oedema and induration around the primary lesion may cause anxiety to those not familiar with it.

Disposal of animal carcases and other control measures are discussed in Chapter Sixteen.

Other Members of the Genus Bacillus (sometimes called anthracoid bacilli or aerobic spore-bearers)

These are a large and varied assortment, having in common a bacillary shape, the ability to form spores and a preference for aerobic conditions. Many of them are only weakly or irregularly Gram-positive, mottled staining being a useful diagnostic feature; and a few are frankly Gram-negative but are included in this genus on other grounds. Sizes and shapes of individual bacilli vary considerably from species to species. In general the spores are narrower than the bacilli, but in a few species they cause bacillary distension as seen in the genus *Clostridium*. Colonial appearances are widely diverse, and in some cases bizarre. Saprophytic existence is the rule, and apart from *B. cereus* food-poisoning (p 304), occasional severe eye lesions (iridocyclitis and panophthalmitis) caused by *B. subtilis* and very rare cases of meningitis, endocarditis, pneumonia and septicaemia in debilitated subjects, these widely distributed organisms can usually be dismissed as non-pathogenic. Their importance in medical bacteriology arises from their frequent occurrence as contaminants of culture media, blood intended for transfusion, other fluids which should be sterile, specimens collected from patients, and foods. Their tiresome ubiquity is due to their ability to grow in widely varied circumstances and to survive, by means of their spores, conditions which kill most other bacteria. However, the bacteriologist can turn these features to good account in testing the efficiency of his methods of sterilization. Heat or irradiation or other physical treatment that can kill organisms of this group–usually represented by *B. subtilis*, the 'hay bacillus', or by *B. stearothermophilus*–is also sufficient to kill all pathogens, including spore-bearers of the next genus to be discussed.

THE GENUS CLOSTRIDIUM

This genus consists of anaerobic Gram-positive bacilli which form spores that in most cases distend their bodies (Fig. 3(*i* and *j*), p 94). Such organisms are widely distributed in nature as soil saprophytes and as intestinal commensals of mammals. They include the causative organisms of three highly lethal human diseases – botulism, tetanus and gas-gangrene.

Clostridium botulinum

OCCURRENCE AND PATHOGENICITY   This species is to be found in soil in many parts of the world. Botulism is due not to bacterial infection of the victim but to eating food that contains the very powerful toxin of *Cl. botulinum* (see p 304). In man this causes little in the way of alimentary disturbances; the first symptoms are difficulties of vision due to muscle paralysis, and these are followed by progressive bulbar paralysis, frequently terminating in death from respiratory or cardiac arrest. The condition is rare, and can be prevented by proper cooking of food as described in Chapter Nineteen.

There are in fact at least five different types of *Cl. botulinum*, producing slightly different toxins. Types A, B and E cause botulism in man, whereas types C and D cause similar natural diseases of animals. Laboratory animals of many sorts are susceptible to the effects of these toxins given by injection.

MICROSCOPY   The individual bacilli, like those of most clostridia, are intermediate in size between those of the genera *Corynebacterium* and *Bacillus*. They are flagellate and have oval spores which are subterminal in position–i.e. near one end of the rod.

CULTIVATION   This species is strictly anaerobic. (Methods of anaerobic culture are discussed on pp 239–40.) It grows best at temperatures somewhat below 37°C, as is to be expected since it is a saprophyte. It has simple nutritional requirements. Like many other members of the genus, when grown anaerobically on common media it forms diffuse, greyish, semi-transparent colonies of irregular shape.

BIOCHEMICAL REACTIONS   The different clostridial species can be distinguished by their patterns of carbohydrate fermentation (cf the enterobacteria, p 124) and by their ability to liquefy coagulated serum and to digest meat.

IMMUNOLOGY   Active immunization is not indicated for a disease that is so rare, and serological diagnosis is out of the question in one that is of such short duration. Antiserum, produced in animals, can be given to counteract the toxin, but its efficacy is low even in those patients who receive it between eating suspected food and developing symptoms. Unless the type of the *Cl. botulinum* strain happens to be known, a polyvalent serum that contains antibodies to the toxins of all types should be used.

ANTIBACTERIAL TREATMENT   Since the organism itself does not multiply in the patient's body, there is no indication for using antibiotics.

Clostridium tetani (the tetanus bacillus)

OCCURRENCE AND PATHOGENICITY   Tetanus spores are particularly common in soil to which animal manure has been added. When introduced into the tissues of man, the horse or various other animals, they may cause tetanus, but only if certain conditions are fulfilled. These are imperfectly understood. Interference with the blood supply to at least a small amount of tissue, together with multiplication of other organisms so that all oxygen is used up, appear to be necessary for the production of an anaerobic environment in which the bacillus can grow. Presence of soil in the lesion increases the risk of tetanus, probably because the calcium salts encourage germination of the spores. However, tetanus may follow puncture wounds or abrasions so trivial that it is hard to see how the necessary conditions are fulfilled. The disease is particularly common in countries in which bare-footed human beings, often with multiple chronic infected lesions of the feet, live in close association with cattle, goats and other domesticated mammals. In such circumstances it is frequently impossible to identify the particular lesion in which the tetanus bacillus is multiplying. Inadequately sterilized dressings or suture materials have often caused post-operative tetanus in the past, and tetanus neonatorum, due to infection of the umbilical stump, is common in communities in which animal dung is used as an umbilical dressing.

Days, weeks or even months after the patient is infected, local multiplication of the organism occurs, with liberation of toxin. This does no harm locally, but travels along peripheral nerves to the central nervous system. The clinical picture resulting from its action there is characterized by severe muscular spasms often involving the jaw ('lockjaw') and by generalized convulsions in response to minimal external stimuli. Patients may die as a result of the direct action of the tetanus toxin on the nervous system, and in the absence of suitable treatment many others succumb to secondary infections, notably of the lungs, by other bacteria.

In the laboratory, most mammals are susceptible to the action of tetanus toxin or to the injection of broth cultures of the organism.

MICROSCOPY   In films from cultures or from pathological material *Cl. tetani* has a typical 'drum-stick' appearance, due to the presence of large, round and strictly terminal spores (Fig. 3(*j*), p 94). However, this appearance can be mimicked by other clostridia, such as the non-toxigenic *Cl. tetanomorphum*, and by some of the aerobic spore-bearers. *Cl. tetani* is usually flagellate and motile (see p 123).

CULTIVATION   A strict anaerobe with an optimal growth temperature of about 37 °C, this species grows on ordinary media as a flat, translucent spreading colony with fine finger-like projections. Its ability to swarm over the surfaces of solid media and the heat-resistance of its spores form the basis of procedures for isolating it from the mixture of organisms often present with it in material from lesions. The material, or a suspension or mixed broth culture made from it, is heated to 65 °C for 30 minutes, in order to destroy all non-sporing organisms, and is then used to inoculate one side of a plate or the bottom of a slope of blood agar; the medium must not be too dry to allow swarming. After a short period of anaerobic incubation the growth begins to swarm across the plate or up the slope, and the advancing edge is subcultured to another plate or slope. If the resultant growth is still mixed, its advancing edge can again be subcultured, and so on.

It is not surprising that in many typical cases of tetanus the organism cannot be isolated. It may not be possible to identify the relevant lesion, the bacilli may in any case be present only in small numbers, they are often heavily outnumbered in the lesion by other organisms including spore-formers, and it is common for the patient to have received antibiotics before the specimen was collected.

BIOCHEMICAL REACTIONS   *Cl. tetani* is unique among medically important clostridia in that it usually fails to ferment any carbohydrates.

TOXIN PRODUCTION   The powerful exotoxin, second in potency only to that of *Cl. botulinum*, can be identified in a broth-culture filtrate by the characteristic spasticity and liability to convulsions that follow its injection into mice and guinea-pigs, and by the neutralization of these effects by specific antitoxin.

IMMUNOLOGY   Immunization is against the toxin, not against the organism itself. Active immunization, sufficiently far in advance and adequately maintained, prevents tetanus. Boosting of active immunity at the time of any appropriate injury, or passive immunization at this stage in those not previously immunized, are of course only applicable to patients whose lesions cause them to seek medical attention. In addition to the hazards of all passive immunization (see p 308), that against tetanus has the defect that toxin already fixed in the patient's nervous system cannot be neutralized; all that can be hoped for is the neutralization of any further toxin formed by the organisms. Tetanus immunization is discussed more fully in Chapter Twenty.

ANTIBACTERIAL TREATMENT   Penicillin and some other antibiotics are effective against *Cl. tetani* in the laboratory, but they have little relevance to the established disease, except in preventing other bacterial infections. However, there is a place for their prophylactic use, along with careful surgical elimination of suitable sites for clostridial germination, in some types of injury, particularly in cases in which temporary protection is needed while active immunity is being induced.

Clostridium welchii (*Cl. perfringens*)

OCCURRENCE AND PATHOGENICITY   This species is commonly present in soil and in the intestines of animals and of man. Together with other organisms of similar habitat, it may gain entry into wounds–from the soil in the case of dirty accidental wounds, but usually from the patient's own intestines, via the skin, in the case of surgical wounds. If there is little or no damaged devitalized tissue in the wound, or if such tissue is promptly and thoroughly excised, clostridial contamination is unlikely to have any ill effects. In the presence of such damaged tissue, gas-gangrene may develop. This condition is due to the multiplication of clostridia (or less commonly of anaerobic streptococci), which digest muscle and subcutaneous tissues. In doing this they liberate gas and an assortment of noxious metabolites as well as their specific toxins. Affected wounds have a foul smell, and the surrounding tissues crepitate when handled because of the presence of free gas. Without appropriate treatment the condition spreads and is commonly fatal. Clostridial cellulitis is a less serious infection, often confused with gas-gangrene (clostridial myositis) because there is much gas-formation and crepitation of the tissues, but differing from it in that there is no destruction of muscle.

Numerous *Cl. welchii* exotoxins have been identified, and strains of this species are classified into six types, A to F, according to the combinations of toxins that they produce. Strains that cause human gas-gangrene belong to type A, and it is therefore with that type that we are chiefly concerned. Types B, C, D and E are all associated with enterotoxaemia in sheep or cattle, and types C and F have been reported as causing rare cases of a similar disease in man, known as *enteritis necroticans*. Finally, certain widely distributed strains which differ slightly from ordinary type A strains (notably in being able to survive prolonged boiling, whereas ordinary strains are killed in about 5 minutes) are responsible for many outbreaks of food-poisoning (see p 303).

Injected cultures of type A strains cause gas-gangrene in guinea-pigs and pigeons, and less readily in mice. Other types vary in their animal pathogenicity.

MICROSCOPY   The bacilli are stouter than those of most clostridia, measuring about 4–8 μm by 1 μm. Capsules may be present in films made from pathological materials but are not formed in culture. Most strains fail to form spores in culture, unless fermentable carbohydrate is absent and the medium is alkaline; but small oval subterminal spores are formed freely in natural conditions. The species is not flagellate.

CULTIVATION   A strict anaerobe with an optimal growth temperature of about 37°C, *Cl. welchii* varies in its colonial appearances, but commonly forms large, round, moderately opaque disks on blood agar, surrounded by zones of haemolysis. The isolation of this and other gas-gangrene organisms from the mixture of bacteria that usually prevails in a gangrenous wound is often a complex procedure, involving a number of special media and techniques which we shall not discuss.

BIOCHEMICAL REACTIONS   See under *Cl. botulinum*.

TOXIN PRODUCTION   Of the many exotoxins formed by this species, the alpha-toxin is common to all types and is believed to be largely responsible for the toxaemia of human gas-gangrene. It is a relatively heat-stable lecithinase (see p 29), and is the basis of the Nagler reaction, by which *Cl. welchii* can be recognized even in mixed culture. Material suspected of containing this organism is streaked across a plate of a transparent medium containing human serum or egg yolk, a small amount of *Cl. welchii* alpha-antitoxin having first been spread over half of the plate. The plate is incubated overnight, and if *Cl. welchii* is present in the inoculum a zone of increased opacity will have been produced by the lecithinase in the medium around and beneath the growth on the untreated side of the plate; but on the other side, although the growth is equally good, there is no increased opacity because the lecithinase has been inactivated by the antitoxin. Other lecithinase-producing organisms exist, but only *Cl. welchii* alpha-toxin and the closely related toxin of *Cl. bifermentans* are inhibited by *Cl. welchii* antitoxin.

IMMUNOLOGY   In view of the nature of *Cl. welchii* infections, there is no indication for active immunization. Passive immunization, both prophylactic and therapeutic, using polyvalent sera against the toxins of all of the common gas-gangrene organisms, is possible but of limited value.

ANTIBACTERIAL TREATMENT   Penicillin, the tetracyclines, chloramphenicol and metranidazole are effective against gas-gangrene bacilli, but the aminoglycosides are not. Surgical removal of necrotic material, in which anaerobes can multiply and to which antibiotics cannot penetrate, is of fundamental importance.

Other Gas-Gangrene Bacilli

Cl. oedematiens (*C. novyi*), *Cl. septicum*, and, less frequently, *Cl. bifermentans*, *Cl. histolyticum* and *Cl. fallax* are all capable of causing gas-gangrene similar to that caused by *Cl. welchii*. In view of the nature of the infection and the similar habitats of the various species, it is not surprising that the same lesion often yields two or more of these species. They are distinguishable by the shapes and sizes of their bacilli, the shapes and situations of their spores, their cultural and biochemical properties and the toxins which they form.

GRAM-NEGATIVE BACILLI: (a) ENTEROBACTERIA

Many species of aerobic, facultatively anaerobic Gram-negative bacilli that ferment (in the strict sense–p 27) glucose and other carbohydrates and are oxidase-negative (see p 107) are commonly present in the human intestine, usually as commensals but some of them as actual or potential pathogens. Such organisms are also widely distributed in nature. They are collectively known by the informal name *enterobacteria*, though it would have been more logical to call them enterobacilli. The name 'coliform bacilli' is used by some to indicate the same range of organisms, but others use it for only part of that range (see p 296).

To save repetition, we shall deal with the common properties of the enterobacteria and the chief procedures used for differentiating between them before we discuss the individual genera *Escherichia*, *Klebsiella*, *Salmonella*, *Shigella*, *Proteus* and *Yersinia*, with brief references to others.

MICROSCOPY   Gram-stained films give little or no help in distinguishing between enterobacteria, all of which are medium sized bacilli, about o·5μm by 1–3μm, with some (at times many) filamentous forms. Spores are not formed. Some of the group–notably the klebsiellae and many *Esch. coli* strains–have easily demonstrable capsules. Possession of flagella can be an important criterion for differentiation–e.g. between the genera *Salmonella* (flagellate) and *Shigella* (non-flagellate) or *Klebsiella* (non-flagellate) and *Enterobacter* (flagellate); or between the species *Yersinia pestis* (non-flagellate) and other yersiniae (flagellate). Direct demonstration of flagella by light microscopy is difficult (p 86), but *motility*, the effect of flagella, is relatively easily detected by direct microscopy of a drop of unstained fluid culture under a microscope, using reduced lighting (see p 20). An alternative non-microscopic method depends on the ability of motile organisms to make their way through a semisolid medium (o·2% agar).

CULTIVATION   Enterobacteria grow well over a wide range of temperatures on or in simple media such as nutrient agar or peptone water (a solution containing 1% commercial peptone and o·5% NaCl) under aerobic conditions, but somewhat less well anaerobically. On aerobically incubated blood agar, colonies are usually rather large (3–4 mm in diameter after 18 hours) and greyish-white, smooth and moderately opaque; however, dry rough surfaced colonies, large mucoid colonies and other variants occur. Haemolysis may occur round the colonies, but is not a useful differentiating feature in this group. Having modest nutritional requirements and being tolerant of bile (understandably, in view of their intestinal habitat), enterobacteria grow on MacConkey's agar (see p 90). This medium, frequently used as a means of separating them from a mixture of other bacteria, also provides a useful distinction between the red colonies of lactose-fermenters (the usual behaviour of *Esch. coli* and klebsiellae) and the straw-coloured colonies of non-lactose-fermenters (salmonellae, most shigellae, proteus and yersiniae).

BIOCHEMICAL REACTIONS   Lactose is only one (though the most useful) of a wide range of carbohydrates that can be employed in fermentation tests for the identification of enterobacteria. If such tests are carried out in liquid media, small inverted tubes or other means can be used to detect generation of gas bubbles during fermentation and so to increase the information derived. For example, fermentation of glucose and failure to ferment lactose, sucrose and various other commonly used carbohydrates are properties common to all salmonellae; but *S. typhi* alone in this genus fails to produce visible amounts of gas during glucose fermentation. Fermentation tests using 6 or 8 sugars or alcohols, supported by some of the other biochemical tests mentioned below, permit provisional or even definitive identification of most enterobacteria to species level.

Among other biochemical tests commonly applied to enterobacterial strains are those for the abilities to produce hydrogen sulphide and indole when growing in peptone water; to split urea with liberation of ammonia (the urease test); to multiply in a medium in which citrate is the only carbon source; to decarboxylate various amino-acids; and, when growing in glucose-phosphate broth, to form acetylmethylcarbinol (the Voges-Proskauer test) and to go on producing acid from the glucose until the pH of the medium is lowered to 4·5 or less (the methyl red test).

ANTIGENIC STRUCTURE   Of the many enterobacterial antigens that have been studied, most can be classified according to their location as H (flagellar), O (somatic) or K (capsular or envelope). (The letters H and O are taken from the German terms *Hauch* and *ohne Hauche*, because flagellate proteus strains form spreading films across culture plates, whereas non-flagellate forms are 'without film'.) The relevance of antigenic analysis to our understanding of the various enterobacterial genera is indicated at appropriate places below.

THE GENUS ESCHERICHIA (See also pp 122–4)
Esch. coli is the only species currently assigned to this genus.

OCCURRENCE AND PATHOGENICITY   *Esch. coli* is a normal inhabitant of the intestine of man and animals, but it not always harmless there. In Britain and other temperate countries the commonest form of entero-pathogenicity of this species to man is gastro-enteritis in infants and other young children. Strains of a limited but growing number of O and K serotypes have been found responsible for this, though by no means all strains of those types are potential pathogens. Many of the recognized outbreaks have occurred in hospital nurseries, and there have often been associated deaths, mainly among premature and debilitated babies. The pathogenetic mechanism of these strains (known as 'infantile entero-pathogenic') is still debatable, but strains of other serotypes ('entero-toxigenic') which cause gastro-enteritis in adults as well as children, mainly in tropical countries, do so by producing enterotoxins similar to that of *Vibrio cholerae* (p 135); and still other strains ('entero-invasive') resemble the shigellae in their ability to invade and destroy intestinal epithelial cells. However, despite the increasing amount of information about *Esch. coli* as an intestinal pathogen, its main contribution to human ill-health is made in the urinary tract; here it is responsible for 80% or more of all infections that occur outside hospital, but a smaller proportion of those acquired in hospital, many of which are due to klebsiellae, proteus, enterococci or other bacteria. *Esch. coli* can also cause biliary tract infections, intra-abdominal abscesses and wound infections (as can various other intestinal bacteria). It is a common cause of meningitis in the first few weeks of life. Its role in the respiratory tract is discussed below, with that of the klebsiellae.

ANTIBACTERIAL TREATMENT   Like most enterobacteria, *Esch. coli* strains are resistant to ordinary levels of penicillins other than ampicillin, amoxycillin and carbenicillin; and they may be resistant to these also, by means of enzymes that destroy them. In general they are sensitive to sulphonamides, trimethoprim, tetracyclines, aminoglycosides, chloramphenicol and various other drugs; but resistance to one or more is common, especially in strains from antibiotic-treated patients. When septicaemia or some other serious infection has to be treated urgently, without waiting for results of sensitivity tests on the causative *Esch. coli* strain, a drug to which it is unlikely to be resistant should be used – e.g. gentamicin. Nitrofurantoin or nalidixic acid may be useful for treating a urinary tract infection (see p 343).

THE GENUS KLEBSIELLA (See also pp 122–4)
This genus has had a particularly confusing taxonomic history, and is still the subject of controversy. Klebsiellae are non-motile, which distinguishes them from the relatively unimportant genus *Enterobacter*; and they have capsules, by means of which, like pneumococci, they can be divided into a large number of types. The more pathogenic members of the genus are included in the first 3 types. Type 3 includes the organism, originally known as Friedländer's bacillus, which in various countries (though not in Britain) is a quite common cause of pneumonia, notably of a form characterized by multiple cavitation of the lung; it can also cause meningitis, otitis and sinusitis. Some use the species name *K. pneumoniae* for this organism, and the names *K. edwardsii* and *K. atlantae* for organisms of somewhat similar pathogenicity that belong to types 1 and 2; whereas others include all of these in *K. pneumoniae*. Most other klebsiellae are classified as *K. aerogenes*, a species that includes strains of many serotypes. These are widely distributed in nature, are commonly found in the human intestine, and occasionally cause urinary tract, wound or other infections. Klebsiellae are often present in large numbers in purulent sputum, a situation in which *Esch. coli* and other similar enterobacteria are also quite common, and it is easy to conclude from this that these organisms are common causes of suppurative respiratory tract infections. However, the usual sequence of events is that the patient has already been treated with antibiotics for a lower respiratory tract infection (or for some other reason), that this treatment has disrupted the normal ecological pattern in the respiratory tract, and that enterobacteria resistant to the antibiotics used have taken advantage of the

situation—often accompanied by yeasts. In such circumstances further antibiotic treatment aimed at the opportunists is likely to complicate the situation still further, whereas stopping all antibiotics usually results in a fairly rapid restoration of the normal bacterial population. Klebsiellae are prominent in this context because of the relatively high frequency of resistance to antibiotics, especially to ampicillin and the cephalosporins, in this genus. (The somewhat similar role of *Pseudomonas aeruginosa* is discussed on p 134.)

THE GENUS SALMONELLA (See also pp 122–4)

Virtually all members of this genus are motile, though non-flagellate variants occur. They are all intestinal pathogens. *S. typhi*, *S. paratyphi A*, *S. paratyphi B* and *S. paratyphi C* cause predominantly febrile illnesses collectively known as enteric fever, discussed below under *S. typhi*. Other members of the genus occasionally produce a somewhat similar picture, but far more commonly they cause the condition known as gastro-enteritis or food-poisoning (see pp 301–2).

The subdivision of this genus is unusual in that it is based mainly upon antigenic analysis. Most strains can be shown to possess two or more somatic (O) antigens and one or more flagellar (H) antigens. On the basis of O antigens alone the species can be divided into ten major and some minor groups, and even then the members of one group are not identical in their O antigenic structure but simply have one or more antigens in common. Each group can then be subdivided according to the H antigenic structure of its members. In this way hundreds of salmonella types have been distinguished and have been allotted binomials which suggest that they are species—e.g. *S. typhi-murium* and *S. enteritidis*. However, antigenic analysis is a much more delicate means of subdivision than those applied to other genera, and the majority of these different salmonellae, which cannot be distinguished by their microscopic or colonial appearances or, in most cases, by their biochemical reactions, are more reasonably described as types rather than as separate species.

Analysis of the H antigenic structure of salmonellae is further complicated by the fact that many types are able to exist in either of two phases differing in their H antigens. Types which are different when in phase 1 may have identical phase 2 H antigens. Thus *S. cholerae-suis* and *S. thompson* have the same phase 2 antigens, designated 1 and 5. Since they happen also to be identical in their O antigens, this means that cultures of these two organisms in phase 2 are indistinguishable. However, an apparently pure phase 2 culture nearly always contains a very small minority of phase 1 forms (and vice versa), and there are ways of extricating a pure culture of the minority phase. In phase 1, *S. cholerae-*

suis has a single H antigen designated *c*, which is distinct from the antigen *k* of phase 1 *S. thompson*.

What is the point of this fine differentiation of salmonellae, which in some cases can be carried still further by detecting variations of phage sensitivity or of biochemical reactions within a single serological type? It is far from being a purely academic exercise, for it greatly increases the precision and certainty with which the sources and methods of spread of outbreaks of infection can be traced. The finding of a salmonella carrier may or may not be relevant to a particular outbreak; the finding of a carrier of a strain identical with that which caused the outbreak is far more likely to be relevant; and that likelihood increases in step with the accuracy with which the identity of the two strains is established.

Salmonella typhi (the typhoid bacillus)

OCCURRENCE AND PATHOGENICITY   Like all salmonellae, this species is entirely parasitic. It differs from many of the others in that man is its only natural host, and that even in the laboratory it is of low virulence for mice and other animals. Although epidemics are usually spread via water supplies or food (as in the examples quoted on p 301), the source of the organism is always a human patient or carrier.

In its early stages enteric fever (whether it is true typhoid or due to one of the other salmonellae—see p 126) is predominantly a septicaemia rather than an alimentary disorder. Having entered the body through the mouth, the organism probably reaches the blood stream via the intestinal lymphatics. After the septicaemic phase it becomes localized, chiefly in the Peyer's patches of the small intestine, in the gall bladder and in the kidneys, but also sometimes in other sites such as the bone marrow, where it may cause osteitis. The clinical picture in the first week of the illness usually consists of progressively mounting fever, headache and severe malaise. Diarrhoea is not common at this stage, and indeed the patient is often constipated. In the second week the nature of the infection is likely to become more obvious with the appearance of the characteristic 'rose-spot' skin eruption and the onset of profuse diarrhoea. Ulceration of Peyer's patches may lead to intestinal perforation or haemorrhage, which are common causes of death in untreated cases. In the convalescent period relapses are common.

CARRIERS   A small proportion of those who recover from typhoid continue to harbour the bacilli in their gall bladders or kidneys, and many excrete them intermittently for many years. Antibiotic treatment often fails to eradicate the organism (see below). Gall-bladder carriers may be rendered innocuous by cholecystectomy, but renal carriage is a more difficult problem. It is highly important that carriers should be aware of their state and should carry out the necessary hygienic precautions. The most infamous example of their harmful potentialities is 'Typhoid Mary', a cook who caused at least six small outbreaks in the New York area between 1901 and 1907, and may also have been responsible for a water-borne outbreak that involved 1300 people. She was then kept under strict supervision for a few years, but escaped and became a hospital cook, causing another 25 cases. The 1937 Croydon outbreak, with 34 deaths among 341 known victims, was traced to a carrier who had been employed to repair a well. By a misunderstanding, water from this well was fed into the main water supply without filtration or chlorination. In contrast to these stories, a mysterious occurrence of a solitary case of typhoid in a small baby in London in the 1950s was found to be due to contact with its grandmother, who had had the disease 30 years earlier and was not known ever to have infected anyone else. (In the biggest outbreak of recent years in Britain, that in Aberdeen in 1964 described on p 302, there was no definite evidence of involvement of human carriers.)

CULTIVATION   Salmonellae, like all enterobacteria, grow well on simple media and are therefore easy to isolate from such specimens as blood or urine. Isolation from faeces is more problematical, because of the large number of other bacteria present; even MacConkey's medium (on which, being non-lactose-fermenters, salmonellae form colourless colonies) is of little use for this purpose, as the salmonellae are often heavily outnumbered by other enterobacteria which grow equally well on this medium. To meet this problem various special *selective media* have been devised, such as *deoxycholate citrate agar* (D.C.A.), which sup-presses the growth of most bacteria other than salmonellae and shigellae. When the number of salmonellae in the specimen is very small even such a medium as this may not permit their detection, and the chances of isolating them are then considerably enhanced by using a *selective enrichment medium*, such as *selenite F broth*. In this, the lag phase (see p 35) of salmonellae is considerably shorter than that of other bacteria. From being a very small minority they may therefore become, within a few hours, a considerable proportion of the population, so that they are easily detected when the broth is subcultured on to MacConkey's agar.

During the first week of typhoid the organism can usually be grown from the blood, either by adding a few ml of blood to a bottle of broth containing bile salts, or by allowing the blood to clot, removing the serum and replacing it by *bile-salt broth* that contains streptokinase to dissolve the clot. Positive blood cultures are less common as the disease progresses; bone marrow cultures may continue to be positive later in the disease than cultures of peripheral blood, particularly if antibiotic treatment has already begun. Faecal culture, which may be positive at any stage, is more often so in the second and third weeks. The bacillus may also be found in the urine after the second week. Repeated examinations of the faeces and urine of all convalescents make possible the early detection and treatment of those who have become carriers.

PHAGE TYPING   Some dozens of *S. typhi* types have been identified by means of Vi phages, so called because they are effective only against strains that still possess the Vi antigen (see below). The typing procedure is essentially similar to that for staphylococci (pp 97 and 210) except that it does not depend upon the specificity of naturally-occurring phages; phages can be 'trained' to detect strains of particular types.

ANTIGENIC STRUCTURE   *S. typhi* has only a single phase 1 H antigen, which it shares with a few other salmonellae but not with any that have the same O antigens; and it has no phase 2. Freshly isolated strains have a surface antigen, designated Vi (for virulence). Some strains of *S. paratyphi B* and a few other salmonellae have the same Vi antigen.

IMMUNOLOGY   There is no conclusive evidence that useful immunity follows natural infection. Active immunization, using suspensions of killed bacilli (see p 309), causes pronounced antibody responses, but whether it also gives a useful degree of protection has been far more difficult to establish, and depends on the method of preparation of the antigen (see p 312). H, Vi and O antibodies can be measured separately in a patient's serum (the *Widal test*, p 260). The value of such measurements is discussed on pp 260–1. In an attack of enteric fever they give useful diagnostic information from the second week of illness onwards.

ANTIBACTERIAL TREATMENT   Chloramphenicol was the first anti-bacterial drug to make a real impact on the treatment of typhoid, being highly effective in controlling the acute illness and greatly reducing the mortality. Unfortunately it fails to eradicate the organism, so that relapse and carriage are common after its use; and in recent years its usefulness has been much reduced in many parts of the world by the emergence of chloramphenicol-resistant strains of *S. typhi*. Ampicillin, while less good than chloramphenicol for controlling the acute illness, has been far more successful in treatment of carriers, eradicating the infection in about 80% of cases; and experience of amoxycillin so far suggests that it is highly effective for both purposes. There have been conflicting reports about the value of co-trimoxazole in this disease.

The Paratyphoid Bacilli
S. paratyphi A, B and C, which also cause enteric fever but usually a

milder form than that due to *S. typhi*, differ from that species and from one another in their biochemical properties and antigenic structure and in their geographical distribution. *S. paratyphi* B is the only one to occur at all commonly in Britain, where it is considerably commoner than *S. typhi*. Like *S. typhi* it can be divided into many phage-types.

Other Salmonellae

Most of the other salmonella types are primarily animal pathogens which occasionally attack man. Since they are mainly transmitted in food and cause vomiting and diarrhoea in man, they are further discussed in Chapter Nineteen. *S. typhimurium*, an organism with many other animal hosts besides the mice from which it takes its name, and *S. enteritidis* are between them responsible for most cases of human salmonellosis in Britain, but many other types make their contributions, with relative frequencies which vary from year to year as the result of changes in imports of human or animal foods and many other factors. In general these organisms are less responsive than *S. typhi* to treatment with antibiotics. A persistent carrier state commonly follows human infection; attempts to prevent or terminate this by giving antibiotics tend to prolong the period of carriage, possibly by inhibiting normal intestinal flora.

THE GENUS SHIGELLA (See also pp 122–4)

OCCURRENCE AND PATHOGENICITY   The dysentery bacilli are obligate parasites, of man or occasionally of chimpanzees or monkeys. They cause illnesses which vary in severity according to the species involved – in the general order *Sh. dysenteriae*, *Sh. flexneri*, *Sh. boydi* and *Sh. sonnei* – from severe abdominal pain, fever, prostration and profuse bloody diarrhoea to a mild intestinal upset with little systemic disturbance. In general their pathogenicity is thought to depend on destructive invasion of the intestinal mucosa, but the fiercer onslaught of *Sh. dysenteriae* includes production of a cholera-like enterotoxin. *Sh. sonnei*, the mildest of the four, is the commonest in Britain and causes many epidemics in institutions. Young children are particularly susceptible. In countries with warm climates and poor standards of hygiene, flies are important in transmission, carrying the organisms from human faeces to food; but direct contact and contamination of toilet fittings, door handles and fomites account for the majority of infections in Britain. It has been shown that *Sh. sonnei* can pass through toilet paper and can survive for several hours on fingers.

CARRIERS   Carriage, which is entirely intestinal, is usually of short duration but may persist for years. In most cases excretion is intermittent, but that of *Sh. dysenteriae* may be continuous.

CULTIVATION   Growth on most media is similar to that of other enterobacteria. Isolation of shigellae from mixed cultures is helped by selective media such as D.C.A. (p 128).

TYPING   Being non-flagellate, shigellae have no H antigens, but they can be divided into serogroups and serotypes based on their O antigens. They can also be typed according to their production of *colicines*–antibiotics of a class produced by many enterobacteria, effective only against limited ranges of other enterobacteria, and therefore classifiable by determining the action of each one on a standard set of test strains. (Colicine-typing can also be carried out the other way round, by testing the susceptibility of the unidentified strain to a set of known colicines–a process similar to phage-typing.)

IMMUNOLOGY   Immunity following natural infection is type-specific and transitory, and it is therefore not surprising that there are no generally accepted procedures for either active or passive immunization, though success has been claimed for some methods.

ANTIBACTERIAL TREATMENT   Many antibacterial drugs are effective against shigellae, but widespread use of almost any of these is liable to be followed by rapid emergence of shigella strains resistant to the drug used and often to various others as well (see p 34–transferable multiple antibiotic resistance). Since many cases, especially of *Sh. sonnei* infection, recover spontaneously and completely within a few days, there seems to be a strong argument for restricting antibacterial treatment to seriously ill or very frail patients and persistent carriers.

THE GENUS PROTEUS (See also pp 122–4)

The members of this genus are commonly found in faeces, in soil and in many other situations. They resemble *Esch. coli* in their ability to cause urinary tract and wound infections. Their ability to swarm over the surfaces of many solid culture media, burying the colonies of other organisms, is a constant source of annoyance to the bacteriologist who is trying to obtain those other organisms in pure culture; he has to resort to special media or make use of such devices as shaking a mixture of organisms up in a bottle with ether, which kills proteus and allows some other organisms, notably staphylococci, to survive. The genus consists of four species, *Pr. mirabilis*, *Pr. vulgaris*, *Pr. morgani* and *Pr. rettgeri*, of which the commonest, in spite of their names, is *Pr. mirabilis* and not *Pr. vulgaris*. They are resistant to various commonly used antibiotics (the range depending to some extent upon the species), and are therefore liable to persist in wounds and other lesions after treatment has disposed of staphylococci or other primary pathogens.

THE GENUS YERSINIA (See also pp 122–4)
This genus contains 3 species of medical interest: *Y. pestis* and *Y. pseudotuberculosis* (both previously classified in the genus *Pasteurella*) and *Y. enterocolitica*.

Yersinia pestis
OCCURRENCE AND PATHOGENICITY   The causative organism of plague (the mediaeval Black Death) is primarily a flea-borne pathogen of rats and other rodents, among which it causes highly lethal epidemics. Transfer to man occurs when an infected rat-flea (*Xenopsylla cheopis*) abandons the dead body of its rodent host. Starving because its proventriculus is blocked by multiplying pasteurellae, it tries to obtain food from a human host. A little blood is aspirated into its proventriculus, mixed with bacilli and then regurgitated into the puncture wound. The human host rapidly becomes ill with *bubonic plague*, developing a marked enlargement or bubo of the regional lymph nodes, usually in the axilla or groin, and then as a rule a septicaemia. If this leads to pulmonary infection, *pneumonic plague*, he becomes a source of droplet spread to other humans. Control of rodents, with particular attention to preventing them from boarding or leaving vessels at ports, has kept Britain and many other countries free of this major scourge for many years.

MICROSCOPY   In tissues and other pathological materials, such as bubo aspirate and sputum, *Y. pestis* is a short, oval, capsulate, non-motile Gram-negative bacillus. With methylene blue and various other dyes it shows bipolar staining–i.e. deeper staining at the ends of the rods than in their centres (Fig. 3(*k*), p 94). In culture the capsule is lost, bipolar staining is less obvious and the bacilli are often longer and pleomorphic.

CULTIVATION   This species is unusual among human pathogens in that it grows best at about 27 °C (see p 28). In other respects its laboratory behaviour is similar to that of other enterobacteria.

Yersinia pseudotuberculosis and Yersinia enterocolitica
Both of these organisms have been isolated from many species of domesticated and wild animals. In man, *Y. pseudotuberculosis* can cause a fulminating typhoid-like septicaemia, which is fortunately rare; *Y. enterocolitica* can cause enterocolitis, resulting in abdominal pain and diarrhoea; and either of them can cause mesenteric adenitis, occurring mainly in children and young adults and frequently misdiagnosed as acute appendicitis. The bacteriological diagnosis in such cases can be

established either by isolating the organisms (both resembling *Y. pestis* in most laboratory properties) from blood, faeces, lymph-nodes or other appropriate material, or by detecting rising levels of specific antibodies in serum. The bacteriologist has to remember *Y. pseudotuberculosis* because natural infection with this organism can produce deceptive lesions in guinea-pigs into which he has injected material suspected of containing tubercle bacilli.

OTHER ENTEROBACTERIA

The organisms classified as *Enterobacter*, *Citrobacter* or *Hafnia* or in various other genera of this group are of interest to the medical bacteriologist only because they are liable to be found in the same situations as potential pathogens and have to be distinguished from them. A few years ago the members of the genus *Serratia* could have been described as harmless organisms forming characteristic red-pigmented colonies. The position is now less simple, however, as *Serratia* strains have sometimes been incriminated as pathogens, mainly in seriously debilitated patients in whom they may even cause septicaemia, and some of them fail to produce the characteristic pigment that is so helpful to the bacteriologist.

GRAM-NEGATIVE BACILLI: (b) THE GENUS PSEUDOMONAS

Members of this genus resemble the enterobacteria in microscopic appearance (apart from having polar rather than lateral flagella, a distinction shown only by special microscopic techniques) but differ from that group in being strict aerobes, in oxidizing carbohydrates instead of fermenting them, and in being oxidase-positive (cf p 107). Many of them produce fluorescent pigments. They are very widely distributed, and include plant pathogens and many saprophytic species. With the exception of the one species described below they are rarely pathogenic to man or of any other interest to the medical bacteriologist.

Pseudomonas aeruginosa *(Ps. pyocyanea)*

OCCURRENCE AND PATHOGENICITY This species, commonly present in the human intestine, has the ability to grow in almost any moist situation over a wide temperature range, needing only oxygen and a modest supply of nutrients. Consequently it can multiply in such preparations as eye-drops, ointments, lotions or even weak disinfectant solutions, and so be applied in large numbers to patients' surfaces or wounds. In such circumstances it can cause serious local or even systemic infections. (See p 50 for the importance of numbers in bacterial infections.) Similarly, it can multiply in the warm moist conditions prevailing inside baby-incubators or ventilating machines and so be inhaled in large doses and colonize the patients' respiratory tracts. Here it usually does little or no harm, but it sometimes causes a necrotizing pneumonia, which may be fatal. Its resistance to most of the antibiotics available for clinical use adds to its capacity for causing trouble, as it is liable to take over when the primary causes of infection in wounds, burns and many other situations have been eliminated by treatment. Its behaviour is much the same in the severely damaged airways of patients with bronchiectasis or cystic fibrosis who have received antibiotics for treatment of more orthodox respiratory tract pathogens. Again, it is usually harmless there but may cause pneumonia. A curious feature of such invasion of the lower respiratory tract is that a strain (apparently almost any strain of this species) which has established itself there undergoes a change that causes it to form mucoid colonies on plate cultures. In the urinary tract, pseudomonas infection is a common and often intractable complication of neurological or other conditions that interfere with bladder emptying. *Ps. aeruginosa* is frequently present in inflamed external auditory canals, and may be pathogenic there, particularly in swimmers and divers.

CULTIVATION   As already indicated, this species grows well on simple media under aerobic conditions. Typically its colonies are rough and irregular (but see the previous paragraph), and are recognizable also by their green pigment (see p 31), which diffuses into the medium and colours it green also. (This pigment-production accounts for the characteristic blue-green colour of pus due to this organism, which is the origin of the older specific name *pyocyanea*; and both colonies and pus share also a distinctive musty smell.)

TYPING   This species may subdivide by *pyocine typing* (analogous to colicine typing–p 131) or by bacteriophage typing.

ANTIBACTERIAL TREATMENT   Widespread resistance is the rule in this species. Antibiotics of the polymyxin group are usually effective in the laboratory but often less so in the patient. Resistance to carbenicillin, the one currently available penicillin effective against this species, is increasingly frequent, and a similar problem is arising with the relevant members of the aminoglycoside group–gentamicin, tobramycin and even amikacin (see p 348). The shortage of reliable drugs for treating them makes it all the more important to minimize the frequency of serious pseudomonas infections, by avoiding the situations that were described above as giving rise to them and by taking care not to transmit pseudomonas strains (especially those that are unusually resistant) from one patient to others. Relatively minor superficial infections should be treated by local application of disinfectants, as use of antibiotics may encourage development of resistance to them. Removal of *Ps. aeruginosa* from the respiratory tract can seldom be achieved by a direct antibiotic attack, but withholding of all antibiotics often permits other more manageable bacteria to displace the pseudomonads.

GRAM-NEGATIVE BACILLI: (c) THE GENUS VIBRIO

Vibrios resemble enterobacteria in being aerobic, facultatively anaerobic Gram-negative bacilli that ferment carbohydrates (cf p 123). They resemble pseudomonads in having polar flagella and in being oxidase-positive (cf p 107). They differ from both in other respects, notably in that their rods are typically not straight but comma-shaped (Fig. 3(o), p 94). They are widely distributed in nature. The species of medical importance are *V. cholerae* and *V. parahaemolyticus*.

Vibrio cholerae (the cholera bacillus)

This species is exclusively a parasite of man. Multiplying in the human intestine, it produces an enterotoxin. This acts on the intestinal epithelium and provokes a sustained outpouring of water and electro-lytes, manifested clinically as a profuse watery diarrhoea. The consequent dehydration may be rapidly fatal, but with prompt, adequate and properly balanced fluid and electrolyte replacement the prognosis is good, since the organism does not invade the host's tissues or blood and its pathogenicity is entirely due to the local action of its toxin. As the 'rice-water stools' are little more than fluid cultures of *V. cholerae*, it is easy to see how the disease can be transmitted directly onto the hands and so into the mouths of attendants, or via food or water supplies if the standards of hygiene and sewage disposal are not good.

Having been endemic in the Indian subcontinent for many cen-turies, cholera spread around the world in a series of devastating pandemics during the 19th and early 20th centuries, but was then restricted in range again until 1961. Up to that date it was predominantly due to what is now called 'classical' *V. cholerae*, which produces severe disease in a large proportion of those infected but is not able to establish a stable relationship with its host–i.e. it is excreted by those incubating or suffering from the disease and for perhaps a few weeks after infection but persistent carriage does not occur. The El Tor biotype of *V. cholerae*, named after the Sinai village where it was first identified in 1906, became established as a cause of a rather mild form of cholera in and around Indonesia during and after the second world war, and then from 1961 onwards it spread westward across Asia into Africa and Europe, reaching Britain as a solitary case (a holiday-maker returned from Tunisia) in

1970, with a few similar cases later. The El Tor vibrio may produce severe disease, but does so less frequently than the classical strain. Its 'success' in spreading so rapidly to virtually the whole world except America can be attributed to the fairly large proportion of those infected who are only mildly affected or symptomless but nevertheless vigorous excreters of the organism, and to its greater capacity for establishing the carrier state.

In the laboratory, cholera vibrios can sometimes be recognized by microscopy of the fluid stools, in which they may be apparent as large numbers of similar slightly curved rods with characteristic darting motility. Their isolation is made easier by their ability to grow in alkaline peptone water (ph 8·0 or more) and to form yellow colonies on TCBS (thiosulphate citrate bile salts sucrose) agar. Their identity is confirmed by agglutination with specific antisera.

Immunization has been widely practised but is of little value. Prevention depends on good general hygiene, with particular reference to protecting water supplies from faecal contamination.

Vibrio parahaemolyticus

This salt-water vibrio is a cause—in Japan a common cause—of acute gastro-enteritis that comes on some 10–20 hours after eating raw or inadequately cooked sea-food, lasting for a day or two. In Britain this organism has been isolated from locally-bred oysters, but imported sea-foods such as prawns are more likely sources. Its isolation from foods, vomitus or faeces is helped by its ability to grow in media containing 3% NaCl and to form green colonies on TCBS agar (as used for *V. cholerae*).

'Anaerobic vibrios' and 'related vibrios'

These names have been used for certain motile oxidase-positive Gram-negative bacilli which are not in fact true anaerobes but grow best in an atmosphere containing 5% of oxygen. They now have the generic name *Campylobacter*. *C.* (formerly *Vibrio*) *fetus* has long been known as a cause of infectious abortion in sheep and cattle; but it is only recently, with the development of selective techniques for their isolation from faeces (using among other things their ability to grow in cultures at 43°C.), that *C. jejuni* and *C. coli* have been incriminated as common causes of severe abdominal pain, diarrhoea and fever in humans, particularly in children. Chickens have in some cases been shown to be the source of infection.

GRAM-NEGATIVE BACILLI: (d) PARVOBACTERIA

Whereas the enterobacteria are a group of essentially similar genera, the name 'parvobacteria' has no sound taxonomic basis; we retain it merely as a convenient collective term for a rather heterogeneous group of organisms that differ in a number of respects from the Gram-negative bacilli that we have described so far. They are smaller bacilli, usually 0.3–0.4 μm in width and are often coccobacillary. They are not intestinal parasites. They are generally exacting in their nutritional requirements, forming much smaller colonies on blood agar than do the enterobacteria. With a few exceptions they also differ from the enterobacteria in failing to grow on MacConkey's medium. Included among them are a number of important pathogens.

THE GENUS HAEMOPHILUS

Members of this genus are characterized by, and classified according to, their need to be supplied with X and V factors (haemin and nicotinamide-adenine dinucleotide, see p 28). Both factors are absent from some forms of nutrient agar, and strains can therefore be tested for their requirements by growing them on such a medium in the presence of filter-paper disks soaked in one or both factors. On blood agar, which contains X factor and a little V factor, enhanced growth of V-factor-requiring organisms occur around colonies or streaks of *Staph. aureus* and various other species which liberate V factor into the medium–a phenomenon known as *satellitism*. Heating of blood agar to produce chocolate agar destroys a substance in the red cells which is inhibitory to V factor, and the amount of this factor present is then sufficient to support a good growth of all haemophilus species.

Haemophilus influenzae (Pfeiffer's bacillus, the influenza bacillus)

OCCURRENCE AND PATHOGENICITY   The species occurs purely as a parasite of man, and is very commonly carried in healthy nasopharynges. Most of these 'respiratory' strains are not capsulate, but a small percentage of healthy people carry capsulate strains, divisible into six types (a to f). Capsulate strains of type b are the commonest bacterial cause of meningitis in young children, and less frequently cause acute epiglottitis (a very severe infection of children, well-known in N. America and increasingly often recognized in Britain), lobar pneumonia, a characteristic cellulitis of face or limbs and various other acute infections, mostly in children. Capsulate strains of the other five types are much less often incriminated as pathogens. Non-capsulate strains are the principal cause of suppuration, either persistent or intermittent during acute exacerbations, in the bronchi of patients with chronic bronchitis or bronchiectasis (see pp 246 and 354–5).

The species owes its name to the claims made by Pfeiffer, who discovered it during the influenza epidemics of 1889–90, that it was the cause of influenza. This suggestion was not finally discredited until the influenza virus was discovered (1933). It still remains possible that in the past this species acted synergically with a virus in producing the disease, as does the closely related *H. influenzae suis* in the production of swine influenza; but in recent human epidemics the bacillus has not appeared to play a significant part.

CARRIERS   At the time when a child develops haemophilus meningitis or epiglottitis there are usually several nasopharyngeal carriers of *H. influenzae* type b in the immediate family circle, but multiple cases of serious illness in the same family due to this organism are unusual.

MICROSCOPY   Members of this species are small non-flagellate, non-sporing and usually non-capsulate Gram-negative bacilli. Films from young cultures grown under favourable conditions usually consist of cocco-bacilli; pleomorphism with filament formation is commoner in cultures on less adequate media.

CULTIVATION   Factors X and V are both required for growth. Colonies on blood agar after 24 hours' incubation vary according to the quality of the medium from minute pin-points to translucent domes approximately 1 mm in diameter. In mixed cultures, satellite clusters of colonies around V-factor-producing colonies of other species are characteristic, and routine addition of a staphylococcal streak to blood agar cultures of respiratory tract specimens can be used as an aid to rapid recognition of the species. Chocolate agar is also a useful primary medium, since colonies formed on it by *H. influenzae* are considerably larger than those formed on blood agar. Capsulate strains can be recognized by growing them on a suitable transparent medium (e.g. *Levinthal's agar*), on which their colonies exhibit iridescence when examined by strong, obliquely transmitted light.

ANTIGENIC STRUCTURE   The six capsulate types have distinct polysaccharide capsular antigens, and with the aid of type-specific rabbit antisera they can be recognized by capsule-swelling tests, by agglutination of the bacilli or by precipitin tests using aqueous extracts of the bacilli.

IMMUNOLOGY   Antibodies to somatic and capsular antigens are common in the blood of adults, and it is thought that acquired immunity is responsible for the restriction of acute infections due to type b strains almost exclusively to young children. Because of the significant mortality from infections with type b, and the disturbingly high rate of permanent disabilities following haemophilus meningitis, active immunization against type b is being developed.

ANTIBACTERIAL TREATMENT   *H. influenzae* is commonly resistant to penicillin; indeed, when Fleming discovered penicillin the first use that he saw for it was as a selective ingredient in media for isolation of this species. Chloramphenicol is the agent of choice for treating haemophilus meningitis and other life-threatening *H. influenzae* type b infections; its action against this species is bactericidal, it has proved highly effective in such situations, and chloramphenicol-resistant haemophili are as yet very rare. On the other hand ampicillin, which has been much used for these infections, had proved somewhat less reliable even before the emergence, from 1974 onwards, of penicillinase-producing *H. influenzae* type b strains against which it is liable to be disastrously ineffective. Long-term prevention or control of haemophilus infections in chronic bronchial disease is a difficult problem; ampicillin, amoxycillin, the tetracyclines and cotrimoxazole are the main weapons for this purpose.

Other Haemophilus Species
H. aegyptius is a name that has been given to the Koch-Weeks bacillus, an organism which was incriminated as a cause of outbreaks of acute conjunctivitis in Egypt and elsewhere before Koch described his 'influenza bacillus'. However, the distinction between the two is a fine one, and it is probably best to regard the Koch-Weeks bacillus as a type within the species *H. influenzae*.

H. para-influenzae (which is virtually non-pathogenic) and *H. parahaemolyticus* (which is haemolytic on blood agar and for which there is circumstantial evidence that it causes acute pharyngitis) differ from *H. influenzae* in that they do not require to be supplied with X factor.

H. ducreyi, the causative organism of the human venereal disease chancroid, require X but not V factor, but it also has other special nutritional needs.

THE GENUS BORDETELLA
Bordetella pertussis (the whooping cough bacillus)
OCCURRENCE AND PATHOGENICITY   Purely a human parasite, this organism causes a well-known febrile respiratory tract infection of childhood, characterized by paroxysms of coughing that end in loud inspiratory whoops. The disease is potentially lethal in infancy. Adults are sometimes affected. The infection is a superficial one of the trachea and bronchi, with epithelial damage and impairment of the normal ciliary clearance mechanism. Some cases of clinical whooping cough are due not to *Bord. pertussis* but to adenoviruses or myxoviruses.

MICROSCOPY   The bacilli resemble cocco-bacillary cultures of *H. influenzae*.

CULTIVATION   Ordinary media do not suffice for primary insolation; for this purpose the medium described in 1906 by Bordet and Gengou is still widely used. It contains glycerol, potato extract and up to 50% of defibrinated horse blood, and must be freshly prepared. It can be 'modernized' by the inclusion of a small amount of penicillin to make it more selective. Several days of aerobic incubation at 37°C are necessary before the typical 'bisected pearl' or 'aluminium paint' colonies of *Bord. pertussis* appear. Once grown in this way, the organism can be transferred to serum agar or blood agar.

Specimens are collected by holding a plate of Bordet–Gengou medium in front of the mouth of a coughing patient ('cough plate'), or by pernasal swabbing of the nasopharynx (see p 244).

IMMUNOLOGY   Natural infection is followed by lasting immunity. Active immunization is discussed on p 311. Agglutinating and complement-fixing antibodies can be detected in the blood from the third week of the disease.

ANTIBACTERIAL TREATMENT   Although *Bord. pertussis* is sensitive *in vitro* to chloramphenicol, the tetracyclines and ampicillin, these drugs have little effect on the disease unless given very early–presumably because after that it is too late to prevent epithelial damage. Antibiotics are valuable, however, in preventing or treating secondary pneumonia.

THE GENUS BRUCELLA

OCCURRENCE AND PATHOGENICITY   The three closely related members of this genus which cause undulant fever in man–*Br. melitensis*, *Br. abortus* and *Br. suis*–are primarily pathogens of goats, cattle and pigs respectively. The human disease, of which *Br. abortus* is virtually the sole cause in Britain, derives its name from the recurrent bouts of fever which are its principal feature. Fatigue, sweating, malaise, headache, anorexia and pains in joints and muscles are other common components of a clinical picture that often causes difficulty in diagnosis. The organism is widely distributed throughout the body, including the blood stream. Multiple small granulomatous nodules and micro-abscesses are found in affected tissues, the bacilli being mainly intracellular. Human infections with *Br. melitensis* occur chiefly in the Mediterranean area (Malta fever), Africa, and parts of the Far East and America. *Br. suis* is found in the U.S.A. and in Denmark. Ingestion of unpasteurized cows' or goats' milk or of milk products may disseminate infection widely in both urban and rural areas, but for those in close contact with farm animals, notably veterinary surgeons and farm workers and their families, and also for laboratory workers there are additional possible modes of infection, by inhalation of the organisms or by their entering the body through skin lesions or even through the conjunctiva.

Contagious abortion of cattle due to *Br. abortus* is one of the very few microbial diseases in which the localization of the pathogens can be explained. The alcohol erythritol enhances the growth of *Br. abortus* in laboratory cultures. In cattle unusually high concentrations of erythritol are present in certain layers of the placenta and in the foetal fluids, and presumably account for the vigorous multiplication of *Br. abortus* in precisely these sites which is a feature of contagious abortion.

MICROSCOPY   The bacilli are small and usually short. They are non-flagellate, non-sporing, non-capsulate (except possibly in some fresh isolates) and Gram-negative.

CULTIVATION   *Br. abortus* requires 5–10% CO_2 in its atmosphere for primary isolation (see p 240). Otherwise all three species are aerobes, with an optimal growth temperature of $37°C$. They are not particularly exacting in their nutritional requirements, but grow slowly, producing translucent and undistinguished colonies. Various special media, including selective media, are available. Isolation from patients is usually attempted by culture of large amounts of blood (up to 40 ml) added to a suitable broth. Appropriate atmospheric conditions must be provided if growth of *Br. abortus* is expected, and incubation should be continued for at least three weeks. Even with these precautions, repeated attempts to isolate *Br. abortus* are often unsuccessful; the other two species are easier to recover from blood. Culture of aspirated bone marrow is sometimes successful when blood-culture has failed. The organism may also be isolated by inoculating the buffy coat from centrifuged blood into a guinea-pig. Similar culture procedures and guinea-pig inoculation are used in isolating brucellae from milk and other animal materials.

SPECIES DIFFERENTIATION   For epidemiological reasons it may be important to be able to identify brucella isolates precisely. Recognition of species, and of biotypes within species, is based on biochemical tests (mostly different from those used for other genera), on susceptibility to a bacteriophage specific for *Br. abortus* and to the inhibitory action of low concentrations of dyes in culture media, and on agglutinability by antisera specific for one or other of the two main antigenic components of the members of this genus. Using these criteria *Br. abortus* can be divided into 9 biotypes and *Br. melitensis* and *Br. suis* into 3 each.

IMMUNOLOGY   Some immunity follows natural infections. An attenuated *Br. abortus* strain has been widely used in Russia for immunization of humans exposed to high occupational risks of brucella infection. Antibodies that appear in the blood of patients with brucellosis can be measured by agglutination, anti-human-globulin (Coombs') or complement-fixation tests; diagnostic use of these tests is discussed on pp 261–2. Skin hypersensitivity following infection or immunization can be detected by using an extract of bacilli–*the brucellin test* (see p 77)–but this test is of little diagnostic value.

ANTIBACTERIAL TREATMENT   On empirical grounds, combined streptomycin and tetracycline treatment is generally recommended. Probably because of the intracellular situation of the organisms, treatment must be continued for several weeks to have a good chance of success, and the course may have to be repeated. Co-trimoxazole has also been shown to be effective in treatment of this disease.

PREVENTION   Transmission of brucellae in milk can be prevented by efficient pasteurization (see p 298). Eradication of the disease is theoretically possible and is near to being achieved in some countries. It depends on vaccination of young animals of appropriate species and slaughter of animals with serological or other evidence of brucella infection. Eradication costs a lot of money (chiefly in compensation to the owners of slaughtered animals); but even in purely economic terms this cost is probably lower, though far more obvious, than that of allowing brucella infection to persist among cattle. Such persistence causes abortions, stillbirths, infertility and reduced milk yield, and inevitably results in transmission to some humans, in whom it produces long periods of obscure ill-health and impaired working capacity.

THE GENUS PASTEURELLA

Among the organisms (small Gram-negative bacilli, mostly oxidase-positive and unable to grow on MacConkey's agar) that remain in this genus after the departure of those now classified as *Yersinia*, there are some that cause haemorrhagic septicaemia and other infections in a wide range of animal hosts. They have been given names that reflected those of their hosts (*Pasteurella boviseptica, P. aviseptica,* etc.) but the differences between them are small and they are now included in a single species *P. multocida.* Such organisms are sometimes found in dog and cat bites of human beings, and such wounds may fail to heal until the pasteurellae are eliminated by suitable antibiotic treatment. Organisms of this and other *Pasteurella* species occur in the sputum of patients with chronic bronchial disease, but their significance there is uncertain.

FRANCISELLA TULARENSIS (*Pasteurella tularensis, Brucella tularensis*)

This small Gram-negative bacillus is an insect-borne pathogen of rabbits and other rodents in many countries, notably in the western U.S.A. and in Russia and Siberia. In such hosts it causes a plague-like illness known as tularaemia. Occasionally humans who handle infected animals are themselves infected, through skin abrasions, and develop a brucellosis-like illness which responds to tetracycline therapy. In the laboratory the organism resembles a pasteurella in some of its properties and a brucella in others, and it has at different times been assigned to each of these genera and to several others.

GRAM-NEGATIVE BACILLI: (e) BACTEROIDES

The classification of anaerobic Gram-negative bacilli is unsatisfactory, largely because they are difficult to maintain in culture and to study. They are commonly fusiform (i.e. spindle-shaped, tapering at both ends) and this fact is reflected in the generic names *Fusiformis* and *Fusobacterium* that have been applied to some of them—e.g. *Fusiformis fusiformis* (pp 94 and 157). However, most of those that are of medical importance are currently included in the genus *Bacteroides*, notably in the species *B. fragilis*. Such organisms are common in the human mouth, nasopharynx and intestine and have been isolated occasionally from a wide variety of human lesions. Since they are strictly anaerobic and form small nondescript colonies, they are easily overlooked. If carefully sought they can be found frequently in pus from intra-abdominal abscesses and in abdominal wounds that are failing to heal, and unless eradicated by suitable antibiotic treatment they may then cause serious generalized infections. They are also sometimes found in pus from cerebral abscesses and other deep-seated lesions. It is not clear whether they cause such conditions or are only secondarily involved. They appear to be primarily responsible for occasional subcutaneous lesions in butchers and other handlers of animals. They are frequently resistant to many of the commonly used antibiotics; erythromycin, lincomycin and clindamycin (all of which are used mainly against Gram-positive cocci) have been employed against them with good results, but metranidazole is currently preferred to antibiotics for treatment of these and most other infections due to strict anaerobes.

ACID-FAST BACILLI
THE GENUS MYCOBACTERIUM

The tubercle bacilli (*Myco. tuberculosis* and *Myco. bovis*), the leprosy bacillus (*Myco. leprae*) and the other members of this genus are distinguished by their acid-fast staining—i.e. their resistance, after being stained with hot carbol fuchsin, to decolorization with acid (see p 146). This property is at least partly dependent upon their high content of certain lipids, notably mycolic acid, but this is not the whole explanation. Mycobacteria are Gram-positive, but some of them are difficult to stain at all by Gram's method or by most other common procedures.

Mycobacterium tuberculosis and Myco. bovis (the tubercle bacilli)

OCCURRENCE AND PATHOGENICITY   Although these two species have different primary hosts (human and cattle), they have much in common and it is convenient to retain the name 'tubercle bacilli' as a means of referring to them collectively. Both are pathogenic to man, but they differ in their pathogenicity to other species as indicated on p 50. Man acquires infections with *Myco. tuberculosis* from his fellow human beings, usually by inhalation, and the resulting disease commonly involves the lungs. The risks of airborne infection are considerably increased by the ability of *Myco. tuberculosis* to survive for months outside the host—e.g. in dust and in books. Human infection with *Myco. bovis* usually results from drinking milk. It has been almost eliminated from this and many other countries by pasteurization of milk and control of tuberculosis in cattle. Because it enters the human body by the alimentary tract, *Myco. bovis* characteristically causes cervical and mesenteric adenitis rather than pulmonary lesions. Either species may attack the meninges, bones, joints, skin and almost any other part of the body, and full discussion of the many possible forms of the disease is beyond our present scope.

It is important, however, to grasp the difference between *primary* and subsequent (variously known as *post-primary, secondary or adult-type*) infections. Infection of a subject who has no previous experience of tubercle bacilli results in a mild acute inflammatory reaction at the point of entry, with carriage of the bacilli to the local lymph nodes. Here a more vigorous reaction occurs, with enlargement of the nodes, which often undergo the caseous necrosis typical of tuberculosis. The small local lesion and the enlarged lymph nodes are together known as the *primary complex*, or, in the case of a lung lesion with mediastinal lymph node enlargement, as a *Ghon focus*. The infection may be arrested at this stage, the bacilli remaining alive for many years inside the lymph nodes, which become fibrotic and calcified. Alternatively, by travelling further along the lymphatic system or by the rupture of a caseous node into a blood vessel, the bacilli may enter the blood stream and be scattered throughout the body. It is likely that such blood stream dissemination occurs on a small scale in many cases, but results only in widespread minute lesions which, like those in the lymph nodes, undergo fibrosis and calcification. Even in the absence of treatment it is only in a small minority of patients that blood stream spread on a larger scale takes place, resulting in small progressive lesions of many organs. This condition is known as *miliary tuberculosis,* and commonly includes meningitis as its principal feature. Before the introduction of streptomycin it was almost invariably fatal within a few weeks.

Quiescent lesions left over from the primary infection may be re-activated later in life, often as a result of some other illness which lowers the patient's resistance. Alternatively, post-primary infection may be exogenous. In either case, the pattern of response is now quite different from that to the first infection (cf. Koch's phenomenon, p 77). As a result of tuberculin-hypersensitivity and probably also of other less well recognized immunological responses to the primary infection, the bacilli are no longer permitted to travel through the tissues to the lymph nodes. They are prevented from doing so by a chronic granulomatous reaction. Slowly progressive lesions result, often involving extensive tissue destruction. Even this form of tuberculosis may lead to rapid miliary dissemination if the advancing lesion erodes the wall of a blood vessel and discharges its contents into it.

MICROSCOPY   Mycobacteria do not form flagella, capsules or spores. Bacilli of this genus are best seen in films stained by the Ziehl–Neelsen (Z.N.) method. In this they are stained with hot carbol fuchsin for 5 minutes and then decolorized. Most mycobacteria other than *Myco. leprae* (see p 149) are resistant to decolorization by 20% sulphuric acid and are therefore called *acid-fast,* but the tubercle bacilli have the distinctive property of being also *alcohol-fast*–i.e. they cannot be decolorized by 95% ethyl alcohol. (As an alternative to using these two reagents separately, *acid-alcohol-fast* bacilli can be detected by washing the stained preparation with 3% hydrochloric acid in 95% ethyl alcohol.) Films are counterstained with methylene blue or malachite green, which stain micro-organisms that have not retained the carbol fuchsin and also host cells and other structures, providing a suitable background against which to see the red mycobacteria. In pathological materials such as sputum and pus, tubercle bacilli are fine, slightly curved bacilli, measuring about 3 μm by 0·3 μm, and often appear beaded. As a rule they are scanty in such preparations, so that a prolonged search may be necessary before they are found. Films from cultures usually show shorter, straight bacilli arranged parallel to one another in 'cords' or 'ropes'.

The finding of tubercle bacilli in pathological material signifies that the patient has an active tuberculous infection. If they are found in sputum, they also indicate that his lesion is 'open'–i.e. is discharging into his respiratory tract–and that he is a danger to those around him; and similar deductions can be made from their presence in any other excreted or discharged material. Because they are of such great significance, and also because they may be present only in very small numbers in a specimen, they must be searched for carefully in the Z.N.-stained smears. Smears from a concentrate of the specimen (see below) may give positive results when no bacilli are to be seen in those from the untreated specimen. It is very important to appreciate that *acid-alcohol-fast bacilli found in smears of pathological material are not necessarily tubercle bacilli.* Their identity must always be confirmed by culture, and if necessary by guinea-pig inoculation.

CULTIVATION   Tubercle bacilli are strict aerobes with a rather narrow range of growth temperature around 37°C, are exacting in their nutritional requirements and will not grow on ordinary media. The widely used *Löwenstein-Jensen medium* is made from eggs, glycerol, asparagine, potato starch and mineral salts; it also contains malachite green which inhibits other organisms and colours the medium so that the slightly yellow, dry, wrinkled colonies of *Myco. tuberculosis* are more easily detected. Solid and fluid culture media of simpler composition are also used. Even on optimal media growth is very slow, and colonies are not visible for a fortnight at least, and often not until several weeks after that.

Most pathological materials to be examined for the presence of tubercle bacilli contain them only in very small numbers, irregularly distributed throughout the specimen and mixed with larger numbers of faster-growing organisms. Various *concentration methods* are used to overcome these problems. They homogenize and liquefy such materials as sputum, so that the tubercle bacilli can be concentrated into a small volume by centrifugation; and they also kill virtually all of the other bacteria present. For this they rely upon the high resistance of tubercle bacilli to various forms of chemical treatment, but there is rather a narrow margin between the minimum treatment that will achieve the desired ends and that which will also kill all of the tubercle bacilli. The *Petroff method* employs 4% sodium hydroxide as digestant and decontaminant. Use of 2% N-acetyl-L-cysteine as digestant, with 2% sodium hydroxide as decontaminant, gives better liquefaction of sputum, and more tubercle bacilli survive this treatment.

Myco. tuberculosis can be distinguished from *Myco. bovis* in culture by differences in its colonial appearance, by its enhanced growth in glycerol-containing media and by its ability to synthesize niacin.

GUINEA-PIG INOCULATION   As well as being cultured, concentrated pathological material is often injected directly into guinea-pigs in order to discover whether it contains tubercle bacilli. The animal is killed after 6 weeks, or earlier if it has developed evident tuberculosis; it is examined post-mortem for a caseous lesion at the site of inoculation (usually flank or thigh), with spread of the disease to regional lymph nodes, liver, spleen and lungs. This method of detecting tubercle bacilli is slow and expensive as compared with culture, and in general should be used only to supplement cultural examination of unrepeatable specimens, such as biopsies, and for other special problems.

Guinea-pig inoculation is also indicated when organisms morphologically and culturally resembling *Myco. tuberculosis* have been grown from a patient who has no clinical evidence of tuberculosis, or whose disease is not typical. A diagnosis of tuberculosis has such serious implications for the patient that it is important to prove beyond doubt the nature of the organism isolated, even if this involves a further six weeks' delay.

IMMUNOLOGY   As we have already indicated, tuberculous infection results in poorly understood immunological responses that modify the course of a subsequent infection but do not prevent it. Various antibodies to different components of the bacilli have been detected in human and animal sera, but they seem to have little to do with resistance to infection and are of no diagnostic value. Active immunization, using an attenuated bovine strain (B.C.G.), is discussed on pp 310–11, and the tuberculin test on pp 266–7.

ANTIBACTERIAL TREATMENT   The prognosis of tuberculous infections, especially of progressive primary infections, was revolutionized by the introduction of streptomycin. However, use of this drug alone commonly resulted in the development of resistance to it by the tubercle bacilli, and the treatment then became ineffective. The use of *p*-aminosalicylic acid (P.A.S.), isoniazid, rifampicin, ethambutol and other drugs in the treatment of tuberculosis is discussed on pp 356–7.

Mycobacterium leprae (the leprosy bacillus, Hansen's bacillus)
OCCURRENCE AND PATHOGENICITY   This organism was first described by Hansen, as early as 1874. It is an obligate parasite of man. It

causes leprosy, a disease which is known in all parts of the world but is now largely restricted to tropical countries, where its frequency seems to be still increasing. The number of patients in Britain at the present time runs into hundreds, but all of these acquired their infections overseas. The method of transmission of the disease has been difficult to investigate, as have many other features, because it has never been possible to grow *Myco. leprae* in non-living culture media, and until 1960 there was no known means of infecting animals. Skin-to-skin contact has been considered the main route of transmission, but two facts–that the bacilli are shed in large numbers from the noses of patients with lepromatous leprosy (see below) and that suitably prepared mice develop the disease after inhaling the bacilli–suggest that airborne infection via the respiratory tract may be important. Whatever the route, infection requires prolonged and intimate contact with an infectious patient. In other words, contrary to general belief, the infectivity of this disease is low. The misconception arises from confusion of terminology, for the disease caused by Hansen's bacillus was at most only one of a number of conditions which went under the name of leprosy in the Middle Ages, and it may have had little or nothing to do with the conditions for which the English translators of the Bible used the same name.

The clinical manifestations of infection with *Myco. leprae* are very diverse and cannot be discussed in detail here. Skin and nerves running close to the skin are primarily affected but much of the disfigurement and disablement associated with this disease is secondary, resulting from repeated and unnoticed trauma to anaesthetic areas. Much of the diversity of clinical manifestations depends on differences in immu-nological response, both between patients and at different times in the same patient. There is thus a spectrum of disease, running from *lepromatous* through *borderline, dimorphous* or *intermediate* to *tuberculoid* leprosy. In lepromatous disease bacilli are numerous in the lesions and are shed in large numbers in nasal and other discharges; the host seems to offer little resistance to the infection, which is progressive and has a bad prognosis in the absence of treatment. At the other end of the spectrum, tuberculoid leprosy is characterized by cell-mediated immunity, de-monstrable by the *lepromin test* which is somewhat analogous to the tuberculin test. The antigen that has long been in use for this test is an extract of lepromatous tissue, and there is an important component of the response to it which takes a week to appear and several weeks to reach its maximum. With the discovery of a species of armadillo which is susceptible to infection with *Myco. leprae* and in which the organism proliferates freely, it has become possible to produce a skin test antigen preparation that is nearer to being a suspension of dead bacilli. Bacilli are scanty in the lesions of tuberculoid leprosy, and there is a strong tendency towards spontaneous healing as a result of the cell-mediated response, but at the cost of a good deal of tissue and nerve destruction.

MICROSCOPY   *Myco. leprae* resembles *Myco. tuberculosis* in its morphology, but it is not alcohol-fast and is less strongly acid-fast. Five per cent sulphuric acid is therefore substituted for 20% in the decolorization of Z.N. films aimed to detect this organism. It is Gram-positive.

For diagnostic purposes, smears are made from scrapings of the nasal mucosa of patients with lepromatous disease, and from subcutaneous material obtained by making small skin incisions into actual lesions and at a number of standard sites such as the ear-lobes and forehead. Staining and microscopy of such smears is useful not only for establishing the diagnosis but also for assessing the effectiveness of treatment, since a satisfactory response is indicated by granularity and fragmentation of the bacilli.

CULTIVATION   The leprologist's equivalent of culture is injection of material from leprosy lesions into the foot-pads of mice. A positive result consists of the development of local granulomatous lesions. Many months later the mice develop, in other sites, lesions that resemble those of human borderline leprosy. Disease of lepromatous type can be produced by injection of material containing *Myco. leprae* into thymectomized irradiated mice, which also develop generalized infections after inhalation of the bacilli, as mentioned above.

IMMUNOLOGY   The main value of the lepromin test, described above, is that a positive result indicates hypersensitivity and hence a good prognosis. The negative result obtained in lepromatous disease indicates a poor prognosis in the absence of suitable treatment.

In Uganda in 1960–64 B.C.G. vaccination of children was found to give a degree of protection against leprosy comparable with that which it gives against tuberculosis. Subsequent reports from other countries have been less encouraging.

ANTIBACTERIAL TREATMENT   Dapsone (diaminodiphenylsulphone) is the mainstay of antibacterial treatment of leprosy, which should be continued for at least 2–4 years. Repository preparations of acedapsone (given at 75-day intervals) have given good results in treatment of leprosy and in prophylaxis of high-risk populations. If sulphone treatment is given at a time when an acute hypersensitivity reaction is taking place, the reaction may be exaggerated and may cause crippling nerve damage.

Rifampicin has been shown to be bactericidal to *Myco. leprae* and so to eradicate the infection in mice, but so far has not been shown to achieve total cure of human lepromatous leprosy.

Other Mycobacteria

As tuberculosis was brought under control, it became apparent that some cases of tuberculosis-like human illness were caused by organisms that came to be known collectively as *atypical mycobacteria*. These mostly differ from tubercle bacilli in growing at 25 °C (as well as at 37 °C) and in being of little or no pathogenicity to guinea-pigs. Most of them are highly resistant to isoniazid, and some are also resistant to streptomycin or P A S or both; treatment therefore may be difficult. *Myco. kansasii* is described as a *photochromogen* because cultures grown in an incubator (i.e. in the dark) and then exposed to light develop a bright orange pigmentation. The *scotochromogens* produce pigment even when grown in the dark. More difficult to distinguish from tubercle bacilli are the non-chromogenic *Myco. intracellulare* (the Battey bacillus), which are now responsible for most cases of mycobacterial cervical adenitis in children in Britain.

Myco. ulcerans and *Myco. marinum*, first reported respectively from Australia and from Sweden as causes of chronic skin ulcers in man, differ from other pathogenic mycobacteria in growing at 30–33 °C but not at 37 °C. They are avirulent for guinea-pigs. Similar organisms causing skin lesions have been reported from East and Central Africa.

There are many mycobacteria which are not known to be pathogenic for man but are so widely distributed as commensals or saprophytes that they frequently cause difficulty in the diagnosis of tuberculosis. They include *Myco. smegmatis*, found in human smegma and urine and sometimes on the skin; *Myco. phlei*, the timothy grass bacillus; *Myco. butyricum*, found in butter; and a large number of unnamed organisms. Such bacilli may even be present in large numbers in tap water. Confusion with the tubercle bacillus can be avoided by the routine use of alcohol in decolorizing Z.N. films, since this decolorizes most non-pathogenic organisms. In general they grow considerably faster than tubercle bacilli in culture and produce at most only local lesions at sites of infection into guinea-pigs.

BRANCHING BACTERIA

Some bacillary species form branched chains, but the branching occurs at the meeting-points of bacilli, not within individual bacilli. True branching, in which the branches are parts of the same cell, is shown by the filamentous fungi (Fig. 4(*b*), p 214) and by certain bacterial groups to which taxonomists have assigned the name *higher bacteria* and a position between other bacteria and the fungi (Fig. 3(l), p 94). These groups include the genera *Streptomyces*, *Actinomyces* and *Nocardia*. The first of these is important to us because its members include many of the important antibiotic-producing organisms (see Chapter Twenty-one). The genera *Actinomyces* and *Nocardia*, sometimes referred to collectively as the actinomycetes, include a number of pathogenic species. They are non-motile, non-capsulate, non-sporing Gram-positive filamentous organisms. The filaments, which are more delicate than those of filamentous fungi, tend to fragment when grown in artificial cultures.

THE GENUS ACTINOMYCES

Members of this genus are micro-aerophilic or anaerobic, are obligate parasites, and, unlike some of the nocardial species, are not acid-fast. *A. israeli* causes human actinomycosis, and the closely related *A. bovis* causes 'lumpy jaw' in cattle. The non-pathogenic *A. naeslundi* can cause confusion, since it is found in human mouths and resembles *A. israeli* in many ways, but it is recognizable by its ability to grow aerobically.

Actinomyces israeli

OCCURRENCE AND PATHOGENICITY   The normal habitat of this species is the human mouth. It can be found around the teeth, gum margins and tonsils of many healthy individuals as well as in the lesions and discharges of actinomycosis, but has not been isolated from sources outside the body.

Actinomycosis is an acute, sub-acute or chronic granulomatous infection, often progressive if not treated. It is characterized by the formation of abscesses which drain to the surface of the body through sinuses that become surrounded by much fibrous tissue. The disease is believed to be endogenous, the *A. israeli* normally commensal in the mouth becoming pathogenic in circumstances which are only partly understood. Trauma, such as dental extraction or fracture of the jaw, may precede the onset of the disease, and it has been suggested that some form of sensitization to the causative organism may also play a part in its production. A small Gram-negative bacillus, dignified with the disproportionately long name of *Actinobacillus actinomycetemcomitans*, is sometimes found in large numbers in closed actinomycotic abscesses, together with *A. israeli*, but its significance is unknown.

The cervico-facial region is involved in over 50% of cases of actinomycosis, the abdomen in 20%, the thorax in 15% and other parts of the body in the remaining few cases. Infection may remain localized, may spread through the tissues in a continuous manner, or may on rare occasions be disseminated through the blood stream. Lymphatic spread apparently does not occur.

MICROSCOPY   On close naked-eye examination of actinomycotic pus small yellow bodies–'*sulphur granules*'–can often be seen. These are in fact colonies of *A. israeli*, and if one of them is crushed between two microscope slides and stained, it can be seen to consist of a tangled mass of Gram-positive branching filaments. This appearance differs from that of a film made from a culture only in that short 'V' and 'Y' forms are common in the latter (Fig. 3(*l*), p 94). In Gram-stained sections of actinomycotic tissue, colonies resembling the sulphur granules are to be seen, surrounded by radiating 'clubs' of Gram-negative lipoid material produced by the host's tissues, probably as a form of protection.

CULTIVATION   *A. israeli* cannot grow aerobically. Some strains are micro-aerophilic and others are strict anaerobes. The addition of 5–10% CO_2 to the atmosphere often stimulates growth. The optimal growth temperature is $37°C$, and growth does not occur at temperatures much below this. Raised, irregular, opaque colonies become visible after 3 or 4 days' incubation on blood agar or serum agar. They adhere firmly to the medium. Good growth also occurs in Robertson's cooked meat medium and the other fluid media for anaerobic growth mentioned on p 240, or in a glucose agar shake culture. This last is set up by inoculating the organism into a tube of melted medium at $50°C$ and dispersing it throughout the medium by shaking. When it has set, the medium is incubated for several days at $37°C$. Colonies of *A. israeli* develop in the depths of the medium, but not within 10 or 15 mm of the surface, where the oxygen tension is too high.

For isolation of this species from pus, sulphur granules should be used as the inoculum. The pus is shaken up with water, and the granules are allowed to sediment. The diluted pus is then removed and the granules are repeatedly washed by shaking them up with more water, in order to rid them of accompanying bacteria.

ANTIBACTERIAL TREATMENT   The prognosis of abdominal and thoracic actinomycosis, formerly often fatal conditions, was radically altered by the advent of antibiotics, to many of which *A. israeli* is sensitive. Penicillin is the agent of choice, but prolonged high dosage may be required, since in chronic cases extensive deposition of fibrous tissue may restrict the amount of antibiotic which reaches the lesion and inadequate dosage may result in the development of antibiotic resistance by the organism. Good results have also been obtained with the tetracyclines.

THE GENUS NOCARDIA

These organisms differ from those of the genus *Actinomyces* in that all of

them are aerobes, many are acid-fast and the majority are soil saprophytes. A few species are pathogenic to man, causing chronic granulomatous lesions.

Nocardia asteroides

This causes a rare pulmonary infection which may be mistaken for
tuberculosis, particularly as acid-fast bacillary fragments may be found in
the sputum. The disease may be carried to the brain or the skin via the
blood stream. Sulphonamides may be effective if given early in the
disease, which is otherwise usually fatal and unaffected by antibiotics.

Nocardia madurae

This is one of the causative agents of the chronic granulomatous, sinus-
forming disease of the human foot known as *Madura foot* or *mycetoma*.
Other forms of the disease are caused by fungi (notably those of the genus
Madurella). Other actinomycetes and streptomycetes have also been
known to produce such a condition. It occurs in tropical areas,
particularly in South India and parts of Africa. The form due to *N.
madurae* is characterized by the presence of white or yellowish granules in
the pus, and responds to treatment with sulphonamides or with dapsone
(see p 149). Such treatment has no effect on the forms due to fungi, which
produce black granules.

SPIROCHAETES

The bacteria included in this group differ markedly in structure from any
of the others that we have described. They consist of spiral filaments, in
many cases too slender to be seen by ordinary microscopy of stained
preparations (see below). They have no flagella, but are motile—often
vigorously so—by means of whip-like flexion movements of their bodies
or by screw-like rotation around their long axes. Partial digestion and
electron-micrography have revealed the presence of one or more fine axial
fibrils intertwined with the coils of their bodies. It seems likely that these
are contractile and are responsible both for maintaining the spiral shapes
of the organisms and for the movements that result in locomotion.

The spirochaetes of medical importance belong to the genera
Treponema, *Leptospira* and *Borrelia*.

THE GENUS TREPONEMA
Treponema pallidum

OCCURRENCE AND PATHOGENICITY   Apart from experimental infections of apes, monkeys and rabbits, this organism is purely a
pathogenic parasite of man. It is transmitted almost exclusively by sexual

154   Bacteria

intercourse or by intra-uterine infection, and causes *syphilis*. The typical ulcerating primary lesion of extra-uterine infection, the *chancre*, appears several weeks after exposure, usually on the skin or mucosa of the genitalia but sometimes around the mouth or anus or elsewhere. It is not certain whether the spirochaete can penetrate unbroken skin or mucosa or depends upon trivial surface lesions for its entry. *T. pallidum* is present in profusion in the exudate from an early chancre, and also in the red macular skin lesions, the moist peri-oral and ano-genital papules (*condylomata*) and the 'snail-track' mouth and throat ulcers of the secondary stage of syphilis, which generally follows within a few weeks of an untreated primary lesion. It is less profuse, but often demonstrable, in the granulomatous lesions of many organs (*gummata*) which characterize the tertiary stage and in the arterial and nervous system lesion of late syphilis. Congenital syphilis, transmitted through the placenta in the latter half of pregnancy, involves many tissues and may kill the foetus.

MICROSCOPY   The organism consists of a delicate thread only about 0.15 μm thick, which is wound into a neat spiral $5–15$ μm long and $1–5$ μm wide with a 'wavelength' of about 1 μm. Being difficult to stain and of low refractility, *T. pallidum* is best seen by dark-ground microscopy (see p 21). A clinical diagnosis of primary or secondary syphilis can be confirmed by examining exudate from the lesion or lesions in this way; *T. pallidum* can be distinguished from the non-pathogenic treponemata (see below) and from other spirochaetes by its delicate structure and by its leisurely motility, which involves flexion and rotation. In dried smears or sections its presence can be demonstrated by the silver-impregnation methods of Fontana and Levaditi, but since these involve the deposition of silver over the bodies of the bacteria, fine detail is obscured.

CULTIVATION   It is doubtful whether *T. pallidum* has ever been grown in laboratory cultures. Spirochaetes have been isolated from lesions and maintained in culture, but these were almost certainly contaminating saprophytes. Nelson devised a medium in which *T. pallidum* can be kept alive for several days, but it does not multiply during that time. It can also survive for several days in refrigerated blood, and could therefore be transmitted by blood transfusion. It can be propagated in the laboratory by intratesticular inoculation of a rabbit and transfer to a new rabbit every 3 weeks or so.

IMMUNOLOGY   The natural history of syphilis, including long periods in which the organism remains latent in the tissues, indicates that some form of partial immunity does develop. Furthermore, reinfection of a person whose tissues already contain live *T. pallidum* does not result in a fresh primary lesion. However, immunity seldom, if ever, progresses to the stage of spontaneous eradication of the organism, and resistance to reinfection disappears following adequate bactericidal treatment of the first infection. Immunization is not practicable. The serological diagnosis of syphilis is discussed on pp 262–5.

ANTIBACTERIAL TREATMENT   Chemotherapy with arsenical compounds, introduced by Ehrlich in 1910, was effective but tedious and not without dangers. It has been entirely replaced by antibiotic treatment. Penicillin is the drug of choice because *T. pallidum* is always sensitive to it and because the possibility of giving a single injection of a long-acting penicillin preparation has overcome the great problem of continuance of treatment at venereal diseases clinics. Other antibiotics can be used for patients who are hypersensitive to penicillin.

Other Treponemata

Yaws or *framboesia* (an ulcerative skin disease occurring in hot countries and affecting mainly those of negro race) and *pinta* (also a disease of dark-skinned races, with non-ulcerative skin lesions and later cardiovascular and nervous system involvement) are caused by spirochaetes respectively named *T. pertenue* and *T. carateum*. Like the causative organism of *bejel* (a highly infectious skin disease occurring in Arabia), they are indistinguishable from *T. pallidum* in their morphology, in the serological reactions that they evoke and in their response to treatment. Since they also cannot be grown in culture, it is impossible to say whether they ought to be regarded simply as variants of *T. pallidum*. The diseases are non-venereal, being transmitted by direct contact or by insects. In addition to their pathological effects, they give rise to problems of serological diagnosis and can cause difficulties for would-be immigrants into countries whose laws exclude those with positive serological tests for syphilis.

Non-pathogenic treponemata are found in the mouth and around the genitalia, but usually differ in morphology from *T. pallidum* and stain more easily by ordinary methods.

THE GENUS LEPTOSPIRA

OCCURRENCE AND PATHOGENICITY   Like the salmonellae, these organisms have been divided serologically into a large number of types. These are now all classified within the single species *L. interrogans*, which is subdivided into 2 complexes. The biflexa complex includes saprophytic strains, which are numerous and widely distributed, particularly in water (even in domestic supplies); and the interrogans complex, consisting of some 130 serotypes arranged in 16 serogroups, includes most of the pathogenic and parasitic strains. These occur throughout the world, but many individual serotypes are geographically restricted. Many are pathogens of animals–e.g. rats (serotype *icterohaemorrhagiae* and many others), mice (*grippotyphosa, hebdomadis*), dogs (*canicola*), and cattle and pigs (*pomona*)–but can survive for long periods in neutral or alkaline (but not acid) water. Their ecology is exceptional, in that they continue to exist by means of living and multiplying in the urinary tracts of convalescent or unaffected carrier members of their various host species. Excreted in the urine, they enter new hosts through skin abrasions or mucous membranes. Man becomes infected in many different ways. In sugar-growing countries, which provide a large proportion of the world's total of cases of human leptospirosis, infection often results from workers scratching their legs and feet on cane-stubble on which rats have urinated. *Icterohaemorrhagiae, canicola* and a number of other serotypes occur in Britain, mostly with rodents as their principal hosts, though *canicola* affects dogs and pigs. Human infection in this country occurs particularly in agricultural workers, and those who handle animals or meat, and sometimes (with *L. canicola*) in those who have been caring for sick dogs, usually puppies. The former relatively high incidence among sewer workers, miners and fish-cleaners is no longer seen. The clinical picture produced in man depends to some extent upon the serotype responsible. Thus *icterohaemorrhagiae* infection typically results in classical *Weil's disease* with fever, jaundice, haemorrhage and renal failure and a high mortality, and *canicola* infection typically produces a milder disease of which the main feature is meningitis. However, many leptospiral infections produce nondescript pyrexial illnesses and some mimic conditions usually associated with other organisms.

MICROSCOPY   The tightly coiled fine spirals, similar in length to those of *T. pallidum*, are often bent into hooks at one or both ends (Fig, 3(*n*), p 94). The organisms are vigorously motile, spinning so rapidly around their long axes that the hooks often have the appearance of closed loops.

CULTIVATION   Leptospires usually grow well just below the surfaces of various fairly simple fluid or semisolid media. The optimal temperature for growth is about 30°C.

Blood culture, by adding a few drops of patient's blood to a few ml of one of the fluid media, is often successful in isolating the organism during the first week of the illness. It can profitably be supplemented by intraperitoneal injection of blood into a young guinea-pig or hamster. If leptospires are present they can be recovered in pure culture a few days later by cardiac puncture of the animal, which also goes on to develop the characteristic and fatal haemorrhagic disease. Leptospires can sometimes be recovered from urine in the second or later weeks of the illness by such animal inoculation, but rarely by culture.

IMMUNOLOGY   Immunity to many or all serotypes follows recovery from natural infection. Artificial immunization has been used successfully in Japan. Complement-fixation tests and various other serological procedures are used in diagnosis.

ANTIBACTERIAL TREATMENT   Treatment with penicillin (in high doses) or one of the tetracyclines is sometimes helpful if used early in the disease but is valueless later on.

THE GENUS BORRELIA

These large, motile spirochaetes with only a few loose, irregular waves are distinctly Gram-negative.

Borrelia vincenti, together with the large tapering bacillus *Fusiformis fusiformis* (see p 143 and Fig. 3(*m*), p 94), is usually present in large numbers in smears from the lesions of *Vincent's angina*–an ulcerative condition of the lips, mouth or throat. Both organisms are also to be found in small numbers in normal mouths and throats. Both are strict anaerobes, difficult to isolate in pure culture, and the laboratory diagnosis of Vincent's angina is usually based entirely upon their abundant presence in the smears. Dilute carbol fuchsin stains them well. Evidence that they are primary pathogens is inconclusive, and since Vincent's angina is often preceded by malnutrition, debilitating disease, poor oral hygiene, injury or mouth lesions due to virus infections, it is possible that these conditions simply allow abnormal multiplication of the two varieties of anaerobic bacteria. However, the clinical picture of Vincent's angina is a distinctive one and almost always responds rapidly to penicillin treatment.

The same combination of organisms is also frequently to be seen in material from lung abscesses and various other lesions involving tissue necrosis. Here there seems to be little doubt that they are purely saprophytes of the dead tissue.

Borrelia recurrentis and *Borrelia duttoni* cause relapsing fever in Europe and in West Africa respectively. Closely related organisms have been described as causing the same disease in other parts of the world. They are transmitted from rodents to man or from man to man by lice or ticks. They can be recognized in the peripheral blood as long, coarse spiral threads, and can be grown in blood-containing media under anaerobic conditions. The relapsing nature of the disease is thought to be due to repeated cycles in which antibody production temporarily checks the progress of the infection but then allows the selective multiplication of antigenic variants of the spirochaete which are unaffected by the antibodies so far produced. The organisms are sensitive to penicillin and tetracyclines *in vitro*, but the erratic and unpredictable behaviour of the disease makes treatment difficult to assess.

MYCOPLASMAS

As far back as 1898 a very small bacterium with unusual properties was shown to be the cause of bovine pleuropneumonia. The many similar organisms that were subsequently isolated from animals, plants, sewage, soil and other sources were for many years known by the cumbrous title of pleuropneumonia-like organisms or PPLO, but are now called myco-plasmas. Their cells, with diameters around 0·25 μm are considerably smaller than those of other bacteria, and of variable shape, as they have no cell walls. They have much in common with the bacterial L-forms described on p 87, including the formation of minute 'fried-egg' colonies on solid media. Indeed, it has often been postulated, but never confirmed, that by derivation they are L-forms of more orthodox bacteria. Even saprophytic mycoplasmas are exacting in their nutritional requirements, and those that are parasitic can be grown only on very rich media, which must contain sterols, usually supplied by incorporating 20% or so of blood or serum into the medium.

Such organisms can be isolated from many human beings and from various sites, notably the respiratory and genito-urinary tracts. The only undoubted pathogen among them is *Mycoplasma pneumoniae*. This was first isolated in 1944 by Eaton and his colleagues from patients with *primary atypical pneumonia*, a condition to which attention had been drawn mainly by its failure to respond like 'ordinary' pneumonia to treatment with the early antibiotics. The organism was at first called *Eaton's agent* and was thought to be a virus, until in 1962 it was grown on a slightly modified PPLO medium and found to have the properties of this group. *M. pneumoniae* infection of humans is common in many parts of the world, and estimates for many different communities suggest that it causes 10 to 30% of all acute lower respiratory tract infections. It appears to be the main, though not the sole, cause of the primary atypical pneumonia syndrome, which occurs both as sporadic cases and in local outbreaks. In about half of the cases in which such pneumonia is due to *M. pneumoniae*, and also in some due to other agents, the patient's blood contains 'cold agglutinins', which agglutinate human red cells at re-frigerator temperatures. The finding of agglutinins for a streptococcal strain known as *Streptococcus MG* is more specific for *M. pneumoniae* infection, but the most definite serological evidence is the development, during the course of the illness, of antibodies which give complement-fixing reactions with suspensions of *M. pneumoniae*. The organism can be cultured from pharyngeal swabs, sputum or blood in many cases, but growth is slow and takes weeks rather than days to produce visible colonies. Since mycoplasmas have no cell walls, they are resistant to penicillin and other antibiotics that interfere with cell-wall development, but treatment with tetracyclines or erythromycin is usually effective in controlling *M. pneumoniae* infections.

Other mycoplasmas frequently isolated from man include *M. hominis*, and strains called T-strains (because they form particularly tiny colonies) or more recently *Ureaplasma urealyticum* (a name based on their characteristic urea-splitting activity). These two species both frequent the human genital tract of either sex, are transmissible by sexual intercourse, and are frequently found in association with genital tract infections. However, it remains uncertain whether they play a part in producing or maintaining these infections.

Suggestions for Further Reading
Bacteriology Illustrated by R. R. Gillies and T. C. Dodds, 4th edn.
(Churchill Livingstone, Edinburgh, London and New York, 1976) and books mentioned in the Preface.

TABLE V
Summary of the More Important Bacterial Causes of Human Disease

Principal diseases

GRAM-POSITIVE COCCI
Staphylococcus aureus — Pustules, boils, abscesses, wound infections and various acute or chronic infections, including septicaemia; food-poisoning

Streptococcus pyogenes — Pharyngitis, tonsillitis, scarlet fever, erysipelas, and other acute infections, including septicaemia

Group B streptococci — Neonatal meningitis and septicaemia

Viridans streptococci — Subacute bacterial endocarditis

Str. pneumoniae — Pneumonia, otitis, sinusitis, meningitis, infection of damaged bronchi

Enterococci — Urinary tract and wound infections, subacute bacterial endocarditis

GRAM-NEGATIVE COCCI
Neisseria meningitidis — Meningitis, septicaemia

N. gonorrhoeae — Gonorrhoea

GRAM-POSITIVE BACILLI
Corynebacterium diphtheriae — Diphtheria

Bacillus anthracis — Anthrax

Clostridia — Botulism and other food-poisoning, tetanus, gas-gangrene

GRAM-NEGATIVE BACILLI
Escherichia coli — Urinary tract and wound infections, infantile gastro-enteritis, neonatal meningitis

Klebsiellae — Urinary tract and wound infections, pneumonia, meningitis, sinusitis, otitis

Salmonellae — Enteric fever, food-poisoning

Shigellae — Bacillary dysentery

Proteus — Urinary tract and wound infections

Yersinia pestis — Plague

Pseudomonas aeruginosa — Infections of wounds, burns, urinary and respiratory tracts

Vibrio cholerae — Cholera

Haemophilus influenzae — Meningitis, epiglottitis, infection of damaged bronchi

Bordetella pertussis — Whooping cough

Brucellae — Brucellosis (undulant fever)

Bacteroides — Intra-abdominal abscesses, wound infections.

ACID-FAST BACILLI
Mycobacterium tuberculosis — Tuberculosis

Myco. leprae — Leprosy

BRANCHING BACTERIA
Actinomyces israeli — Actinomycosis

SPIROCHAETES
Treponema pallidum — Syphilis

Leptospires — Leptospirosis (including Weil's disease)

MYCOPLASMA
Mycoplasma pneumoniae — Primary atypical pneumonia

10

Rickettsiae, Coxiella and Chlamydiae

The rickettsiae, *Coxiella burnetii* (the sole species in that genus) and the chlamydiae belong to the borderland between the bacteria and the viruses, though they are closer to the former. They resemble bacteria in containing both RNA and DNA, in having muramic acid in their cell walls, in having enzymes and demonstrable metabolic activities, in multiplying by binary fission, and in their sensitivities to many antiseptics and antibiotics. They resemble viruses in being unable, so far as we know, to reproduce except inside host cells—with the exception of *R. quintana*. Being similar in size to the smallest bacteria and the largest viruses, they are visible by light microscopy. Unlike viruses they can be stained by Gram's method. However, the reactions are weak (Gram-negative except for *C. burnetii*—see below) and they are better stained by other methods, such as those of Giemsa, Castaneda or Macchiavello. They are killed by heating to 60°C for 30 minutes (except for *C. burnetii*—see below), or by low concentrations of phenol or formalin. Many of them can survive for long periods outside their hosts at usual atmospheric temperatures. They are sensitive to many antibiotics, but in general only the tetracyclines and chloramphenicol are sufficiently potent against them to be of therapeutic value, and these drugs are merely inhibitory. The sulphonamides inhibit some of the chlamydiae but actually enhance the growth of rickettsiae, whereas this is inhibited by *p*-aminobenzoic acid (see p 40).

RICKETTSIAE

Dr. Howard Taylor Ricketts died of typhus fever while investigating its cause and transmission, and the micro-organisms causing this and a number of closely related diseases have been given the generic name *Rickettsia* in his honour. They are primarily intestinal parasites of blood-sucking arthropods, such as ticks, mites, rat-fleas and lice, to which they are not usually harmful and indeed may in some cases be necessary for survival. They are pathogenic to man, and to many animals in the laboratory though their natural host ranges are more restricted. Man becomes infected by direct inoculation into bites, by contamination of bites or scratches with arthropod faeces or by inhalation of dried arthropod faeces.

MICROSCOPY   Rickettsiae range from 0·3 to 1·5 μm in length and from 0·25 to 0·5 μm in breadth. They are pleomorphic, forming cocci, bacilli and filaments. They can be stained as described above.

ISOLATION AND CULTIVATION   These procedures are restricted to specialized laboratories because they are technically difficult and because of the high infectivity of rickettsiae for man. Material suspected of containing rickettsiae is injected into guinea-pigs, rats or mice (the choice depending upon the organism expected), and these animals are examined for clinical changes, for development of specific antibodies, and for the presence of rickettsiae (visible microscopically or transmissible to other animals or to chick embryo yolk-sacs) in their tissues. Tissue culture, as for viruses, has also been used. Yolk-sac culture is used for production of vaccines and of antigen preparations for the more specific serological tests.

SEROLOGICAL INVESTIGATION
1 The Weil-Felix reaction.   This is the mainstay of rickettsial diagnosis. Its discovery was the result of a fortunate accident. In 1916 Weil and Felix found that certain proteus strains recovered from the urine and the blood of patients with typhus fever were agglutinated by the patients' sera. This is now known to be due to the sharing of carbohydrate antigens by the causative organism of typhus (*R. prowazekii*) and the proteus strains, of which the most strongly agglutinated was given the name *Proteus* OX 19. The technique of the test is similar to that of the Widal test (see p. 260). The antigenic suspensions are made from non-flagellate variants of the proteus strains since the relevant antigens are of O (somatic) type. By the end of the first week of an attack of epidemic typhus it is usual for the *Proteus* OX 19 suspension to be agglutinated by a 1:100 or greater dilution of the patient's serum, and much higher titres are reached by the end of the second week; a suspension of *Proteus* OX 2 is agglutinated only by low serum dilutions or not at all. The findings in endemic typhus are similar. In Rocky Mountain spotted fever and related tick-borne rickettsial infections both *Proteus* OX 19 and *Proteus* OX 2 are strongly agglutinated; in scrub typhus negative results are obtained with both of these strains but a third, *Proteus* OX K, which gives negative

results in the other diseases, is strongly agglutinated (see Table VI, p 164).

Since the antigenic suspensions for the Weil–Felix test are easily prepared and distributed, its use is not confined to specialized laboratories.

2 More specific serological tests.   Patients with rickettsial infections also form species-specific and even strain-specific antibodies which can be detected by using rickettsial suspensions in agglutination and complement fixation tests. By these means it is possible to distinguish the individual members of the groups of diseases detected by the Weil–Felix reaction, but the difficulty of preparing rickettsial suspensions limits the use of such tests.

THE INDIVIDUAL RICKETTSIAL DISEASES
Epidemic Typhus (classical, famine or European typhus)
This is purely a human disease, due to *R. prowazekii* and transmitted by the human body louse. After being ingested in human blood by the louse and multiplying in its intestine, the organism appears in large numbers in its faeces and enters the body of the next human victim by contamination either of a louse-bite or of the scratches which he inflicts on himself in response to the bites. A severe febrile illness follows, characterized by a widespread rash and cerebral disturbances. The death-rate in the absence of antibiotic treatment is high, especially in older patients.

Louse infestation is a product of overcrowding and poor hygiene, and typhus epidemics are consequently associated with war and famine. Spread can be prevented by 'delousing' threatened populations, their clothing and their bedding by spraying them with an insecticide. A formalin-killed yolk-sac culture of *R. prowazekii* has been widely used as a vaccine for active immunization, and a live attenuated vaccine is now available.

Brill's Disease
This is a recrudescence of typhus in a mild atypical form in a patient in whose tissues *R. prowazekii* has remained dormant, sometimes for many years, following a previous typical attack. The Weil–Felix test may give negative results in this condition.

Endemic Typhus (murine typhus)
This is primarily a disease of rats, due to *R. typhi* (*mooseri*) and transmitted by the rat-flea and the rat-louse. Sporadic cases of human infection occur throughout the world in places where the rat population is high. The resultant disease is much less severe than epidemic typhus.

The Spotted Fevers

These are tick-borne diseases of man, horses, dogs and rodents. The ticks themselves are the main reservoirs for the causative organisms, passing them on from generation to generation via their eggs. All of the human diseases are characterized by fever and rashes, but they vary in severity. Rocky Mountain spotted fever, caused by *R. rickettsii*, has a mortality comparable to that of epidemic typhus, whereas at the other extreme Mediterranean fever or 'fièvre boutonneuse', caused by *R. conorii*, is a mild illness.

Scrub Typhus (tsutsugamushi fever)

This occurs in Japan, Malaya and the Pacific area. The causative organism, *R. tsutsugamushi*, is transmitted to man by mites, which become infected by biting field mice, rats and other rodents, and which then pass on the infection to succeeding generations of mites. Mite larvae are common on scrub in low-lying damp areas; human beings who walk there are liable to be bitten unless they wear protective clothing and use insect repellants. The resultant disease resembles epidemic typhus with the addition of a local black-scabbed ulcer or eschar at the point of entry of the organism.

Rickettsialpox

Yet another mite-borne disease transmitted to man from rodents is caused by *R. akari*. There is again an eschar at the point of entry, but the disease is mild. It occurs in Russia, Korea and America.

TABLE VI
Summary of the Rickettsial Diseases and Q fever

Diseases	Organism	Reservoir	Vectors	OX 19	OX2	OXK
				Weil-Felix reaction		
Epidemic typhus	R. prowazekii	Men	Lice	+ + +	(+)	−
Brill's disease	R. prowazekii	—	—	Usually −	−	−
Endemic typhus	R. typhi	Rats	Fleas, lice	+ + +	+	−
Spotted fevers	{ R. rickettsii	Men, horses,		+ +	+ +	−
	{ R. conorii etc.,	dogs, rodents	Ticks			
Scrub typhus	R. tsutsugamushi	Rodents	Mites	−	−	+ + +
Rickettsialpox	R. akari	Mice	Mites	−	−	−
Trench fever	R. quintana	Men	Lice	−	−	−
Q fever	Cl. burnetii	Various animals and birds	Ticks, droplets, dust, milk	−	−	−

Trench Fever

This louse-borne disease of grossly overcrowded and dirty populations gained its name during the first world war and was prominent again in some areas during the second world war. Its main contemporary interest is that its causative organism, *R. quintana*, which has never been insolated from any host except man and the louse, has been shown to be capable of extracellular multiplication in the lumen of the louse gut and has been grown on non-living culture media.

COXIELLA BURNETII

A somewhat influenza-like febrile illness, with variable manifestations that usually include patchy pneumonic consolidation, was first recognized as an entity in 1935 in Queensland, Australia. It was named Q fever, not because of its place of origin but because of the original query about its aetiology. When the agent responsible for it was identified, it was named *Rickettsia burneti*, since in many respects it resembles the rickettsiae. However, it differs from them in being more resistant to heat, desiccation and antiseptics; in staining positive by some variants of Gram's staining method; in its base-pair ratio (see p 84); in its mode of transmission to man (see below); in the pattern of illness that it produces; and in various other respects. It therefore now has its own genus. It is found throughout the world, and affects various birds and wild animals as well as the domesticated goats, sheep and cattle from which man usually acquires his infection. It is carried between animals largely by ticks, but human infection is usually by inhalation of dust or droplets contaminated from the excreta or other products of infected animals, or by ingestion of infected milk. Its spread is therefore greatly assisted by its resistance to desiccation, and by its ability to survive heat treatment only slightly less than that generally recommended for the pasteurization of milk. Slaughterhouse men and farm workers are among those most at risk, but there are now many records of accidental infection of laboratory workers. There is serological evidence that subclinical infection is common in rural communities, in Britain and elsewhere. An important but fortunately uncommon sequel of clinical or subclinical infection is chronic endocarditis, usually superimposed on existing heart-valve abnormalities and resembling the bacterial endocarditis produced by viridans streptococci.

The laboratory diagnosis of Q fever depends upon isolation of the organism from the patient's blood, sputum, urine or cerebrospinal fluid by intraperitoneal inoculation into guinea-pigs or by inoculation into chick embryo yolk-sacs; and upon specific agglutination and complement-fixation tests. For the latter, two different antigenic preparations of *C. burnetii* are used—phase 1, grown in arthropods, and phase 2, from yolk-sac culture. In acute Q fever there is a rise only of antibodies to phase 2, whereas in Q fever endocarditis there are usually high titres of antibodies for both phases.

Tetracyclines are the most useful antibiotics for treatment of Q fever, but their effects are unreliable, especially in endocarditis. Addition of either lincomycin or co-trimoxazole is said to enhance their efficacy.

CHLAMYDIAE

Some of the properties of these organisms have been mentioned in the first paragraph of this chapter. They share a common antigenic component not found in rickettsiae; they are not arthropod-borne; and they also differ from rickettsiae in being spherical, with no bacillary or filamentous forms, and in having an unusual type of intracellular developmental cycle. The infective forms are about 0·25 μm in diameter, but on entering the host cell they develop into larger bodies, up to 2 μm in diameter. Division of these large forms produces mainly more large forms during the first 24 hours, but by about 48 hours many small forms appear, and these are liberated from the cell and can infect new cells. Clusters of chalamydiae form basophilic intracellular inclusion bodies, whereas those formed by viruses (see p 177) are acidophilic. Chlamydiae of the *psittacosis group* (otherwise known as *Chlamydia psittaci* or Subgroup B) are bird pathogens that sometimes infect man. The *lymphogranuloma venereum* (LGV) and *trachoma and inclusion conjunctivitis* (TRIC) agents (collectively known as *Chlamydia trachomatis* or Subgroup A) are purely human parasites so far as is known, though closely related organisms have been isolated from rodents.

The tetracyclines are of value in treatment of all chlamydial infections, and sulphonamides may also be useful in lymphogranuloma and in the TRIC group.

The Psittacosis Group

Psittacosis in the strict sense is an infection of psittacine birds (parrots, etc.), or of man with chlamydiae derived from such birds. Similar infections of many other kinds of birds, including pigeons, ducks, turkeys and gulls, are collectively known as *ornithosis*; when transmitted to man they tend to produce illnesses milder than psittacosis. Human infection usually results from inhalation of dust containing dried droppings from infected birds (which may be apparently healthy or only mildly ill). Less commonly it follows a bite from such a bird, or is acquired from a laboratory culture. Droplet transmission between human beings is possible. Human infection may be subclinical, or may produce pictures varying from a mild influenza-like illness to a severe and sometimes fatal pneumonia. Respiratory tract carriage of the organism may persist long after recovery from the disease.

The incidence of human psittacosis in Britain appears to have increased following the removal of restrictions on importation of psittacine birds.

The organisms may be isolated from the patient's blood in the first week of the illness or from the sputum at any stage, by yolk-sac culture (see p 173) or by intraperitoneal or intranasal inoculation of mice.

All of the chlamydiae share a heat-stable carbohydrate antigen, and antibodies to it, detectable by complement-fixation tests, are formed in all of the diseases. Species-specific antibodies are also formed, and it is possible to differentiate between the serological responses to the various chlamydiae by studying sera which have first been treated with a preparation of the group-specific antigen to remove its corresponding antibody. Such differentiation is useful only as a means of showing whether antibodies present might be relevant to the present illness; there is no question of using serological tests to distinguish between the illnesses produced by different groups of chlamydiae, since there is no possibility of clinical confusion between them.

Lymphogranuloma Venereum (LGV)

This is purely a human disease, transmitted as a rule by sexual intercourse, though non-venereal infection can occur—e.g. through the conjunctiva. It is largely confined to tropical and sub-tropical countries. In its common form it produces ulcerative genital lesions with regional lymph-node suppuration (called 'climatic bubo' when the inguinal glands are involved). Generalized dissemination follows, with fever and diffuse aches and sometimes with conjunctivitis, arthritis or encephalitis. Chronic infection leads to anal and genital strictures and elephantiasis.

Basophilic inclusions may be visible in microscopic preparations made from bubo pus or biopsy material from glands. Yolk-sac culture, tissue culture or intra-cerebral inoculation of mice may lead to isolation of the organism in some cases. Serological diagnosis depends on complement-fixation tests as described for psittacosis. The *Frei test*, a test for hypersensitivity similar in principle to the tuberculin test (see pp 77 and 267), is used in the diagnosis of lymphogranuloma, but since its antigen is a heat-inactivated suspension of lymphogranuloma agent which contains the group-specific factor, a positive result may follow infection with any of the chlamydiae; such reactivity may persist for many years.

The TRIC Group

Trachoma is a form of conjunctivitis in which formation of fibrous tissue in the conjunctiva and cornea commonly leads both to lid deformities and to blindness; indeed, it is the world's commonest cause of blindness. It is a disease of communities with poor hygiene, especially in the Middle East and in Africa. It is mainly transmitted by direct and close contact—e.g. mother to baby—or by flies.

Inclusion conjunctivitis is a similar but milder condition, of world-wide distribution. Its causative organism is indistinguishable in the laboratory from that of trachoma. It has its primary habitat in the human genital tract. Carriage there may be asymptomatic, but is frequently associated with the common venereally transmitted condition known as 'non-gonococcal urethritis' (N.G.U.) or 'non-specific urethritis' (N.S.U.). Neonatal conjunctivitis ('inclusion blenorrhoea') is a result of contamination of the infant's eyes, during delivery, with chlamydiae from the mother's genital tract. 'Swimming bath conjunctivitis' is a similar condition in older children or adults, believed to be due to transmission of the organism from the genitalia of one bather to the conjuctivae of another via the water.

TRIC agents can be demonstrated in conjuctival scrapings in many cases of these diseases, either as basophilic inclusions or as particles that take up specific fluorescent antibodies; and they can be isolated by yolk-sac or tissue culture of scrapings or pus.

Suggestions for Further Reading
See Preface.

11

Viruses

In the very early days of bacteriology it became apparent that some undoubtedly infectious diseases had no detectable bacterial causes. Pasteur, for example, demonstrated the infectivity of rabies and the possibility of preventing it by immunization, but he could not find its aetiological agent. He suggested that this might be because it was very small. Then in 1892 the Russian botanist Ivanovsky transmitted tobacco mosaic disease to healthy plants by means of a bacterium-free filtrate of sap from affected plants–work which was corroborated by the Dutch bacteriologist Beijerink. Six years later Loeffler and Frosch showed that foot-and-mouth disease of cattle was also transmissible by means of a bacterium-free filtrate. From that time onwards it was generally accepted that some diseases are due to living agents even smaller than bacteria. For many years their further study was hampered by lack of suitable techniques. By light microscopy it was possible to detect single particles of some of the larger viruses ('elementary bodies') and others could be seen as cytoplasmic or intra-nuclear aggregates of particles ('inclusion bodies') inside infected cells. A certain amount could be learned by transmission experiments in living animal hosts. But virology, and in particular animal virology, did not really get into its stride until it became possible to grow viruses in fertile hens' eggs and in tissue culture, and to study their structure by electron microscopy.

Before continuing with this chapter it may be helpful to look again at the summary of the properties of viruses given on p 19. Since viruses have no metabolism of their own and cannot reproduce themselves, it is arguable whether they should be described as living organisms. For this reason, viruses which are able to invade host cells and to multiply there are often described as *active* rather than alive, and those which have lost the ability to do these things are then described as *inactivated* rather than dead.

STRUCTURE AND GROUP CLASSIFICATION

Increased knowledge of virus structure has made possible their logical classification, and although there is not complete agreement as to the best system, the one on which Table VII is based is widely accepted. The character used in delineating the main groups include:

1 *The nature of the nucleic acid in the genome.*   This is either RNA or DNA but not both.

2 *The symmetry of the capsid.*   This is determined by the shapes and mutual attractions of the units, called *capsomeres*, of which the capsid is composed. In some virus groups these protein 'building bricks' are such that the capsid is an icosahedron–a hollow near-spherical structure with 20 identical triangular faces. Such a capsid is said to show *cubic symmetry*, and the classification of these viruses into groups is based on the numbers of capsomeres that they possess. In other groups the capsomeres arrange themselves in a spiral thread, forming a hollow cylinder, and such a capsid is said to show *helical symmetry*. In either case, if the virus is intact the genome is inside the capsid. Analysis of capsid structure depends on interpretation of fine details in two-dimensional electronmicrographs, and these need to be good quality pictures of satisfactory virus preparations. It is therefore understandable that even among virus groups that are of medical interest there are some of which the capsid designs are as yet incompletely understood or unknown. The complex tadpole-like design of many bateriophages is described on p 211.

3 *The presence of an envelope.*   In some virus groups the *nucleocapsid* (i.e. nucleic acid core + capsid) is surrounded by a loose membranous envelope consisting of lipids, proteins and carbohydrates. Some of these components closely resemble those of host cells, and are believed to be derived from host cell membrane as the virus is liberated from the host cell. Many enveloped viruses are described as *ether-sensitive* because they are inactivated by treatment with ether (or with other lipid solvents). Presumably this means that lipid components of their envelopes are necessary for their activity. Closely associated with the envelopes of the myxoviruses are numerous projecting spikes, and these are connected with haemagglutinating activity of these viruses.

4 *Particle size.*   Viruses are measured in nanometres (nm–see p 19). The size of virus particles used to be determined by filtration through membranes of known pore-size, by measuring their rate of sedimentation in a high-speed centrifuge, or by density-gradient centrifugation; though the last of these, which involves finding the depth to which the particles can be centrifuged through a fluid that increases in density from top to bottom, is primarily a means of measuring the specific gravity of particles rather than their size. All of these procedures are still useful as means of purifying virus preparations, but for the determination of virus particle size they have been largely superseded by electron-microscopy.

TABLE VII

Classification of the more important viruses affecting man

Nucleic acid	Capsid symmetry	Enve-lope	Group	Approx. size (nm)*	Members of the group†	Principal diseases caused
RNA	CUBIC	−	PICORNAVIRUSES	20–30	Enteroviruses: polioviruses coxsackieviruses echoviruses Rhinoviruses	Poliomyelitis Aseptic meningitis Aseptic meningitis Common cold
		−	REOVIRUSES	60–80	Reoviruses Rotaviruses	Gastro-enteritis
		+	TOGAVIRUSES	20–80	Alphaviruses Flaviviruses	Encephalitides Yellow fever, dengue Rubella (German measles)
	HELICAL	+	ORTHOMYXOVIRUSES	80–120		Influenza
		+	PARAMYXOVIRUSES	100–200	Parainfluenza viruses	Croup, other respiratory infections Mumps Measles
					Respiratory syncytial virus	Bronchiolitis
		+	RHABDOVIRUSES	80 × 180 80 × 660		Rabies Marburg disease
	UNKNOWN	?	ARENAVIRUSES	110		Lymphocytic choriomeningitis Lassa fever
		+	CORONAVIRUSES	80–160		Common cold
DNA	CUBIC	−	PAPOVAVIRUSES	50		Warts
		−	ADENOVIRUSES	80		Respiratory infections
		+	HERPESVIRUSES	120		Herpes simplex Chickenpox, shingles Cytomegalic inclusion disease
					Epstein-Barr virus	Infectious mononucleosis
	COMPLEX	−	POXVIRUSES	200 × 300		Smallpox
UNCLASSIFIED			HEPATITIS VIRUSES	25–28 42	A virus B virus	Hepatitis A Hepatitis B

* Most viruses are roughly spherical, except rhabdoviruses (bullet-shaped) and poxviruses (brick-shaped).

† Virus names merely derived from the names of diseases shown in the next column (mumps virus, measles virus, etc.) are not listed in this column.

MULTIPLICATION

Viruses do not reproduce themselves; they are replicated by host cells. The essence of this process is that the virus nucleic acid enters a host cell and takes control of its mechanisms for nucleic acid and protein synthesis, diverting them to production of virus components. In the laboratory such a take-over can be achieved by nucleic acid alone, free from capsid or envelope. Indeed, the host range of such naked nucleic acid may be far wider than that of intact virus; e.g. intact polioviruses can infect only primate cells, whereas poliovirus RNA, freed from its capsid protein, can be made to infect chicken cells and to cause them to manufacture complete polioviruses–which, being now complete, cannot invade further chicken cells. The outer coat protects the nucleic acid when it is not in the host cell, makes possible its entry into the fresh host cells, and determines the range of hosts into whose cells such entry is possible. (It also largely determines and is the main target for the host's immunological responses to the virus.) The first step towards invasion of fresh host cells is attachment and *adsorption* of viruses to their surfaces. For some and possibly for all groups of animal viruses adsorption depends on an antigen-antibody-like precision of fit between parts of the virus surface and receptor areas on the surfaces of the host cells–hence the limitation of host range imposed by the outer coat of the virus, and probably also the fact that the various tissues of a host differ in their susceptibility to a given virus. Much remains to be discovered about adsorption mechanisms, but some facts are clearly established. It is known, for example, that adsorption of myxoviruses is a function of projections associated with their envelopes (see p 193) and that their host-cell receptors are muco-proteins, whereas receptors for polioviruses are lipoproteins. Once adsorbed, viruses gain admission to animal cells by a process resembling phagocytosis (in contrast to the self-injecting mechanism of bacterio-phages–see p 211). The nucleic acid loses its coat and is released into the cells. At this stage and for some hours afterwards no infective virus can be recovered from the host cells, and the virus is said to be in *eclipse*. During this period the take-over is proceeding, and the cells, acting on instructions given by the invading nucleic acid, are forging enzymatic tools with which to make new viruses. Where these viruses are made and assembled depends upon the group to which the virus belongs. Some are made within the host nucleus and some within the cytoplasm, though the correlation that might be expected–DNA viruses in the nucleus and RNA viruses in the cytoplasm–does not in fact exist. Some viruses appear to be made entirely in one part of the cell, whereas for others the nucleic acid core is made in one site and capsomeres are transported ready-made from other sites (within the same cell). The degree of disturbance of the host cell's metabolism also varies, as does its fate. For example, myxoviruses are released from the cell surface by a budding process, acquiring their envelopes as they emerge, and the cell can continue to produce and release them for a long period; whereas polioviruses accumulate inside the host cell, kill it and are released in large numbers when it bursts.

CULTIVATION
Laboratory Animals
In earlier days the isolation and recognition of viruses depended on the availability of suitable laboratory animals. Thus the proof that influenza is a virus disease had to await the discovery that it is transmissible to ferrets. Animal inoculation still has a place in the investigation of virus diseases, as is indicated in later sections of this chapter, but wherever possible it has been replaced by the methods described below, which are simpler and more economical of time, space and money, and which often give more useful information.

Chick Embryos
Fertile hens' eggs are fairly readily available, require a minimum of attention and have the advantage over laboratory animals that their reaction to viruses is not complicated by the possession of acquired immunity. They must be only a few days old when incubation begins, and are inoculated with virus a week or so later, provided that inspection by bright transmitted light ('candling') confirms that the embryos are still alive. After a small hole has been drilled in the shell of an egg, viruses are introduced, according to their nature, into the allantoic or amniotic cavity or on to the chorio-allantoic membrane. The amniotic cavity is used for primary isolation of influenza and mumps viruses, but for subsequent cultures of influenza viruses that have adapted to growth in the egg it is technically easier and generally satisfactory to use the allantoic cavity. When grown on the chorioallantoic membrane, the pox and herpes viruses produce characteristic lesions which, like bacterial colonies on a plate culture, permit the identification and the enumeration of the organisms in the inoculum. (The yolk sac is used for growing rickettsiae, C. burnetii and chlamydiae—see p 162 and 165–7; their multiplication in this site may lead to the death of the embryo.)

Tissue Culture
When it became possible to grow mammalian tissues in test tubes, a new method was available for artificial propagation of viruses. However, it was at first of limited value because the cells were in the form of tissue particles suspended in fluid and were therefore difficult to examine. Furthermore, their susceptibility to virus infection was hard to predict.

Today it is possible to grow tissues as *monolayers* (sheets of single-cell thickness) attached to the inner surfaces of the glass or plastic of culture tubes or bottles, and they can then be examined microscopically at any stage without being disturbed. Furthermore, standard 'cell lines', mostly of human or simian origin and in many cases derived from neoplastic or foetal tissues, have been developed and distributed throughout the world, so that different laboratories can use tissue cultures of comparable and predictable virus susceptibilities. Monolayers need nourishment, and this is usually supplied by bathing them in nutrient fluid. However, it is then virtually impossible to separate out pure virus lines from a mixture, just as it was difficult to obtain pure bacterial cultures until solid media were introduced (see p 88). The virological equivalent of plating out bacteria to obtain separate colonies is to seed a monolayer with virus inoculum and then cover it not with fluid but with a nutrient agar. Any one virus particle and its progeny are then restricted to the cell originally entered and those in its immediate vicinity. If these cells are damaged (see below, C.P.E.), a visible plaque of degeneration may appear in the monolayer. As with a bacterial colony, the appearance of the plaque may be characteristic of infection with a particular virus, and subculture from a single plaque is likely to yield a pure strain.

The multiplication of virus in tissue culture can be detected by:

(1) *cytopathic effect* (C.P.E.)–i.e. degenerative changes in the infected cells which can be seen when a monolayer is examined microscopically. Viruses of many different groups produce such effects, and to some extent the nature of the virus can be deduced from the type of change which occurs in the cells;

(2) functional changes in the cells which can be detected by tests of such metabolic activities as acid production;

(3) the presence of detectable antigens, *haemagglutinins* (see below) or other virus components or products in the fluid bathing the cells;

(4) acquisition by the cells of the power to adsorb red blood cells on to their surfaces (*haemadsorption*). This results from infection by some of the myxoviruses, and the consequent formation of virus-containing buds on the surfaces of the infected cells;

(5) resistance of the cells to infection by other viruses (*interference* –see below);

(6) attachment of virus-specific fluorescent antibodies to virus particles or virus antigens within the cells.

Though monolayer culture has many useful features, simple suspensions of cells in suitable nutrient fluids may suffice for virus propagation and for carrying out tests that depend on changes in cell metabolism.

Organ culture is another form of tissue culture that has given valuable results (see p 188). Portions of intact ciliated epithelium from the respiratory tract of a human embryo can be kept alive on a culture medium for several weeks, and their cilia continue to beat. Some respiratory-tract viruses that cannot be grown in any other form of tissue culture (as well as many that can) are able to infect such portions of epithelium and demonstrate their presence by damaging the cells – notably by stopping their visible ciliary activity. It seems probable that the development of similar cultures of other intact tissues will lead to the discovery of other new viruses. As well as being useful for primary isolation and subsequent maintenance of viruses that cannot be grown in other ways, organ cultures of respiratory epithelium have made possible some most elegant studies of precisely what viruses do when they infect tissue that was functioning normally prior to their arrival.

HAEMAGGLUTINATION

Myxoviruses and members of several other virus groups have the ability to agglutinate red blood cells of various species. This property, which in some cases at least is related to the organism's method of entering host cells (see p 172), has the following laboratory applications:

(1) Such viruses can be detected in fluids by their ability to agglutinate human or other suitable red cells.

(2) Some of them endow infected tissue culture cells with the power of haemadsorption, as indicated above.

(3) The haemagglutinins are antigens, and infected hosts are stimulated to form antibodies. These can be demonstrated and measured by their specific inhibition of the *in vitro* haemagglutinating activity of the responsible virus, and their presence in a patient's serum is evidence of infection with that virus (see p 185, haemagglutination-inhibition test).

There are 3 kinds of virus haemagglutination:

(*a*) Myxoviruses attach themselves, by means of some of their projecting spikes (see p 193), to mucoprotein receptor areas on the cell surfaces, and since each virus may adsorb on to several cells, the cells are agglutinated into masses. In the course of a few hours neuraminidase released from other surface projections of the virus (see p 193) destroys all the mucoprotein substrate and the agglutinates disintegrate. The red cells cannot then be further agglutinated by fresh viruses of the same kind, but the original viruses are still able to agglutinate fresh red cells.

(b) The poxviruses and some others produce lipoprotein haemagglutinins which are distinct from the viruses themselves and can be separated from them by centrifugation.

(c) The haemagglutinins of the togavirus group, like those of the influenza group, are integral parts of the organisms, but they do not permanently alter the surfaces of red cells and their attachment can be repeatedly broken and renewed.

INTERFERENCE

Host cells infected with one virus may be resistant to infection with a second virus. This phenomenon of interference does not depend on the two viruses being closely related, and in some cases it is not even necessary for the first virus to be active; after inactivation by heating or by exposure to ultra-violet light it may still protect the host cells containing it from subsequent infection by an active virus. Interference is sometimes due to an activity of the host cells–the production of *interferon*, discussed on p 55. This does not prevent a second virus from entering the cells, but having entered it fails to multiply; the cell ribosomes are prevented from making virus proteins but can continue to make normal cell proteins. In other cases it is thought that interference is a direct result of the activities of the first virus; it may have destroyed all of the receptor areas on the surfaces of the cells so that further viruses are unable to attach themselves, or it may have taken complete control of the enzyme systems of the cells and directed them to its own reproduction, so that a second virus may enter the cells but finds no available enzymes. However, it is possible for two viruses to exist and multiply together in the same cell–e.g. herpes simplex and vaccinia, in the nucleus and the cytoplasm respectively.

It is easy to see in theory the possible relevance of the interference phenomenon to the prophylaxis of virus diseases, but its possibilities have not yet been widely exploited. Oral administration of live poliovirus vaccine (see p 315) owes part of its effectiveness to the fact that the vaccine virus established itself in the recipient's intestine to the exclusion of wild poliovirus strains. Conversely, pre-existing natural enterovirus infections may impair the success of such oral vaccination with live poliovirus.

TRANSMISSION AND PATHOGENESIS OF VIRUS INFECTIONS

Most of the viruses pathogenic to man are primarily human parasites, but some have other animal species as their principal hosts. Transmission is in accordance with the general outline given in Chapter Six. Droplet infection is of pre-eminent importance: it is the common mode of spread of diseases which involve the respiratory tract predominantly (e.g. the common cold and influenza) or in addition to other parts of the body (e.g. measles), and also of many diseases which have no apparent connection with the respiratory tract (e.g. smallpox). Infection with a poliovirus or other enterovirus is acquired by ingestion. Most of the togaviruses are arthropod-borne (hence their earlier name of arboviruses) and enter their human hosts via bites inflicted by their vectors. Other viruses introduced through the skin are those of rabies (via bites from infected animals) and hepatitis B (via transfusions and syringes). A few viruses are transmitted by direct contact—e.g. those of infectious warts.

Viruses generally invade and multiply in cells around their portal of entry into the host's body. Some do no more than this and produce only local lesions—e.g. in the skin, those of warts; in the upper respiratory tract, those of the common cold. Generally, however, there is lymphatic and blood-stream spread from the site of primary infection to other parts of the body. In some cases further multiplication in some central site and further blood-stream dissemination precede the arrival of the viruses at their final target organs. On reaching these final destinations they again have to invade cells and multiply sufficiently to cause local tissue damage before the typical lesions of the disease appear. The incubation periods of virus infections (and of infections of other types) can sometimes be explained in terms of these different cycles of multiplication which precede development of the final disease-patterns.

Invasion of host cells does not necessarily result in their destruction. In some cases a symbiotic relationship is established between them and the viruses. Such latent infection is difficult to detect, but it may be revealed when some external stimulus upsets the relationship. This is clearly illustrated by the liability of some people to recurrent herpes lesions on the lips or elsewhere. These may recur repeatedly in the same sites in the course of other virus or bacterial infections. They may also be provoked by widely different stimuli such as strong sunlight.

Inclusion Bodies

These are accumulations of virus material up to 30 μm in diameter, which are formed within host cells in some virus infections. Such structures were recognized in association with some diseases long before it was possible to isolate the viruses, and many of them were named after their discoverers—e.g. those found in rabies are called *Negri* bodies and those in smallpox and vaccinia are called *Guarnieri* bodies. Their appearances and situations are often sufficiently characteristic to be of diagnostic value. Those of herpes, poliomyelitis, yellow fever and adenovirus infections are found within the nuclei of the infected cells, whereas others, such as those of poxvirus infections and rabies, are cytoplasmic.

Most of them contain active viruses and are intracellular 'colonies', but some intranuclear inclusions seem to be merely deposits of material left over from previous virus synthesis.

RESISTANCE TO VIRUS INFECTIONS

The outcome of a first encounter between a potential animal or human host and a potentially pathogenic virus depends on many of the rather ill-defined factors discussed in Chapter Seven under the headings 'Non-specific defences' and 'Innate immunity'. In our present context 'potentially pathogenic' means among other things that the virus has surface components with affinities for receptors on the surfaces of at least some of the host's cells – in other words, that it has a key or keys with which to unlock their doors.

Once the infection is established, the host's ability to survive it and to recover from it depends in part on how much damage the virus can do to his cells and on the number and functions of those cells that are susceptible to it, and in part on the host's ability to prevent the virus spreading from cell to cell. In many primary acute virus infections recovery begins too soon to be attributable to antibody formation; furthermore, many common virus infections may run normal courses in patients with B-lymphocyte deficiency who cannot mount normal antibody responses (see p 78). Destruction by phagocytes, the fate of many bacterial invaders, probably plays little part in the disposal of viruses until they have been prepared for it by the action of antibodies. The only readily identifiable mechanism for an early response to a primary virus infection is interferon production, but virulent viruses are liable to be poor stimulators of this mechanism and relatively insensitive to it (see p 55).

When antibodies are produced they cannot deal with intracellular viruses or prevent direct spread between contiguous cells, but they may prevent viruses in the blood or extracellular fluid from invading fresh cells. Possible mechanisms for achieving this include (i) clumping of virus particles; (ii) obstructing attachment to cells by coating the relevant parts of the virus surface or by mechanical interference with the approach of the virus to the cells; (iii) coating the virus particle so that when it has entered the cell its nucleic acid cannot be liberated. Any of these processes could help to eradicate an existing virus infection and also to prevent reinfection. IgA antibodies have a special role in connection with virus infections that are limited to mucous membranes, since these are the only class of antibodies found in mucous secretions (see p 61).

Cell-mediated immunity is an important component of acquired resistance to at least some virus infections. The main evidence for this statement comes once again from patients with B-lymphocyte deficiency. In some types of this disease the T-lymphocytes are also deficient, whereas in other types they are normal (see p 78). In the first group, resistance to common virus infection is poor and smallpox vaccination may be lethal. In the second group, recovery from measles, rubella, chickenpox and various other common virus infections, including smallpox vaccination, may be normal and may be followed by normal subsequent resistance to reinfection.

The principles and practice of immunization are discussed in Chapter Twenty.

Virus Mutation

While it also has wider applications, the subject of virus mutation is particularly relevant to that of our present section – resistance to virus infections. From most animal viruses mutant strains can be readily isolated which differ from their parent strains in antigenic structure, host range, pathogenicity or other properties. Such changes are of great immunological and epidemiological importance.

(1) *Changes of antigenic structure.*   The influenza A group of viruses is notorious for its antigenic plasticity. As an epidemic or pandemic travels, there is often a continual change in the nature of the virus, with two important consequences. One is that those who have been attacked by the virus may fail to 'recognize' it when it returns to their community in a second wave; their antibodies may be of only limited relevance to its structure by that time. The other consequence is that prophylactic immunization may be ineffective unless the vaccine used is prepared from a very recent isolate.

(2) *Changes in host range and pathogenicity.*   These two properties are often interdependent. Thus from a virus which is pathogenic to man it may be possible to select out by animal passage a mutant which becomes adapted to living in an animal host, and which then has little or no pathogenicity for man. At least some strains of vaccinia virus were derived from smallpox viruses in this way. Similarly the 17D strain used in immunization against yellow fever was derived from a virulent strain and has been artificially adapted to grow in hens' eggs. These are two among many possible examples of viruses which are valuable immunizing agents because in the course of host-adaptation they have lost their pathogenicity to man and show no tendency to recover it when reintroduced to him. It is, of course, vitally important to ensure that the attenuation of strains used for such purposes is irreversible (see p 316). Loss of virulence is not necessarily linked with change of host range; for

example, some strains of poliovirus used in live vaccines were isolated from human sources but were found to be avirulent, and it is presumed that they were mutants of virulent strains. It is obvious that an avirulent mutant is only of value as an immunizing agent if it is still antigenically much the same as the parent strain.

Not all changes in the heritable characteristics of viruses are to be attributed to mutation. Sometimes infection of a cell by two related viruses results in the production of new viruses having some of the properties of each 'parent'—a process known as *recombination*. This may occur naturally among influenza viruses (for example) and has been used in the laboratory as a means of 'synthesizing' influenza vaccine strains that have the important antigenic components of current epidemic strains but without their virulence.

CHEMOTHERAPY

Most antimicrobial drugs owe their therapeutic usefulness to the fact that they interfere with the metabolic processes of the pathogens but not to any serious extent with those of the host's cells. Clearly there is not much scope for such discrimination in virus infections, though the action of interferons shows that it is possible. Much hard work has gone into the search for antivirus agents, but so far it has had little success. *Methisazone* (a thiosemicarbazone) has been shown to reduce the incidence of smallpox among contacts if given to them soon enough after exposure, but it is ineffective against the established disease. It has been reported to be of some value in control of eczema vaccinatum and progressive vaccinia, two rare complications of smallpox vaccination (see p 315). It is effective only against poxviruses, and its action is to disorganize the late stages of their replication. *Idoxuridine* (IDU), one of a series of halogenated deoxyuridine derivatives that interfere with DNA synthesis, gives good results when applied in aqueous solution to herpetic corneal ulcers. Dissolved in dimethyl sulphoxide, which allows it to penetrate skin, it has been used successfully in treatment of skin lesions due to viruses of the herpes group and even of herpetic whitlows. Although highly toxic and unstable, it has been given intravenously to patients with life-threatening disseminated herpes infections or herpes encephalitis, possibly with some benefit. *Cytosine arabinoside* (ara-C), also a toxic drug, has been used for infections of this kind, but without much success; its analogue *adenosine arabinoside* (ara-A) is less toxic but as yet of uncertain usefulness. The value of *amantidine* in prophylaxis against influenza A viruses is still debatable. It is ineffective against other viruses. No antibiotics that can be used against virus infections have been discovered. *Interferon* is discussed on p 55 and p 176.

SENSITIVITY OF VIRUSES TO OTHER AGENTS

PHYSICAL AGENTS   Viruses differ considerably in their ability to survive outside the body under ordinary atmospheric conditions. Poxviruses can survive in dust for weeks or even months, whereas those of influenza, mumps and measles are extremely labile at room temperatures. Heating to 60°C will inactivate most viruses in 30 minutes, those of poliomyelitis and hepatitis B being important exceptions. Nearly all viruses can be preserved for long periods if they are rapidly frozen to −70°C and kept at that temperature. Many, but not all, can be preserved by lyophilization (see p 37). The majority can tolerate pH variations within the range 5–9. All are inactivated by ultra-violet light and by X-rays, though there are quite large variations in the dosage required by different viruses.

GLYCEROL   Many viruses, notably those of poliomyelitis, rabies and vaccinia, remain infective for months or years in glycerol concentrations which rapidly kill non-sporing bacteria. Glycerol is therefore used as a preservative in virus vaccines.

DISINFECTANTS   Phenols and cresols are relatively ineffective against viruses. The compounds listed as oxidising agents in Table I (p 39) are more active against them, but may have to be used in concentrations much higher than those which kill vegetative bacteria; hypochlorite solutions are widely used as disinfectants in virology laboratories. Formaldehyde inactivates viruses, but its action is slow, and glutaraldehyde is generally preferable.

LABORATORY DIAGNOSIS OF VIRUS INFECTIONS

In many forms of microbial infection the possibility of aiming treatment at the causative agent itself is the main incentive for its rapid identification. In virus infections treatment is mostly symptomatic and seldom directed at the virus. Methods of identifying viruses have in general been slow, and diagnostic virology has tended to be an academic subject, concerned with eventual understanding of virus infections rather than with immediate clinical and therapeutic problems. However, quite apart from the hope of developing antivirus chemotherapy, there are several reasons for wanting to know as soon as possible the identity of a virus that is causing disease. This information may lead to precise diagnosis, more accurate prognosis and the possibility of anticipating a need for special forms of treatment; it may spare the patient an unnecessary exposure to the hazards of antibiotic treatment (see p 322) for an imagined bacterial infection; and it may indicate steps that should be taken to prevent spread of the disease in the community. In an increasing number of virus infections it has become possible to identify the pathogen with reasonable certainty within hours of the specimen reaching a suitably equipped laboratory, instead of having to wait for days or weeks.

Proof that a potential pathogen is present in the body of a patient should never be mistaken for proof that it is causing his illness. In virology as in other forms of microbiology the finding of such an organism has to be interpreted in the light of available information as to how often it can be recovered from healthy people and how likely it is to produce the type of illness from which the patient is suffering. Even a rising level of antibodies in the patient's blood specific for the organism in question is evidence only that it has been present, not that it has been acting as a pathogen – though the case against it is stronger if the pattern of antibody rise suggests that it arrived at the right time to initiate the illness.

In the majority of virus infections the organisms are most easily found early in the illness or even in the prodromal period, before the symptoms appear. Decisions about the best times to collect specimens, their nature and the sites from which they should be taken depend on knowledge of individual virus diseases; some of the necessary information is given in later sections of this chapter. Rapid diagnosis depends on microscopic or serological demonstration that virus particles or antigens are present in material from the patient. Isolation of the virus by growing it in tissue culture, in eggs or in animals takes longer but may be more sensitive and more conclusive and may make possible more precise identification. Measurement of the patient's antibody responses may give indirect supporting evidence for the diagnosis or may be the only grounds on which it is based, but such responses take time.

Microscopy

Only rarely is ordinary light microscopy useful in virological diagnosis; examination of stained smears or tissue sections may show characteristic histological changes, or the presence of pathognomic inclusion bodies (see p 177) or even that of individual particles (elementary bodies) in poxvirus infections (see p 207). Electron microscopy can be far more informative, since a much wider range of viruses can be seen and recognized; but electron microscopes are expensive and relatively rare. Fluorescence microscopy needs little special apparatus, and immuno-fluorescence techniques (see p 21) are increasingly applied to the rapid identification of viruses and virus antigens inside host cells. The main technical problem in this field has been the production of antisera of such precise specificity that presence of fluorescence in the microscopic preparation can be confidently interpreted as meaning presence of the appropriate virus antigens in the material.

Serological Demonstration of Antigens in Lesions

Both complement-fixation and gel-diffusion precipitation tests (including C.I.E.–p 69) are used to detect virus antigens in such material as vesicle fluid or suspensions of crusts from skin lesions. Antisera for such purposes are prepared by immunizing rabbits. These tests give quick results–the precipitation test may be positive within an hour. Their use in smallpox diagnosis is discussed on p 207. Reversed passive haemagglutination, as used for antigen detection in hepatitis B (p 209) can give a positive result within 30 minutes.

Virus Isolation

The first essential is to ensure that the viruses survive the period between collection of specimens and setting up of cultures, since it is not usually practicable to set these up at the bedside or in the clinic. Some viruses are relatively robust; for example, poxviruses in material from lesions or polioviruses in faeces require no special precautions during transport so far as their own survival is concerned, though precautions must be taken to prevent infection of those who transport the specimens. Most viruses are unstable at normal room temperatures, and materials containing them should be kept at about 4 °C (on ice or in a refrigerator) if the delay before culture is likely to be an hour or two, or at lower temperatures (e.g. in an insulated flask partly filled with solid CO_2, or in a deep-freeze at -20 °C or better still at -40 °C or below) if a longer delay is anticipated. However, sub-zero temperatures should be used with discretion, as they are lethal to some viruses–notably respiratory syncytial virus. Repeated freezing and thawing must be avoided. Drying is another hazard to virus survival, especially when the specimens are swabs with only a little material on them; such specimens should be placed in a fluid transport medium (e.g. 0·2% bovine albumin in buffered salt solution).

Most clinical specimens contain bacteria which can interfere with virus isolation, and which therefore must first be killed (usually by incorporation of antibiotics into the nutrient media of tissue cultures) or removed (e.g. by filtration).

The methods of isolation appropriate to individual viruses are indicated in later sections. If animal inoculation is used, viruses are detected and identified by the diseases and particular lesions which they produce. They may be identified in hens' eggs by the lesions which they produce on the chorioallantoic membrane, or by the presence of their antigens in fluid from the cavities. However, because of the convenience and low cost of tissue culture, this method of isolation is used in preference to animal inoculation or hen's egg culture whenever the nature of the virus permits it. The identification of viruses in tissue culture has been discussed on p 174). The immunofluorescence method mentioned there may make it possible to identify the infecting agent within the first few days of culture, long before it is detectable by most other methods.

Diagnostic Serology

In virology, even more often than in other branches of microbiology, tests with known antigenic preparations are used to detect and measure antibodies in patients' sera, and conversely animal antisera of known specificity are used in identification of viruses.

Subject to the qualifications given on pp 257–8, a patient whose serum contains antibodies that react with a particular virus can be assumed to have encountered that virus, but the encounter was not necessarily a recent one. Serological proof that an illness was caused by a particular virus depends on the demonstration that the level of antibodies against that virus in the patient's blood underwent a substantial increase (at least 4-fold—see p 258) in the weeks immediately following onset of the illness. In other words, for serological diagnosis of virological (and most other microbial) diseases it is always desirable and often essential to examine *paired serum specimens*, one taken at the beginning of the illness and one taken a few weeks later. This is commonly forgotten by those in charge of the patients. There is no difficulty about remembering the acute-stage specimen, when the patient is ill and the doctor is worried; but that specimen is worthless without a second, collected in most cases when all anxiety is passed and the patient may no longer be in hospital or under the doctor's care. A virologist's deep-freeze is often a repository for acute-phase sera which wait in vain for their partners! When no acute-stage specimen has been taken, a single specimen taken later may be of value, either by giving negative results for the suspected organism and thus casting doubt on or excluding the suspected diagnosis, or by showing a level of antibodies high enough to suggest recent infection. In some diseases demonstration of an appropriately timed fall in antibody level may be confirmation of the nature of a recent illness.

The serological methods most widely used in clinical virology are *complement-fixation* tests, *neutralization* tests and *haemagglutination-inhibition* tests (described below) and *immunofluorescence* (described on pp 21 and 72).

COMPLEMENT-FIXATION (C.F.) TESTS These are in outline the same as those used for detecting antibodies against bacteria (see pp 70 and 262). As antigens, fluids from tissue cultures or from the allantoic cavities of hens' egg cultures of appropriate viruses are commonly used. Tests using such antigens are in general less precise in their specificity than are neutralization and haemagglutination-inhibition tests, and these latter methods are more valuable for distinguishing between related virus types.

NEUTRALIZATION TESTS   The theory of these is simple. The activity of a virus suspension can be demonstrated, according to the nature of the virus, by inoculating it into animals, into hens' eggs or into tissue cultures. If a serum sample contains adequate amounts of neutralizing antibody for the virus in question, then a dose of virus suspension + serum will fail to produce the effect which is produced by the suspension alone. The amount of antibody can be determined by discovering how much the serum can be diluted before it ceases to neutralize the suspension. Antibodies in the blood of patients or of immunized animals will efficiently neutralize only those viruses that are identical with or closely related to the one that provoked their formation. Conversely, virus isolates can be identified by their susceptibility to neutralization by antisera of known specificity.

HAEMAGGLUTINATION-INHIBITION (H.A.I.) TESTS   These are similar in principle to the neutralization tests, but the activity of the virus which is studied and which is inhibited by specific antibodies is the agglutination of red cells. Such tests can be used for antibodies against any of the assorted viruses which produce one or other of the three kinds of haemagglutination listed on pp 175–6; and for recognizing particular virus types within groups of haemagglutinating viruses.

NOMENCLATURE AND SUBDIVISION OF VIRUS GROUPS

Attempts to introduce Linnaean binomials for viruses have not been acceptable to many virologists because of the difficulty of applying the concepts of genera and species to these organisms. In the widely accepted system of classification and nomenclature that we are using, virus composition and structure are the chief criteria for primary division into major groups, as we indicated at the beginning of this chapter. Recognition of smaller groups and subgroups relies to a varying extent on similarities of habitat, pathogenicity, mode of transmission, antigenic composition and laboratory behaviour. This diversity of criteria is reflected in the names that have been compounded for the groups and subgroups—e.g. picornaviruses = small RNA viruses; enteroviruses = = intestinal viruses; polioviruses = viruses of poliomyelitis. In some cases such names are retained although they are no longer true descriptions of all viruses currently grouped under them, and they should therefore be regarded as convenient labels rather than as statements about the members of the groups. (Cf bacterial nomenclature, p 85.)

Fine subdivisions into types, designated by letters or numbers, depend on demonstration of antigenic diversity among viruses that are similar in their other properties, including in many cases possession of common group antigens.

Our descriptions of medically important viruses in the next few pages are arranged according to the order in which they are listed in Table VII, p 171. Many of the groups described include animal viruses with which this book is not concerned.

PICORNAVIRUSES (SMALL RNA VIRUSES)

These are small icosahedral RNA viruses without envelopes. They include two groups that are of considerable importance in medicine–the enteroviruses and the rhinoviruses–and the virus of foot and mouth disease of cattle, which attacks man on rare occasions.

(a) ENTEROVIRUSES (INTESTINAL VIRUSES)

These viruses are primarily inhabitants of the human intestine, though they are also commonly found in the upper respiratory tract. They occur throughout the world, their frequency in temperate climates being higher during the warmer part of the year. They are excreted in faeces, in which they can sometimes survive for many days even in the presence of antiseptics such as cresols. Not much is known about their transmission, but flies can certainly play a part. Infection occurs via the mouth, and the viruses establish themselves in the lymphoid tissue of the upper respiratory and alimentary tracts before travelling via the blood stream to other parts of the body, such as the central nervous system where many of them can produce lesions. Symptomless carriage of enteroviruses is common, and therefore mere isolation of such an organism, unsupported by a rise in appropriate antibody levels, is not evidence of its involvement in the patient's illness. Enteroviruses can be divided into polioviruses (3 types) and coxsackieviruses and echoviruses (about 30 types each).

Polioviruses (viruses of poliomyelitis)

Some features of the epidemiology of poliomyelitis have been discussed on p 58. It is caused by three antigenically distinct types of poliovirus, of which type 1 is responsible for the majority of epidemics. Infection is often *subclinical*, or results only in a mild febrile illness which has no distinctive features and which is due to viraemia following preliminary multiplication of the organism in lymphoid tissue. In a minority of cases this febrile phase may be followed after a few days either by an *aseptic* (i.e. *non-bacterial*) *meningitis* or by true *paralytic poliomyelitis*–a condition due to virus multiplication in cells of the central nervous system and particularly in the anterior horn cells of the spinal cord. Recovery from poliovirus meningitis is rapid and complete, whereas paralytic polio-myelitis may be fatal (particularly if the brain stem is involved) or may leave severe permanent disabilities. Certain types of coxsackie or echoviruses sometimes cause either meningitis or paralytic poliomyelitis clinically indistinguishable from the illnesses produced by polioviruses.

VIRUS ISOLATION   Polioviruses can be isolated by growing them in human or monkey tissue cultures. They are recoverable from throat swabs or washings during the first few days of illness and from the faeces for some weeks longer. They are also to be found in affected parts of the central nervous system in fatal cases, and in the faeces of symptomless carriers. Their isolation from faeces is made easier by treatment of the specimen with penicillin and streptomycin to kill bacteria and with ether to kill viruses of other groups. Polioviruses are pathogenic to monkeys and apes.

DIAGNOSTIC SEROLOGY   Neutralizing and complement-fixing anti-bodies appear in the blood following infection. As a rule they are specific enough in their action to indicate the type of the infecting organism, though there may also be rises of antibodies to other types previously encountered.

IMMUNITY   Natural infection results in lasting immunity, but only against the type involved. Active immunization is discussed on pp 315–16.

Coxsackieviruses (prototype isolated in Coxsackie, U.S.A.)
These are distinguished from other enteroviruses by the fact that they are pathogenic to newborn mice. They are divided into two groups, A and B, according to the lesions which they cause in these animals. They are further divided into about thirty types according to their antigenic composition. Group B contains fewer types than group A but they are more often incriminated as pathogens. Diseases caused by coxsackie-viruses include *aseptic meningitis*; *epidemic myalgia* or *Bornholm disease*, a febrile illness associated with severe pain in the chest muscles and elsewhere; an un-named *fever with an accompanying rash*; *herpangina*, an acute pharyngitis with vesicle formation; *hand, foot and mouth disease*, characterized by vesicles in all the 3 sites indicated (not the same as foot and mouth disease, p 186); and *myocarditis* of newborn babies. Also they are among the miscellaneous viruses that cause *colds* (see p 188). Individual types are associated with particular forms of disease. Diagnostic procedures are similar to those used for poliomyelitis, except that inoculation of newborn mice is used as well as tissue culture, and that

virus may be recovered from the cerebrospinal fluid in cases of meningitis, whereas such recovery is rare in poliovirus infection.

Echoviruses (= **e**nteric **c**ytopathogenic **h**uman **o**rphan viruses) The presence of these viruses in human faeces was first recognized because of their cytopathic effect in tissue cultures; since they did not appear to 'belong' to any disease they were described as orphans. However, it has since then been established that at least some of the thirty or so types can cause *aseptic meningitis, febrile illnesses with or without rashes, diarrhoea* or *mild upper respiratory tract infections.* Isolation procedures are as for polioviruses. Virus may also be recovered from the cerebrospinal fluid in cases of meningitis. Diagnostic serology is seldom practicable until the virus has been isolated, because of the number of viruses in the group, the lack of any common antigen and the impossibility of predicting which type is involved in a particular illness.

(b) RHINOVIRUSES AND THE COMMON COLD
The all-too-familiar symptom-complex known as coryza or the common cold was for many years an insoluble problem to virologists. Coxsackie or echoviruses could be incriminated as causing a few cases, and so could some of the myxoviruses (influenza, para-influenza and respiratory syncytial viruses) and some adenoviruses. But most colds remained unexplained until 1960, when the rhinoviruses were discovered as a consequence of growing tissue cultures in a slightly acid culture medium at 33 °C (a better approximation to human nose temperature than 37 °C). Some rhinoviruses (H strains) grow only in human cells; the rest (M strains) will also grow in monkey cells. Still more rhinoviruses were discovered when organ culture was introduced (see p 175), and over 100 types have now been distinguished. They conform to the description of picornaviruses, and are similar in size and structure to the enteroviruses. Other viruses have also been identified as causing colds, notably the coronaviruses (p 199), and it is now possible to isolate causative agents from most patients with colds, and indeed quite often to isolate several from one patient. The next obviously desirable step – production of vaccines that will prevent colds – seems to be a long way off. This is because of the embarrassingly large number of different cold-producing viruses (with the further complication that mycoplasmas are also involved – see p 175). Immunization with a vaccine prepared from one strain may protect the recipient against infection with that strain, but it leaves him still liable to the attacks of some hundreds of other viruses that can give him colds. Immunity resulting from natural infection is equally strain-specific.

REOVIRUSES   (= RESPIRATORY ENTERIC ORPHAN VIRUSES)

The original members of this group of relatively large icosahedral RNA viruses without envelopes are frequently to be found in the human respiratory or intestinal tract, often in association with mild inflammatory diseases, but have never been shown to be responsible for these conditions.

Apparently similar viruses, which have been called orbiviruses or duoviruses but are now generally known as *rotaviruses*, have been found by electron microscopy in the faeces of many patients (mostly infants) suffering from gastro-enteritis, in many different countries. These viruses are believed to be responsible for the gastro-enteritis.

TOGAVIRUSES (arboviruses)

This group consists of icosahedral RNA viruses of variable size (20–80 nm), which differ from the two previous groups in having lipid-containing envelopes. There are more than 300 of them, mostly transmitted by arthropods such as mosquitoes, ticks and sandflies (i.e. arthropod-borne) and so formerly known as *arboviruses*. They have little resistance to physical or chemical agents, and are unstable outside the bodies of their hosts except at very low temperatures (e.g. $-70°C$) or when lyophilized.

Togavirus diseases are most common where animal hosts and insect vectors are plentiful – e.g. in tropical forests. Individual species show quite sharp geographical localization – e.g. eastern and western equine, Venezuelan, Japanese B and Murray Valley encephalitis viruses are found respectively on the east and west sides of North America, in Central and South America, in East Asia and in Australia. Among the many animals and birds known to act as hosts for togaviruses are monkeys, deer, horses, cattle, sheep, pigs, poultry and pigeons. One virus species may have more than one major host – e.g. birds as well as horses are commonly infected with the equine encephalitis viruses. Only for a few species – e.g. dengue – is man the sole known host. He plays an important part in the cycle of transmission of some others – e.g. yellow fever – but with the majority human infection is incidental, the disease being maintained chiefly in other hosts. One virus species may have more than one cycle of transmission (e.g. in yellow fever, see below). The arthropod vectors are blood-suckers, and their infection depends on the occurrence of viraemia in the vertebrate hosts. The viruses multiply within the bodies of the vectors but cause no disease in them.

Human infection may be subclinical or may produce pictures varying from a mild generalized febrile condition to a severe illness with localization of its main effects–to the brain in the encephalitides and to the liver and kidneys in yellow fever. Such localization is often preceded by a more generalized febrile illness, presumably resulting from virus multiplication at some site other than the point of entry or the final target organs.

Most togaviruses are haemagglutinators. Haemagglutination-inhibition and complement-fixation tests are used to divide them into subgroups containing antigenically-related members. Most of those that are pathogenic to man are included in the *alphavirus* and *flavivirus* subgroups (corresponding to the arbovirus groups A and B). Infection-neutralization tests are used in species identification.

Alphaviruses

These include the organisms of *eastern equine, western equine,* and *Venezuelan encephalitis* and others which cause encephalitis or dengue-like illnesses (see below). They are mosquito-borne.

Flaviviruses

Some of these are mosquito-borne—e.g. *St. Louis, Japanese B* and *Murray Valley encephalitis*; *dengue* and the somewhat similar *West Nile fever*; and *yellow fever*. Ticks are the vectors of *Russian spring-summer encephalitis, louping ill* and some haemorrhagic febrile illnesses which occur in Russia and in India.

DENGUE   This disease of tropical and subtropical lands is characterized by fever, severe and widespread pains (hence its other name of 'break-bone fever') and rashes. It is rarely fatal, except in outbreaks of a severe haemorrhagic form of the disease in S.E. Asia. Man is the only known vertebrate host for the virus, and it is transmitted by *Aedes aegypti* (the vector of yellow fever) and related mosquitoes.

YELLOW FEVER   This is a febrile illness causing hepatic and renal necrosis and haemorrhages in various sites. It occurs mainly in equatorial Africa and South America, and caused the death of many early explorers of such regions. Monkeys of many species are susceptible to it, and the 'jungle yellow fever' cycle, maintained by *Haemagogus* mosquitoes in South America and by various *Aedes* species other than *A. aegypti* in Africa, does not include man unless he penetrates into the jungle and allows himself to be bitten. 'Urban yellow fever' has man as its host and *A. aegypti* as its vector. Fortunately this mosquito species, which breeds mainly in small accumulations of water around human habitations, is relatively easy to control, and the urban cycle can therefore be broken. However, the virtually uncontrollable jungle cycle remains as a menace to human beings who enter the jungle, and to nearby communities which allow their *A. aegypti* population to recover.

Vaccination with the egg-adapted 17D strain of yellow fever virus is safe and is effective for 10 years or more following a single injection.

LOUPING ILL   This is the only arthropod-borne togavirus infection known to occur in Britain. It is primarily a disease of sheep, causing cerebellar damage and the characteristic ataxic movements from which its name is derived. It is transmitted by a tick, *Ixodes ricinus*, which sometimes bites man, who may then develop a mild encephalitis.

Sandfly Fever Virus
Sandfly fever is an acute illness with high fever, muscle aches and pains behind the eyes. Recovery is invariable, rapid and complete. The causative agent is an arthropod-borne togavirus not belonging to either of the two previous groups. The disease occurs around the Mediterranean sea and in parts of Africa, India, Russia and China. The vector is the sandfly *Phlebotomus papatasii*.

Laboratory Diagnosis of Infections with Arthropod-borne Togaviruses

ISOLATION   Nearly all of these viruses can be detected and isolated by intracerebral inoculation of suckling mice, in which they cause encephalitis. Most of them also grow readily in the yolk-sacs or on the chorio-allantoic membranes of fertile hens' eggs or in tissue culture. Virus isolation may be possible from the blood of patients in the very early days of the illness, especially in yellow fever, but otherwise it may be impossible unless the patient dies and tissue from the brain or other affected organs can be used.

DIAGNOSTIC SEROLOGY Haemagglutination-inhibition, complement-fixation and neutralization tests are used to detect antibodies in patients' sera. The first two tests are likely to give results which indicate only the subgroup to which the infecting organism belongs, though they can be made more specific by studying the ability of various antigenic suspensions to remove the antibodies. Neutralization tests are more likely to indicate the species of the organism.

Rubella Virus
The virus of rubella (German measles), first isolated in 1962, is now classified as a togavirus on morphological grounds, but differs from those already discussed in being purely a parasite of man, with no arthropod or other vector. Rubella infection in childhood may be too mild to attract any attention, or it may be recognizable by the presence of lymphadeno-

pathy and a maculo-papular rash. In adults there may be more con-
stitutional disturbance, and joint pains are a common feature in women,
but the illness is still mild, brief and followed by a high level of lasting
immunity. However, when a non-immune woman becomes infected
during early pregnancy and the infection is transmitted to the foetus, the
story is strikingly different. The foetal tissues may become very heavily
infected with virus, and this infection is liable to persist throughout
pregnancy (if the foetus survives) and for months or years after birth,
despite the presence of maternal IgG and foetal IgM antibodies against
the virus. If the infection occurs early in pregnancy, foetal cells may be
damaged at important stages in their differentiation. Some such foetuses
die, and others are born with congenital abnormalities, of which cataract,
heart abnormalities and deafness are the most important. Probably 50%
or more of foetuses infected during the first month of pregnancy have
some consequent abnormalities (not necessarily serious), but the risks are
less with later infection and by the fourth month are much reduced.
Infected babies may be born with large livers and spleens and may be
profuse excreters of virus during their early months of life, so constitut-
ing a potential danger to other pregnant women and their foetuses.

It is clearly desirable that all women of child-bearing age should be
immune to rubella. In Britain at least 80% of them are immune as a result
of natural infection, which gives far more solid and lasting immunity than
any vaccine at present available. There is thus a strong case for allowing
rubella to persist in the community. This is the basis for the current
British practice of making rubella immunization available to all girls
between the ages of 11 and 13 years and to adult women whose serological
tests indicate absence of rubella antibodies. Live attenuated vaccine is
used, given subcutaneously. Since it is not certain whether these vaccine
strains are themselves hazardous to foetuses, non-immune women should
be warned against becoming pregnant within 2 months after
immunization–and of course women who are already pregnant should
not be immunized until after delivery.

If a woman who is not known to be immune is exposed to the risk of
rubella infection, or develops an illness that might be rubella, during the
early months of pregnancy, her blood should be tested for
haemagglutination-inhibiting antibodies before there is time for them to
rise as a result of the infection–i.e. the blood sample should be collected
within 14 days of exposure or within the first day or two of the illness.
Such a test is likely to show that she is immune. If it does not, a further
sample should be taken 16 days or more after exposure or 7–10 days after
the onset of symptoms, and this may show an antibody rise, indicating
that she has been infected and that the foetus is at risk. To establish that
she has not been infected, it is necessary to obtain negative results from

samples taken over the next few weeks. If no early sample is available, the interpretation of antibody levels found in a late sample may be difficult, but may be made easier by determining whether the antibodies are IgG or IgM (see p 257). The purpose of all these antibody tests is to determine whether there is a risk of foetal infection and consequent malformation, and much anxiety on this score can be avoided by checking the rubella antibody level as part of the routine early care of a pregnant woman, rather than waiting until there is a known risk of infection. There is at present nothing that can be done to prevent or treat the infection in an exposed non-immune pregnant woman, and passive immunization of the mother with human gamma-globulin has been shown to be of negligible value as a protection to the foetus.

MYXOVIRUSES (ORTHO- AND PARA-)

These two groups of enveloped RNA viruses with helical symmetry derive the shared part of their names from their affinity for mucus. By means of spikes projecting from their envelopes they are able to attach themselves to mucoprotein receptors on the surfaces of host cells (see p 175). The same mechanism is responsible for the phenomena of haemagglutination by virus suspensions and of haemadsorption by virus-infected cells (see p 174). Other more mushroom-shaped projections consist of neuram-inidase, which allows the viruses to penetrate through surface mucus to host cell surfaces and also accounts for the reversal of haemagglutination described on p 175. The envelopes of myxoviruses have high lipid contents and disintegrate when treated with ether, releasing the filamen-tous nucleocapsids which are then no longer infective. Naturally occurring filamentous forms of the influenza virus, however, are fully infective.

(a) ORTHOMYXOVIRUSES

These are the influenza viruses. Human influenza is an acute febrile illness of world-wide distribution, occurring as sporadic cases or in epidemics or sometimes in pandemics. Transmission is mainly by droplets, and the incubation period is only a day or two because the respiratory epithelium is both the portal of entry and the final target organ. The illness itself is also typically of short duration (though recovery of full health may be slow, particularly in the elderly). As a rule it is not a serious illness, though severe and even fatal pneumonia due to the virus itself can occur, and in some outbreaks there is a high incidence of secondary bacterial infection of the damaged bronchial epithelium and lungs, notably by *Staph. aureus*, and this too can be rapidly fatal. Except during epidemics it is often difficult or impossible to make a clinical diagnosis of infection by an influenza virus rather than by one of the other viruses that attack the respiratory tract, and many sporadic cases or small outbreaks of 'flu' are not in fact influenza.

Influenza viruses are relatively stable at room and refrigerator temperatures and can survive for some weeks in dust.

ANTIGENIC STRUCTURE   Influenza viruses are divided according to their ribonucleoprotein (S) antigens into three types–A, B and C. Strains belonging to these types can be recovered from various animals and birds as well as from man, and these may well be important sources of new strains causing human outbreaks. Most epidemic strains belong to type A, and the antigenic structure of this type is particularly complex and unstable; at least 18 possible surface protein (haemagglutinin and neuraminidase) antigenic components are known, and these are possessed by different strains in various combinations and proportions. Furthermore, a prevailing strain may undergo progressive minor antigenic changes, as described on p 179 ('antigenic drift'), and from time to time a much bigger change occurs, producing what is from the point of view of the host community a new virus to which there is little or no existing herd immunity. These changes are of great importance in the planning of immunization programmes. Individual strains are described by a complicated code; for example, A/Hong Kong/1/68(H3,N2) was the first type A strain isolated in Hong Kong in 1968 and possessed haemagglutinin antigen 3 and neuraminidase antigen 2. Type B strains undergo some antigenic variation, but type C strains are stable.

VIRUS ISOLATION   The viruses can be found in the throat during the first few days of illness. They can be grown in the amniotic cavities of fertile hens' eggs, where they are detected by their formation of haemagglutinins, or they can be grown in monolayers of human or monkey cells, in which they cause cytopathic changes and endue the cells with the property of haemadsorption.

DIAGNOSTIC SEROLOGY   Haemagglutination-inhibition tests are valuable for precise identification of virus isolates, but they are too highly strain-specific to be suitable for routine diagnostic examination of patients' sera. For this purpose it is better to employ complement-fixation tests, using type-specific antigens of which each will detect antibodies formed in response to infection with any virus strain belonging to one type (A, B or C). Such an antigen is formed when any virus of the appropriate type is grown in hens' eggs, and being soluble it can be separated from the virus particles. Since influenza antibodies are to be found in the blood of healthy people, it is particularly important in this disease to look for a *rising* titre of antibodies, though an unusually high titre in a single specimen may be diagnostic of recent infection.

IMMUNITY As already indicated, immunity following natural infection with a type A virus is highly strain-specific and therefore of limited value. Similarly, active immunization, using injections of inactivated virus, gives adequate protection only against strains closely related to those used. (See also p 180.)

(b) PARAMYXOVIRUSES

These are larger than orthomyxoviruses, do not undergo recombination, and in some cases are unable to agglutinate red cells.

Parainfluenza Viruses

These include the various myxoviruses formerly called Sendai, croup-associated or haemadsorption viruses. They cause minor respiratory ailments, and can be distinguished from viruses of sundry other groups found in similar conditions by the haemadsorption phenomenon which they cause in tissue cultures. They are divisible into 4 antigenic types.

Mumps Virus

Mumps occurs mainly in childhood, when it produces acute and painful inflammatory swelling of one or more salivary glands, the parotids being most commonly involved. About 20% of post-pubertal males who have this disease develop orchitis. Central nervous system involvement is not uncommon, and may occur in the absence of parotitis; it may take the form of an aseptic meningitis or of menigo-encephalitis, but is rarely serious. Transmission of mumps virus is thought to be mainly by droplets. There is no certain explanation for the long incubation period–commonly 18–21 days or more–but it seems probable that generalized dissemination, along the lines indicated on p 177, precedes localized disease.

In most of its properties the mumps virus has a general resemblance to the influenza virus. It differs in that it rapidly becomes inactive at room temperature, is able to lyse chick red cells, and has a distinct and stable antigenic structure. It can be isolated during the first few days of illness from the mouth, from the salivary ducts or in appropriate cases from the cerebrospinal fluid. It grows in the amniotic cavities of hens' eggs, or in monkey kidney tissue culture; in the latter it induces the formation of syncytia (giant cells). Complement-fixation tests of patients' sera are of greater diagnostic value than haemagglutination-inhibition tests. Active immunization, using either formalin-killed viruses from chick embryo tissue cultures or live attenuated strains of mumps virus, has been reported to give good protection, but the duration of this protection and the indications for such immunization are not yet established. Passive immunization with human convalescent gammaglobulin is of some value in preventing orchitis. In most cases permanent immunity follows natural infection.

Measles Virus
In most parts of the world measles is a common, usually mild disease of children, characterized by fever, respiratory tract infection and a diffuse macular rash; a small number of deaths occur, either from measles virus encephalitis or from secondary bacterial infection of the respiratory tract. However, isolated communities in which the disease is not endemic are liable to severe outbreaks affecting all age groups and with mortality rates as high as 25%. Infection is spread by droplets, and the virus multiplies in the respiratory tract epithelium before being spread via the blood stream. Subacute sclerosing panencephalitis (SSPE) is a rare fatal disease of children or adolescents who have had measles some years earlier; it is apparently due to reactivation of measles virus latent in the brain.

The measles virus has the characteristic structure of a myxovirus, but its known haemagglutinating activity affects only monkey red cells and it has no neuraminidase. Like many paramyxoviruses it can lyse red cells. It can be grown, with difficulty, in human or monkey tissue cultures, in which it causes the formation of multinucleate cells and syncytia (giant cells). Rising levels of complement-fixing and haemagglutination-inhibiting antibodies may be found in patients' sera, but a single finding of a high level means little because of the likelihood of past infection. These problems are of little practical importance, since laboratory confirmation of the diagnosis is seldom required. Lasting immunity follows natural infection. Passive immunization with human gammaglobulin is indicated when young or delicate infants have been exposed to infection. Active immunization is discussed on pp 316–17.

Respiratory Syncytial (R.S.) Virus
Because it survives for only a short time outide the host and cannot tolerate freezing, this common pathogen of the human respiratory tract escaped detection until 1957. It is now known to be widely disseminated in Britain, the U.S.A and many other countries during winter months, presumably by means of droplets, and to be a major cause of respiratory tract infections. In adults these affect only the upper respiratory tract and are not serious, but children may be more severely affected and in particular infants may develop *bronchiolitis* (the syndrome characteristic of this virus) and bronchopneumonia, which may be fatal. The virus can be detected in nasopharyngeal exudate by immunofluorescence. It grows

in human or monkey tissue cultures, and as its name implies it shares with mumps and measles viruses the property of causing the infected cells to fuse into syncytia but it does not cause haemagglutination. Complement-fixing and neutralizing antibodies are formed in response to infection with this virus, even in very young patients.

RHABDOVIRUSES
Rabies Virus
The causative agent of rabies is a helical enveloped RNA virus which differs from the myxoviruses in that its virions are bullet-shaped (typically) or rod-shaped or filamentous.

All mammals are susceptible to this grim disease. It is transmitted chiefly through bites inflicted by its victims upon other animals; vampire bats are exceptional in that they can carry and pass on the virus without themselves having the disease. Human infection is usually the result of a bite from a rabid dog. However, even a lick may be sufficient to transmit the virus, which multiplies in the salivary glands and may be present in large amounts in the saliva. The incubation period of the disease varies from less than 2 weeks to several months. The virus is believed to travel from its point of entry along the nerves or perineural lymphatics to the brain, and the incubation period is to some extent dependent on the length of this journey, being short if the bite is on the face. After multiplying in the brain, where it does extensive damage, the virus travels to the salivary glands and other parts of the body, probably again along the nerves. The outstanding clinical feature of the disease is a violent and painful spasm of the throat on attempting to swallow, with a consequent fear of drinking (*hydrophobia*). Once established, the disease is incurable and invariably fatal.

The virus is highly resistant to most disinfectants, which are therefore of little value for application to bites that might contain it. Surgical debridement, thorough washing with soap and water, and local injection of antiserum are probably the most useful forms of local treatment.

DIAGNOSIS   If the animal causing the bite is available, it is important to determine whether it really has rabies. If it is dead, microscopic examination of its brain tissue is likely to reveal the typical Negri cytoplasmic inclusion bodies in the nerve cells, and the virus can also be demonstrated and identified by immunofluorescence or by electron microscopy. Mice inoculated with infected brain tissue or saliva develop typical nervous system signs in about a week. If the animal is still alive and fails to become paralysed within 10 days, it is not rabid. The diagnosis can be made by mouse-inoculation of specimens from the human patient, but by the time that this is possible it is too late to do anything about treatment. Patients do not live long enough for serological tests to be useful.

IMMUNIZATION   Passive immunization with animal anti-rabies serum given systemically (as well as locally—see above) may prevent rabies if treatment is started soon after the patient is bitten—preferably on the first day. The long incubation period also permits active immunization to be used as a means of treatment. This was first done by Pasteur. Although he did not know the nature of the rabies organism, he so modified it by drying infected rabbit spinal cords that it was harmless and yet an effective antigen when given by subcutaneous injection. Patients could be given further injections of such cord preparations dried for progressively shorter periods, until they were able to tolerate a preparation containing fully virulent virus. Both Pasteur's live vaccines and inactivated vaccines such as that introduced by Semple had the disadvantage that repeated injections of tissue from the central nervous system were liable to cause allergic encephalitis. A vaccine produced by growing the virus in embryonated duck eggs and inactivating it with beta-propiolactone has been widely used; it is a fairly potent immunizing agent (though far from being ideal, as a course of injections is still required), and it rarely produces undesirable side-effects. An effective vaccine prepared in human diploid cell culture is now available, and has the advantages that fewer injections are required and that adverse reactions are minimal.

CONTROL   In countries where there is rabies, stray dogs should be destroyed and all others actively immunized. Quarantine regulations and some other aspects of control of this disease are discussed on p 273.

Marburg Virus
In 1967 a sudden outbreak of an unrecognized disease occurred in a group of laboratory workers in Marburg, West Germany, and then similar outbreaks affected laboratory workers in Frankfurt and in Belgrade. It was discovered that all of the patients had been dealing with tissues from the same batch of African green monkeys, and that the monkeys were carrying the virus which caused the disease. Further outbreaks of the disease were subsequently recognized in other places.

    The disease is severe, with a mortality rate of over 20%. The illness consists of fever, headache, muscle pain, diarrhoea and vomiting, with a maculopapular rash and evidence of liver, kidney and central nervous system involvement.

    The virus particles are similar to but much longer than those of rabies virus. The virus can be grown in tissue culture, and forms inclusion bodies resembling Negri bodies; it can be demonstrated and identified by immunofluorescence or by electron microscopy. Antibodies can be detected in patients' sera by complement-fixation tests or by immunofluorescence.

ARENAVIRUSES
These are medium-sized enveloped RNA viruses characterized by granularity of appearance in electron micrographs.

Lymphocytic Choriomeningitis Virus
A virus that causes endemic infection in wild mice and is excreted in their urine and faeces is occasionally transmitted to man, by inhalation of contaminated dust or eating of contaminated food. The resultant human illness may be influenza-like, but characteristically it is an aseptic meningitis with a high lymphocyte count (up to 1000 per μl) in the cerebrospinal fluid. The virus may be isolated from the patient's cerebrospinal fluid or blood by tissue culture or by intracerebral inoculation into mice. Antibodies can be detected in patients' sera by complement-fixation tests.

Lassa Fever Virus
A similar virus causes the much more serious human illness first described in Lassa, Nigeria, in 1969, and subsequently seen in outbreaks in other parts of Africa. Rodents may again be the source of the virus. Common features of the disease, which has a mortality rate of up to 45% in some outbreaks, are fever, sore throat with ulceration of the mouth and pharynx, vomiting, abdominal or chest pain, headache, cough and diarrhoea. Leucopenia and proteinuria are common. The virus can be isolated in tissue culture, and antibodies can be detected in sera by a complement-fixation test, but this is rather insensitive and liable to give false positive results.

CORONAVIRUSES
These pleomorphic enveloped RNA viruses take their name from their crown-like ring of petal-shaped projections. Many distinct types within this group attack the human respiratory tract, usually producing illnesses indistinguishable from common colds produced by rhinoviruses. Coronaviruses were first discovered by inoculating tracheal organ cultures with material from the respiratory tracts of patients with such illnesses, but can now be grown and identified in simple tissue cultures. Infection can also be confirmed by demonstrating rising antibody titres in complement-fixation tests.

PAPOVAVIRUSES (VIRUSES OF PAPILLOMAS, POLY-OMAVIRUS AND MONKEY VACUOLATING VIRUS)

These are small icosahedral DNA viruses without envelopes. A virus of this morphology is found in common human warts, and since such warts are transmissible to other humans by means of cell-free filtrates they are presumed to be due to the virus. It has not been certainly grown in tissue culture or transmitted to other species. Morphologically similar viruses have been demonstrated by electron-microscopy in (but not yet grown from) brain tissue of patients with progressive multifocal leuco-encephalopathy, a rare form of encephalitis occurring in the terminal stages of neoplastic diseases or sometimes in association with other diseases in which the reticulo-endothelial system is extensively involved. The other members of this group are all animal viruses. Among those which are found in and are the causative agents of benign papillomas in their various host species, the rabbit papilloma virus is unique in that it can also cause malignant tumours. The polyoma virus, isolated from the tissues of leukaemic mice, produces a wide range of malignant tumours when injected into newborn mice, hamsters and other rodents. The monkey vacuolating virus or simian virus (SV) 40, isolated from monkey kidney tissue cultures, also causes malignant tumours when administered to newborn hamsters; and a 'hybrid' virus, formed when adenovirus type 7 is grown in monkey kidney cells that are infected with SV 40, produces malignant tumours in newborn hamsters more rapidly than does SV 40 itself. These animal viruses are of no direct medical importance, but are mentioned here because their behaviour clearly suggests the possibility that similar DNA viruses may be involved in the aetiology of human malignant diseases. (See also pp 202 and 204.) Such speculation is not limited to this group of viruses, as some RNA viruses also cause malignant tumours in animals – notably the first two viruses ever shown to do so, the fowl leukaemia virus and the Rous sarcoma virus.

ADENOVIRUSES

These also are icosahedral DNA viruses without envelopes. They are larger than the viruses of the previous group, and nearly all agglutinate red cells of one or more animal species. Those isolated from humans share a group complement-fixing antigen but can be separated into 33 types by haemagglutination-inhibition and neutralization tests. Some types are not known to be pathogenic, but some (notably types 3, 4, 7, 14 and 21) cause *acute febrile illnesses with inflammation of various parts of the respiratory tract*, of which *sore throat* is a frequent component. Epidemics of such infection may occur, and have been particularly noted among large communities of new recruits to the U.S. forces, where they have been sufficiently troublesome to stimulate research into means of active immunization. *Conjunctivitis* is often associated with the respiratory tract infections ('pharyngo-conjunctival fever'). Type 8 has been incriminated in many countries as a cause of *epidemic keratoconjunctivitis*, notably among shipyard workers and others exposed to abnormal risks of minor corneal abrasions. Outbreaks of this condition have also resulted from cross-infection between patients who were being investigated and treated at the same ophthalmological clinics. There is evidence that enlargement of Peyer's patches as a result of adenovirus infection may lead to *intussusception* in children. The viruses can be recovered from appropriate sites in these infections by growing them in human tissue cultures. Both group and type-specific antibodies appear in the blood following infection; complement-fixation tests for the former are used to provide evidence of adenovirus infection and neutralization tests to indicate the type of virus involved.

HERPESVIRUSES

These are icosahedral DNA viruses which are larger than those of the two previous groups and have envelopes. They multiply inside the nuclei of host cells, producing intranuclear inclusion bodies. The group includes the herpes simplex virus (and their simian equivalent, the monkey B virus, an occasional cause of fatal central nervous system infection in humans who work with monkeys or monkey tissues); the varicella-zoster (chickenpox and shingles) virus; the cytomegalovirus; and the Epstein-Barr virus of infectious mononucleosis.

Herpes Simplex Viruses

These are probably man's commonest virus parasites. Rarely, infants are infected from their mothers during birth, and severe generalized infection may result. Far more commonly primary infection occurs early in childhood, often without any more specific manifestations than mild fever and malaise, but sometimes in the form of *aphthous stomatitis* (herpetic gingivo-stomatitis), an acute febrile illness with vesiculation and then ulceration of the oral mucous membranes. Primary infection in eczematous children may cause *eczema herpeticum*, in which large numbers of vesicles appear on the eczematous skin. *Herpetic whitlow* is a painful and often destructive finger infection, resulting from direct inoculation of herpes virus into the skin of the finger—sometimes the finger of a doctor, dentist or nurse attending to a patient with herpes. Other possible results of primary infection include mild *aseptic meningitis*, a more severe *encephalitis* and various manifestations of *genital infection*. However, in most cases the primary infection is inapparent, but despite antibody formation by the host the virus establishes itself in a latent state in his tissues. From time to time this host–parasite relationship is disturbed (see p 177) and a crop of vesicles may appear on the skin near the lip margin, near the nose of elsewhere–commonly recurring many times, possibly as a result of widely different stimuli, and nearly always occupying the same site in a given patient. This is by far the commonest disorder caused by this virus, and is known as *herpes simplex* (or as *herpes labialis* when in its commonest site, or as *herpes genitalis* when on the genitalia, or as *herpes febrilis* on the frequent occasions when the stimulus is a febrile illness). Herpetic lesions, either primary or recurrent, may involve the cornea or conjunctiva or both (*kerato-conjunctivitis*). Treatment of such lesions and of other herpetic infections is discussed on p 180.

Two types of herpes simplex virus can be distinguished serologically and by some of their cultural features–notably by the pocks that they produce on chorio-allantoic membranes. Type 1 is responsible for virtually all oral and nervous system infections, whereas type 2, which is transmissible by sexual intercourse, is found mainly in the genital tract. Women with carcinoma or precancerous changes of the cervix uteri have antibodies to the type 2 virus in their blood more commonly than do women from appropriate control groups. It is therefore possible that the virus, though seldom isolated from such lesions, is responsible for inducing neoplastic changes. Alternatively, it may be transmitted in company with a carcinogenic agent.

Herpesvirus may be detected in material from lesions by electron microscopy or by immunofluorescence. It can be grown on hens' egg chorio-allantoic membranes or in tissue culture, in which it forms inclusion bodies and is cytopathogenic. Detection of rising levels of neutralizing and complement-fixing antibodies may be of diagnostic value in primary infections, but such antibodies are common in the blood of healthy adults.

Varicella-Zoster (V.Z.) Virus

Chickenpox (varicella) is a highly infectious and usually mild illness, occurring mainly in childhood and characterized by a vesicular eruption. The lesions, unlike those of smallpox, appear in crops on successive days, so that new ones are still appearing when others are well advanced. The trunk is usually affected before the face and limbs. *Shingles* (zoster) is a much less common condition, and almost confined to adults. Its main features are severe pain in the distribution of one or more nerve roots and clusters of vesicles in the same distribution. The pain is due to virus infection of the appropriate posterior horn cells. These two diseases are due to the same virus. An attack of chickenpox commonly confers lifelong immunity against that disease; but the virus may remain latent for years after the attack and then, reactivated by irradiation or a neoplasm or more often without any known cause, it may produce an attack of shingles. It may then go on to produce chickenpox in the susceptible close contacts of the shingles patient—usually, of course, in children.

Despite the clinical resemblance between chickenpox and the poxvirus diseases, the V.Z. virus is morphologically not a poxvirus but a herpesvirus. Furthermore, characteristic giant cells with intranuclear inclusions (Tzank cells) are seen on microscopic examination of material from the skin lesions that V.Z. virus produces, and are also found in herpes simplex lesions, but not in those of poxvirus infections. When laboratory help is requested in the diagnosis of chickenpox, the usual chief requirement is to establish as quickly as possible that the patient does not have smallpox. Means of making this differentiation rapidly are considered below under 'Laboratory diagnosis of smallpox'. The V.Z. virus can also be differentiated from both poxviruses and herpes simplex virus by its failure to produce lesions on the chorio-allantoic membranes of eggs. It can be grown in human-embryo tissue culture, where it produces cytopathic effects and intranuclear inclusions. It has not been transmitted to laboratory animals. Immunofluorescence and immunodiffusion can be used to detect virus antigen. Complement-fixing antibodies for V.Z. virus antigen can be detected in patients' blood following either chickenpox or shingles, but levels are higher after the latter—a finding which fits in with the concept that shingles is a disease produced by the chickenpox virus in subjects who are already partly immune.

There is no specific drug treatment for chickenpox, but local application of idoxuridine accelerates healing of shingles lesions. Hyperimmune human immunoglobulin (i.e. having a high titre of V.Z. virus antibodies) can be used in prevention of chickenpox or treatment of shingles in patients with reduced immunological competence. The possibility of active immunization against V.Z. virus has received little attention.

Cytomegalovirus

This is another of man's common parasites, and many other animal species have their own equivalent viruses. The names cytomegalovirus and cytomegalic inclusion disease are derived from the characteristic changes found in infected cells, whether in the body or in tissue culture—namely, marked cellular enlargement and the formation of intranuclear inclusions.

Primary infection, which occurs mainly during adolescence and adult life, may be asymptomatic and detectable only by an antibody rise, or may cause a mild fever or occasionally hepatitis, pneumonitis or heterophil-antibody-negative infectious mononucleosis (see below). The virus may also be associated with localized or more generalized disease in debilitated elderly patients or in those with impaired immunological mechanisms, particularly those on immunosuppressive or cytotoxic drugs. Primary infection acquired during pregnancy may be transmitted to the foetus; such intra-uterine infection may be asymptomatic or may have various clinical manifestations, including severe brain and other neurological damage, liver and spleen enlargement and deranged erythropoiesis.

Cytomegalic inclusion disease can be diagnosed in the laboratory by finding typical infected cells, with 'owl's eye' inclusions, in the patient's saliva or urine or in portions of infected tissue. The virus can be grown in human embryo tissue culture, and antibodies can be detected by complement-fixation tests or immunofluorescence. It is important to remember that the mere presence of this virus in the human body does not mean that it is causing disease.

No effective drug therapy or vaccine is available for use against this virus.

Epstein-Barr (E.B.) Virus

In 1962 Burkitt drew attention to the occurrence in certain parts of Africa of an assortment of malignant tumours in children which had many features in common. Their epidemiology was such as to suggest that they are transmitted by insects, and this idea led to a vigorous pursuit of a possible virus agent, both in material from the African tumours and in that from similar conditions since recognized in many parts of the world. As in other attempts to find causative agents for tumours and leukaemias, the results were confusing because too many viruses were found. Presumably some of them at least were innocent 'passengers' in the tissues examined. The most convincing contender for the role of the Burkitt's lymphoma virus is the herpesvirus detected in cell-cultures from lymphoma tissue by Epstein and Barr in 1964. The same virus has been shown to be associated with nasopharyngeal carcinomas in Chinese patients, and its role in the aetiology of these malignant conditions is still a matter for debate and vigorous research. Meanwhile a quite different field of research was opened up when a technician developed infectious mononucleosis (glandular fever) after working with the E.B. virus, and was observed to produce antibodies to that virus during her illness. Subsequent studies showed that many patients with infectious mononucleosis produce such antibodies. Those who do so nearly always also give positive Paul Bunnell tests: these depend on the presence of antibodies that are called heterophil because they react with cells from another species (in this case, sheep or horse red cells). It now appears that the E.B. virus is responsible for most heterophil-antibody-positive and some heterophil-antibody-negative cases of infectious mononucleosis; its role in a particular case can be confined by using immunofluorescence to detect virus-specific antibodies. In some (usually heterophil-antibody-negative) cases of this disease rising antibody titres can be demonstrated instead for cytomegalovirus or other viruses. (See also p 224).

It is now clear that the E.B. virus resembles other herpesviruses not only in its morphology but in its epidemiology. Natural infection is common in childhood, and indeed almost universal in many communities, but is usually asymptomatic. A substantial minority of those infected have persistent buccal infection with shedding of virus, and are therefore a source of infection to others, particularly by kissing. Persistence of virus can also be demonstrated in some of the circulating B-lymphocytes of some such people. Infectious mononucleosis occurs mainly in those whose primary infection has been delayed to the age-range 15–25 years, and is uncommon in children or in older adults. The mononuclear cells in the blood which give the condition its name are T-lymphocytes, presumably proliferating in response to the presence of the virus. Activation or reactivation of latent E.B. virus infection may follow immunosuppression.

POXVIRUSES
The information necessary for replication of a virus is coded on its nucleic acid. A small virus contains only a small amount of nucleic acid and it is therefore limited to a few structural components and a simple structure. By virus standards the poxviruses are large, and their enveloped particles, which appear brick-shaped on electron-microscopy, have a relatively complex structure that is not yet fully elucidated.

Members of this group of DNA viruses cause skin lesions in various bird and animal species. The viruses of greatest interest to us are those of smallpox, cowpox and vaccinia. *Contagious pustular dermatitis* ('orf') is a poxvirus infection occasionally transmitted to man from sheep or goats. *Molluscum contagiosum* is a transmissible human disease which produces multiple warty skin nodules in many parts of the body.

Smallpox (Variola), Cowpox and Vaccinia Viruses
Smallpox, which is said to have killed 60 million people in the 18th century, was still endemic in many countries and liable to appear anywhere in the world until a few years ago. In the last decade, however, a vigorous World Health Organization eradication programme has almost eliminated the disease except in Ethiopia and Somalia. Two distinct types of smallpox have long been recognized—the *classical* or *Asiatic* type (*variola major*), with a mortality rate of up to 40% in some outbreaks, and the much milder *alastrim* (*variola minor*), caused by a different strain of

smallpox virus and now probably extinct. Either type begins as a systemic febrile illness. A few days later macular skin lesions appear which turn into papules, then vesicles and then pustules, and become crusted about 10 days after their first appearance. In severe cases they may be confluent and haemorrhagic. The mucous membranes of the mouth and elsewhere may also be involved. During the 12-day incubation period which precedes the onset of fever the virus, which enters the body through the mucous membranes of the respiratory tract, is thought to multiply first in the local lymph nodes draining the point of entry and then more generally throughout the reticulo-endothelial system before reaching the skin.

Variola virus survives for long periods in dust at room temperatures, and even heating at 100°C for 5 minutes fails to inactivate it if it is dry.

Cowpox is a disease of cattle. Its lesions resemble those of smallpox, but the infection causes little or no systemic disturbance, either to cattle or to humans who acquire it from them—and are thereby immunized against smallpox, as Jenner discovered (see p 11).

Vaccinia is the condition resulting from infection with the virus currently used for immunization against smallpox (see p 315). The origins of this virus are uncertain. It may well be that some of the strains now used were derived from smallpox viruses and some from cowpox viruses, both types having been so modified by animal passage that they are now identical. Vaccinia virus is maintained at the desired level of pathogenicity for man—able to produce local lesions but not progressive disease—by passaging it alternately in the skin of a rabbit and in that of a calf or sheep. 'Calf lymph', the material commonly used for smallpox vaccination, is made by collecting fluid from artificially induced pox lesions on the skin of a calf or sheep, and mixing it with four times its volume of 50% glycerol. It is then stored at −10°C, and the glycerol slowly destroys any contaminating bacteria. Alternatively, the vesicle fluid is first treated with phenol (to which the virus is resistant) before the glycerol is added. The lymph remains potent for some weeks if constantly refrigerated, but the virus rapidly becomes inactive if kept at room temperature.

DIFFERENTIATION OF VARIOLA AND VACCINIA VIRUSES Microscopically, antigenically and in most other ways these viruses are indistinguishable, but it may be epidemiologically important to know whether a patient with a pox-type rash is suffering from variola major, variola minor or only vaccinia. This information can be obtained by growing the virus on hen's egg chorio-allantoic membrane. There are differences between the lesions (pocks) produced there, after 3 days' incubation at 37°C, by the viruses of smallpox, vaccinia, cowpox (a less common source of diagnostic confusion) or herpes simplex. Vaccinia viruses, unlike those of smallpox, multiply and form pocks in eggs incubated at 39°C. The laboratory distinction between variola major and variola minor is difficult.

LABORATORY DIAGNOSIS OF SMALLPOX Rapid diagnosis may be of great importance in this disease, and for this reason electron microscopy is a valuable means of distinguishing poxvirus infections from those due to other viruses, notably chickenpox. Fluid or crusts from skin lesions are used for this purpose. Such material can also be stained and examined by light microscopy for elementary bodies and Guarnieri inclusion bodies. Gel-diffusion tests for antigen (see p 68), using rabbit anti-variola serum, may clearly indicate a poxvirus infection within a few hours of being set up; or by using serum from zoster patients in parallel tests it may be possible to make a firm diagnosis of chickenpox instead. Variola antigen may be detectable in the patient's serum also. The virus may be isolated, and its type determined, by chorio-allantoic membrane culture of material from lesions, or of blood collected in the pre-eruptive stage of the illness. Complement-fixation, gel-diffusion and haemagglutination-inhibition tests for antibodies in the patient's serum are virtually always positive in smallpox, but not until the end of the first week at the earliest; interpretation of early tests are complicated by pre-existing antibody levels in patients vaccinated within the past year or so.

PROPHYLAXIS The use of vaccinia virus for active immunization is discussed on p 315, and the chemoprophylactic use of methisazone on p 180.

HEPATITIS

Since the early days of World War 2 (a time at which blood transfusion was undertaken on an unprecedented scale) it has been possible to distinguish on epidemiological grounds between two clinically similar types of hepatitis, both clearly due to viruses or virus-like agents even though these agents could not be seen or cultured:

(1) *Infective hepatitis*, a world-wide disease, often occurring in epidemics, and mainly affecting children and young adults; usually transmitted by faecal excretion and oral ingestion (the faeco-oral route), with flies, food, water and other vectors often involved; and having an incubation period of 2–6 weeks.

(2) *Serum hepatitis*, usually transmitted by transfusion or injection of human blood, plasma or serum (even of the minute amounts transferred by drawing up several doses of a vaccine into a syringe and using it to inject a series of patients, with minimal reflux when changing needles); and having an incubation period of 6 weeks to 5 months.

Both types have a spectrum of severity ranging from subclinical infection through to acute liver necrosis with death of the patient; intermediate degrees of liver damage may be followed by complete recovery or (in the case of serum hepatitis at least) by chronic hepatitis, leading on to cirrhosis in some cases.

This epidemiological classification, while useful in the understanding of the hepatitis problem as a whole, was often difficult to apply to the individual case, particularly in the absence of an epidemic or of any information as to the probable source of infection or time of exposure. The situation became more complicated when it was discovered that the difference in mode of transmission of the two types was by no means clear-cut, since infectious hepatitis can be transmitted in blood and serum hepatitis can be acquired by ingestion, as well as by application of minute amounts of infected material to minor abrasions of the skin, or probably even by sexual intercourse or by use of a common tooth-brush.

The first advance towards a classification of cases of virus hepatitis according to aetiological agents resulted from a totally unconnected investigation. In 1964 the blood of a certain Australian aborigine was found to contain an antigen (subsequently known as *Australia antigen*) which gave a precipitin reaction with the serum of a much-transfused haemophiliac. The same antigen was subsequently found in the blood of many patients with hepatitis of the long-incubation type. Hepatitis associated with the presence of this antigen is now called hepatitis B, and the antigen has been renamed hepatitis B or HB antigen. Its nature is further discussed below. Recognition of an agent associated with short-incubation hepatitis followed in 1973, and the condition for which it is responsible is now known as hepatitis A. As tests have been developed which make it possible to classify most cases of hepatitis as either A or B, it is becoming clear that there are still some cases which do not fit into either category and which cannot be attributed to the E.B. virus, the cytomegalovirus or any other known agent.

Hepatitis A and B Viruses

HEPATITIS A VIRUS is a small virus (25–28 nm), of cubic symmetry and morphologically similar to the enteroviruses. It appears to have been successfully transferred from man to marmosets and to chimpanzees, but has not been grown in culture. It can be found in electron-micrographs of faeces of patients in the early stages of hepatitis of the short-incubation (infective hepatitis) type, and antibodies to it appear in the blood of such patients shortly afterwards, often persisting for many years. Such antibodies can be detected by complement fixation and various other procedures. There is no longer any room for doubt about the role of this organism as the cause of most cases of short-incubation virus hepatitis, but a great deal remains to be discovered about the virus itself.

HEPATITIS B VIRUS, having been detected some 9 years earlier than hepatitis A virus, has been more fully studied. Electron-micrographs of sera from patients with long-incubation hepatitis, and from some other people who are symptomless carriers of the virus, show 3 characteristic types of particle – 42 nm double-shelled spherical particles believed to be the viruses proper (formerly known as Dane particles); 22 nm spheres; and filaments of similar diameter. The latter two types are thought to consist of capsid material, since they share an antigen (the original Australia antigen) found on the surfaces of the 42 nm particles and known as hepatitis B surface antigen (HBsAg). A second antigen, found only after disruption of the 42 nm particles, is known as hepatitis B core antigen (HBcAg). This cannot be found in patients' blood, but a third antigen (HBeAg) can be found there, and its presence correlates with the presence of 42 nm particles in the blood and with a high level of infectivity. Serological tests for antigens are far more practicable than electron microscopy when testing large numbers of blood samples for the presence of the virus. Of the various tests that have been devised, the one most commonly used at present is a passive haemagglutination procedure, in which red cells coated with anti-HBs antibody (from the serum of a convalescent patient) are exposed to the serum under test and are agglutinated if it contains HBsAg. Subgroups of HBsAg and HBeAg have been defined and are useful in epidemiological studies.

HBsAg and HBeAg are detectable in serum during the last few weeks of the long incubation period, before the onset of clinical hepatitis, and as a rule for some weeks afterwards, HBsAg persisting longer than HBeAg and each of them disappearing at about the time that its corresponding antibody becomes detectable. These antibodies are long-lasting, but anti-HBc antibody, which appears earlier, is transitory, and therefore its presence indicates recent infection with hepatitis B virus. In some patients, and also in some carriers who have never had clinical hepatitis, the virus may persist for years, as indicated by positive tests for HBsAg and HBeAg and by infectivity of their blood to any who may be exposed to it. All potential blood donors must therefore be screened to exclude the possibility of their being carriers of hepatitis B virus. Furthermore, *all* samples of human blood should be regarded and treated as potential sources of hepatitis B infection for medical and nursing staff, laboratory workers and all others exposed to them, until tests for HB antigens have excluded this possibility – though clearly the risk is greater if the samples come from jaundiced patients. The assortment of people among whom persistent carriage of hepatitis B virus is particularly common includes children with Down's syndrome, patients with lepromatous leprosy, patients undergoing haemodialysis, drug addicts and those who have been tattooed. The carriage rate in the community in general is of the order of 1:1000 in Britain, but as high as 5–10% in some countries, notably in the tropics.

PROPHYLAXIS   Active immunization is not yet possible against either of these viruses, but is the subject of vigorous research, since both diseases are common, liable to be severe and virtually untreatable. Injections of pooled normal human immunuglobulin provide passive protection for 4–6 months against hepatitis A; they are valuable as a means of controlling an outbreak of this disease in a closed community, such as a school, and usually prevent the disease even if not given until a few days after exposure. Such injections are also widely and effectively used to protect travellers going to countries where this disease is common. Normal human immunoglobulin is not effective, however, in preventing hepatitis B, but special hyperimmune immunoglobulin (prepared from sera with high titres of anti-HB antibodies) has been found to protect against it when given after a known exposure, such as an accident with a contaminated needle or scalpel.

BACTERIOPHAGES

Bacterial cultures on solid media sometimes have a 'moth-eaten' appearance, due to the presence of many small areas in which the bacteria have been lysed. This phenomenon was first studied by Twort in 1915. He found that bacterium-free filtrates of a suspension of such a culture of staphylococci could produce similar lysis in other staphylococcal cultures. In 1917 d'Herelle, working with fluid cultures of dysentery bacilli, discovered a similar lytic activity, and concluded that it was due to very small living agents parasitic upon the bacteria. He called them *bacteriophages*, a name which has persisted and is often abbreviated to *phages*.

Bacteriophages are in fact a group of viruses. They have been demonstrated in connection with many bacterial species, but show a high degree of host-specificity, so that any one phage is usually limited not only to a single bacterial species but to certain strains of that species. As we have seen (e.g. pp 97 and 129), this specificity is of practical value in the subdivision of species for epidemiological purposes.

Bacteriophages can be recovered from such natural sources as faeces, sewage and polluted water. Their presence can be demonstrated by applying bacterium-free filtrates of such materials to cultures of susceptible bacteria, but they are also carried inside bacteria which have only a latent infection and do not undergo lysis (lysogenic bacteria, described more fully later).

Phages differ in size and form, but as a group they have the greatest structural complexity of any viruses. The nucleic acid is DNA in most of those that have been studied, including those that have been the subject of the most intensive investigation, the T phages of *Esch. coli*. Such a phage is tadpole-shaped, its head consisting of a DNA core surrounded by a protein coat that corresponds to the capsid of an animal virus. Taking the T2 phage as an example, the head is about 100 nm long and consists of a short tube, hexagonal in cross-section and about 60 nm across, closed at its ends by caps that are two halves of an icosahedron. From one of these ends emerges a thin hollow tubular tail, with an end-plate and terminal fibres that are the means by which the virus becomes attached and adsorbed to the cell wall of its bacterial host. Such adsorption is possible only if the phage, which is non-motile, happens to come into contact with a bacterium of a strain with the appropriate specific receptors on its surface, and if various other conditions are fulfilled. Once adsorbed, the phage digests a small area of bacterial cell wall and then contracts, injecting its DNA into the bacterial body.

Bacteriolysis

If a large excess of phages is added to a bacterial culture, so that many phages are adsorbed on to each bacterium, the cells may be disrupted because many small areas of their walls are dissolved at once–'lysis from without'. If the infection is not so heavy, the bacteria survive this external assault, but intracellular phage multiplication may then occur, beginning within a few minutes of the injection of the phage DNA. Instead of synthesizing its own DNA, the bacterial cell provides that for new phages, and also supplies them with their protein coats. Within an hour or less, many phages have been formed, which then lyse the cell and are released–'lysis from within'.

As we have already indicated, bacteriolysis by phage can be studied in cultures either on solid or in fluid media. A bacterial 'lawn' can be produced by inoculating the whole surface of an agar plate with the bacterial strain to be studied. Before this culture is· incubated, fluid preparations of various phages can be spotted on to it in marked positions. The culture is then incubated overnight, and lytic action of bacterio-phages is shown by failure of bacterial growth in the areas on to which the preparations were spotted. If the number of effective phage particles is small, each one produces a separate small defect in the bacterial lawn–*a plaque*–roughly analogous to a single bacterial colony; but a large number of effective phage particles will produce confluent lysis of the whole area covered by the original spot. Bacteriolysis in a fluid culture becomes apparent far more rapidly, a broth culture of a susceptible bacterium becoming crystal clear within 30 to 60 minutes of the addition of a phage preparation; but of course only one phage preparation can be tested for lytic action on any one culture in this way, whereas the lawn procedure on a solid medium allows the testing of many preparations simultaneously on a single plate.

Lysogeny

Infection of a bacterium by phage is not necessarily followed by phage multiplication and bacteriolysis. Sometimes when phage DNA enters a host cell it does not derange its synthetic activities but is integrated into the bacterial chromosome. Such a phage is described as *temperate*, as distinct from *virulent* or *lytic*, and the integrated non-lytic form in which it persists in the cell is called *prophage*. In this form it is reproduced synchronously with the bacterium and handed down to all the progeny of the original cell. This relationship is described as *lysogeny* and the host bacterium as *lysogenic* because in certain circumstances propagation and release of the phage may occur, and it may then cause lysis of other bacterial strains. Such propagation may occur spontaneously, and it can also be induced by using ultra-violet light or various chemicals. A lysogenic bacterial strain is also resistant to lysis by another preparation of the same phage as that which it is carrying.

Transduction and Lysogenic Conversion

The role of temperate phages in the *transduction* of genetic material from one bacterial strain to another has already been mentioned (p 33). *Lysogenic conversion* is somewhat different, in that the phage does not transfer a property from one strain to another but the phage's own DNA confers new properties upon strains with which it enters into a lysogenic relationship. Thus certain phages, when they lysogenize non-toxigenic *C. diphtheriae* strains, render them toxigenic (p 112).

Suggestions for Further Reading

Virus Hunters by Greer Williams (Hutchinson, London, 1960) for the history of virological reasearch.
Notes on Medical Virology by Morag C. Timbury, 6th edn. (Churchill Livingstone, Edinburgh, New York and London, 1978).

12

Fungi

Fungi are eukaryotes (see p 17). The microscopic fungi are a large and varied group, classified mainly according to their methods of sexual reproduction. However, the few species that are pathogenic to man are mostly included in the *fungi imperfecti* because they have no known sexual phase to their life-cycle. The study of fungi is called *mycology*, and diseases caused by fungi are known as *mycoses*.

The fungi with which we are concerned can be divided into four groups:

(1) *Filamentous fungi or moulds* form branching tubular filaments or *hyphae* which are interwoven into a felt-like *mycelium*. Hyphae vary considerably in thickness, but even the finest are much coarser than bacterial filaments. They may be divided by transverse partitions called *septa*. In cultures some of the mycelium is embedded in the medium, some lies on its surface and some is raised into the air, giving to the colonies a fluffy appearance such as is seen also in naturally occurring surface growth of moulds. These fungi produce asexual spores of many kinds, including *arthrospores*, formed by the breaking up of hyphae into short lengths; *chlamydospores*, formed by local hyphal dilatations; and *conidia*. These last may be single-celled micro-conidia, about 2–6 μm in diameter, or considerably larger macro-conidia, containing a number of cells; in either case they are borne on special hyphal structures called *conidiophores*.

(2) *Yeasts* are single round or oval cells which reproduce by forming small lateral buds that enlarge and develop into new cells. Their colonies on culture media resemble those of bacteria.

(3) *Yeast-like fungi*, such as the medically important genus *Candida*, also reproduce by budding. However, the buds tend to elongate into filaments (*pseudohyphae*) which remain linked together in chains that

have some resemblance to mould mycelium. They can be differentiated by the facts that pseudohyphae do not form arthrospores or conidia and do not branch, though two or more buds may arise from the same end of a single filamentous cell and so give an appearance of branching.

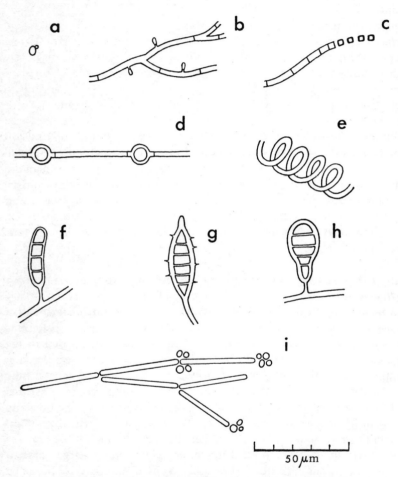

Figure 4   Some morphological features of fungi.

(a) The same yeast as in Fig. 3(p), to emphasize the difference of scale.
(b) Branching septate mycelium with lateral microconidia.
(c) A hypha breaking up to form arthrospores.
(d) A hypha showing chlamydospores.
(e) A spiral hypha.
(f, g and h) Macroconidia of *Trichophyton*, *Microsporum* and *Epidermophyton*.
(i) Pseudohyphae of a yeast-like fungus with yeast forms at junctions.

(4) *Dimorphic fungi* have a yeast morphology in tissues or when growing in cultures at 37°C, but form mycelium when growing saprophytically in the soil or in cultures at ordinary room temperatures.

Although many pathogenic fungi will grow on ordinary bacteriological culture media, they grow better and with less risk of bacterial overgrowth on special mycological media. The commonest of these is *Sabouraud's glucose agar* medium, which used to depend for its suppression of bacteria upon its high glucose content (4%) and its acidity (pH around 5·4). Since this acidity also discourages the growth of some pathogenic fungi, the medium is now commonly used at a neutral reaction with the addition of chloramphenicol to suppress the bacteria. Cycloheximide is often included as well in order to suppress non-pathogenic fungi, but it also inhibits some of the rarer pathogens. On such a medium, most of the pathogenic fungi grow as well at room temperatures as they do at 37°C.

The fungi of medical importance are more conveniently discussed according to the diseases that they cause than according to any taxonomic arrangement.

CANDIDIASIS (MONILIASIS)
Candida (or Monilia) albicans

This is a yeast-like fungus commonly present in the upper respiratory, alimentary and female genital tracts and on the skins of healthy people. From time to time it becomes pathogenic, often as a sequel to malnutrition, general debility, diabetes, antibiotic suppression of the bacterial flora which normally inhibit proliferation of these and other fungi, steroid therapy, immunosuppression or other predisposing factors. It can then cause a wide variety of disorders, including the following:

(1) *Thrush*, a superficial infection of the mucous membrane of the mouth, characterized by white adherent patches of pseudomycelium. This affects mainly small children or elderly patients.

(2) *Vulvo-vaginitis*, with white discharge and much irritation, affecting mainly adults and more common during pregnancy.

(3) *Chronic paronychia* of housewives, barmaids, fruit packers and others whose hands are constantly in water.

(4) *Dermatitis*, usually affecting warm moist skin folds (e.g. intra-gluteal or sub-mammary) or obese subjects. The skin becomes red, exudative and irritant.

(5) *Bronchial candidiasis*, a rare condition in Britain, in which the fungus invades the bronchial walls and lungs and may go on to

produce a generalized infection. This must be clearly distinguished from the multiplication of *C. albicans* in the bronchi which often follows vigorous antibiotic treatment of bacterial infections, and which usually ceases spontaneously when treatment is stopped, though on rare occasions it may develop into a true bronchial candidiasis.

(6) *Candida enteritis*, almost always a consequence of suppression of the normal bowel flora by broad-spectrum antibiotics.

(7) *Candida endocarditis*, formerly a rare disease mainly of drug addicts and diabetics (who presumably introduced the organism into their blood when giving themselves injections), but more recently a serious and all-too-common complication of heart-valve replacement.

LABORATORY INVESTIGATION   The oval yeast cells, 2–5 μm in diameter, and the larger pseudohyphae are strongly Gram-positive and are easily recognized in stained films. Alternatively they may be demonstrated in skin and nail scrapings by the methods described below for the dermatophytes. Their mere presence in clinical specimens means little, and even their presence in abundance is significant only if the specimen is fresh, as they multiply rapidly at room temperatures. They give visible growth on blood agar after overnight incubation at 37°C, but are more easily recognized on Sabouraud's medium, on which they form moist creamy colonies. *Candida* species show characteristic submerged growth with budding (*blastospore* formation) when inoculated into the depths of a plate of corn-meal agar, and *Candida albicans* can be differentiated from other species of the genus by its formation of chlamydospores in such circumstances, by its carbohydrate fermentation reactions, and by its formation of germ-tubes within a few hours of inoculation into neat human serum. *C. tropicalis* and other species of this genus are also sometimes pathogenic to man.

TREATMENT   The first step is to remove the predisposing cause, if possible—in particular, to stop or change antibiotic therapy if candidiasis threatens to be troublesome. Local applications of 1% gentian violet is effective in the treatment of thrush, and an antibiotic *nystatin*, which has no useful antibacterial action, is valuable for the treatment of accessible candida infections, such as vulvovaginitis and the intestinal candidiasis that sometimes follows treatment with wide-spectrum antibacterial agents. Since it is poorly absorbed from the intestine and cannot be given parenterally, nystatin is of no value for generalized candidiasis. The antibiotic *amphotericin B* is an alternative to nystatin for local and oral administration and can also be given intravenously for treatment of generalized infections, or these can be treated by oral administration of *5-fluorocytosine*. However, these and all other available drugs for treatment of systemic fungal infections have unpleasant and sometimes serious side-effects.

RINGWORM (THE DERMATOMYCOSES)

Fungi of the genera *Trichopyton, Epidermophyton* and *Microsporum*, collectively known as the *dermatophytes*, cause superficial infections of the keratinized layers of the skin, hair and nails but never attack deeper tissues. There is considerable overlap in the clinical syndromes which they produce, but *Epidermophyton floccosum* (the only species in this genus) does not attack hair and *Microsporum* species do not attack nails. Infection is commonly from man to man. For example, *tinea pedis* (athlete's foot), usually due to *T. rubrum* or *T. mentagrophytes*, is frequently transmitted via wet floors around swimming pools and bath-rooms; and *tinea capitis* (scalp ringworm) due to *M. audouini*, which affects children before puberty, is readily transmitted by direct contact or via infected combs and brushes. Other species are acquired from animals – e.g. *M. canis*, which affects dogs, cats and other animals and is transmitted to human beings, particularly children, in close contact with them. Human infections with such animal pathogens tend to provoke vigorous local reactions and to be self-limiting.

LABORATORY INVESTIGATION   Scales are collected from skin lesions by scraping with a blunt scalpel; swabbing the skin first with 70% alcohol may help to reduce bacterial contamination. The scales should be placed in a folded piece of paper (preferably black) for transmission to the laboratory. Infected hairs are carefully extracted from their follicles, using forceps; dull, broken hairs should be taken, and recognition of hairs infected with *Microsporum* species is helped by the fact that they fluoresce in U.V. light. Full thickness clippings of affected nails are taken for examination, together with debris from under the nails.

Portions of these specimens are placed on slides in drops of 20–30% KOH, covered with coverslips and warmed gently. This treatment dissolves the host cells, and the highly refractile fungal elements can then be seen, using a microscope with a dry objective. Nail clippings usually need preliminary softening in KOH in a test tube before they can be made into microscopic preparations. In skin or nails all of the dermatophytes form branching hyphae and arthrospores, and are indistinguishable from one another. Hyphae also abound in and around the roots of hairs, but spores predominate further up the hairs. In those infected with *Microsporum* and some *Trichophyton* species, the spores are closely applied to the outside of the hairs (ectothrix), whereas those of other *Trichophyton* species are within the hairs (endothrix).

Material that has not been treated with KOH is inoculated on to

Sabouraud's or other suitable media and kept at room temperature. Colonies take 1 to 3 weeks to appear, and species recognition depends on the fluffiness, texture and colour of the colonies and on the liberation of pigment into the medium, and also on the microscopic appearances of the growth. Among the most important distinctive features are the macro-conidia, which may be cylindrical (*Trichophyton*), spindle- or boat-shaped (*Microsporum*) or pear-shaped (*Epidermophyton*). The number, shape and distribution of the macroconidia and the presence or absence of other structures such as chlamydospores and spiral hyphae help in species identification (see Fig. 4, p 214).

TREATMENT   In some dermatophyte infections, notably athlete's foot, secondary bacterial infection may have to be dealt with before the fungal infection can be controlled. Ointments of benzoic, salicylic or undecylinic acid or combinations of these were for many years the best treatments for skin ringworm; surgical removal was often the only effective way to deal with infected nails; and infected hair was removed by X-irradiation. The introduction of the antibiotic *griseofulvin* radically changed the situation. This antibiotic, which is valueless in treatment of bacterial or monilial infections, cures most forms of ringworm. Taken by mouth for a number of weeks, it is incorporated in newly-formed cells of the skin and its appendages, and makes them unsuitable media for the growth of most dermatophytes. These cells then gradually replace the existing kerati-nized epithelial layers, hair and nails, causing the dermatophyte infection to die out. Nail infection is the form of ringworm that most commonly fails to respond to such treatment.

Pityriasis versicolor
This common and benign form of skin ringworm produces red, scaling patches on the body and limbs. It is caused by *Pityrosporum furfur* (*P. orbiculare*), a yeast-like fungus which is readily recognized in KOH preparations of scales by its characteristic mixture of round budding cells and short irregular lengths of mycelium. If confirmatory culture is required, olive oil or other suitable lipid must be added to the medium. A closely similar lipophilic organism, *P. ovale*, is commonly found on human skin, particularly in association with dandruff. Pityriasis versi-color usually responds well to treatment with a sulphur ointment.

ASPERGILLOSIS
Members of the genus *Aspergillus* are common saprophytic moulds, such as grow on stored foods. They are recognized by their conidiophores. These are swollen ends of hyphae from which radiate large numbers of sterigmata (short lengths of narrower hyphae) ending in short chains of

spores. Species of this genus are occasionally pathogenic to man, but since they are common saprophytes and multiply rapidly at room temperature, their presence in clinical specimens is significant only if these are very recently collected. The conditions produced include:

1 *Otomycosis.*   A chronic condition in which the external auditory meatus is filled with fungal growth, usually of *A. niger*. Treatment is complex and difficult.

2 *Pulmonary aspergillosis.*   This term is used to cover several different conditions. It is believed that some patients develop a hypersensitivity to aspergilli, which leads to asthmatic bronchial spasm and even patchy collapse of the lungs as a result of the mere presence of the fungus on the bronchial mucosa. In other patients, the fungus grows in the bronchi in much the same way as it does in the ears and may also invade the lung parenchyma. Amphotericin B may be effective in treatment of such cases. In yet other cases an aspergillus, usually *A. fumigatus*, invades a lung abscess cavity or lung tissue damaged by infarction, and forms a giant colony. This lies free within the lung, surrounded by air, and does not invade healthy lung tissue. Such a mass is called an *aspergilloma*. Treatment is by surgical removal.

THE DEEP MYCOSES

Apart from candidiasis, fungus infections that involve deep structures are rare in Britain. In the absence of suitable treatment they are commonly fatal, but good results have been obtained with amphotericin B in each of the conditions described below, and other effective treatments for some of them are indicated in the appropriate paragraphs.

Cryptococcus neoformans (*Torula histolytica*)

This is a true yeast found in soil throughout the world. It is an occasional cause of disease in man and animals. Human infection begins as a local cutaneous or pulmonary lesion but usually becomes generalized, its commonest feature being a form of subacute or chronic meningitis which is liable to be mistaken for a brain abscess or tumour. The yeasts can be seen by microscopic examination of the cerebrospinal fluid, and their characteristic large capsules are well demonstrated if indian ink is first added to the fluid to provide a dark background. They grow well on Sabouraud's glucose agar, forming creamy colonies and differing from other saprophytic yeasts in that they grow rapidly at $37°C$. 5-fluorocytosine is a valuable alternative or addition to amphotericin B in treatment of cryptococcosis.

Blastomyces dermatitidis

Blastomycosis, the disease caused by this dimorphic fungus which is thought to have its main habitat in soil, was formerly believed to be restricted to eastern parts of the U.S.A. and Canada and was known as N. American blastomycosis. However, there is increasing evidence of its occurrence in S. America and in many parts of Africa. The fungus probably enters the human body via the respiratory tract. It may then cause chronic lesions of skin, bones, viscera and meninges. The organisms can be seen in their yeast state in the lesions, and can be grown on ordinary mycological media. Hydroxystilbamidine is often effective in treatment.

Paracoccidioides brasiliensis

Paracoccidioidomycosis (formerly known as S. American blastomycosis, and indeed apparently restricted to S. America, with its highest reported incidence in Brazil) is due to another dimorphic fungus, of which the natural habitat is not known. Initial ulcerative lesions of the oral or nasal mucous membranes may be followed by systemic spread, mainly to lymphatic tissues. Surprisingly for a fungus infection, sulphonamides are of some value in controlling (though not usually curing) the disease; even amphotericin B is not reliably effective.

Histoplasma capsulatum

This is another dimorphic fungus found in soil, notably in parts of the U.S.A. In endemic areas symptomless human infection is common, as judged by the frequency of skin hypersensitivity to an extract of the organism called histoplasmin. Miliary lung lesions, similar to those of tuberculosis but healing spontaneously, are often found in such people. In a few subjects the infection progresses to involve lymph nodes and other organs, causing a febrile and often fatal illness.

Coccidioides immitis

This is also a dimorphic fungus found in the soil. It is largely restricted to certain areas of the south-west of the U.S.A. Almost all of the inhabitants of those areas are infected, most of them without symptoms but with the development of a coccidioidin hypersensitivity. A very few of those infected develop a generalized tuberculosis-like illness with a bad prognosis.

Hormodendrum pedrosoi, H. compactum, Phialophora verrucosa

These and certain other filamentous fungi cause a disease incongruously named *chromoblastomycosis* (the only colourful element being the brown fungal bodies seen in microscopic preparations from lesions and the disease not being a blastomycosis or yeast infection). This disease is world-wide but mainly tropical. The organisms, which are to be found in soil and on trees and plants, enter the skin, usually of a forester or farm worker, as a result of some minor penetrating injury. Very slowly the surrounding skin becomes thickened and crusted, and the lesion gradually extends, possibly to involve the surface of a whole limb or more. In the soft material underlying the crusts are to be found many rounded brown structures, 10 μm or so in diameter, usually divided into compartments in a 'hot cross bun' manner. Inoculated on to Sabouraud's glucose agar, these give the black or brown colonies of one of the causative fungi. Generous excision of all affected skin was the only effective treatment before the introduction of amphotericin B.

IMMUNOLOGY OF THE MYCOSES

IMMUNITY In general, no detectable immunity follows natural infections of human beings by fungi. Histoplasmosis and coccidioidomycosis are exceptions to this rule, but even for these no method of artificial immunization has been worked out.

SEROLOGICAL TESTS   Tests for specific agglutinins and precipitins in patients' blood may provide useful information in suspected candidiasis, aspergillosis and other mycoses, but they have to be interpreted with due allowance for the frequency of such antibodies in the blood of healthy people. Measurement of complement-fixing antibodies for the appropriate organisms is of diagnostic and prognostic value in the deep mycoses due to dimorphic fungi.

SKIN TESTS FOR HYPERSENSITIVITY   Delayed-type hypersensitivity to fungal extracts can be demonstrated in a number of mycosis by procedures similar to the tuberculin test (see p 267). Like most tests of this nature, they indicate only whether the patient has at some time been exposed to the relevant organism. The trichophytin and aspergillin tests are therefore of limited value because of the ubiquity of their respective fungi. Positive reactions to blastomycin, paracoccidioidin, histoplasmin and coccidioidin are more informative.

Suggestions for Further Reading

Manual of Clinical Mycology by N. F. Conant and others, 3rd edn. (Saunders, Philadelphia, London and Toronto, 1971).

Medical Mycology by C. W. Emmons and others, 3rd edn. (Lea and Febiger, Philadelphia, 1977).

Also Section V of *Bacteriology Illustrated*—see p 159.

13

Protozoa

Protozoa are unicellular eukaryotes (see p 17), in most cases considerably larger than bacteria but still of microscopic dimensions. They all have nuclei clearly differentiated from their cytoplasm. They vary greatly in shape, structure and habitat. The phylum is divided into *Sporozoa, Mastigophora, Sarcodina* and *Ciliophora*.

All four of these subphyla are represented among man's parasites. Only a few of them are pathogenic, but since they include the causative organisms of malaria, trypanosomiasis and amoebic dysentery they make a formidable contribution to human illness and mortality.

SPOROZOA
THE GENUS PLASMODIUM

Malaria was formerly endemic in Britain and other temperate countries but is now mainly restricted to the tropics and subtropics. The four plasmodial species that are pathogenic to man – *P. vivax, P. falciparum, P. malariae* and *P. ovale* – respectively cause *benign tertian, malignant tertian, quartan* and *ovale* malaria. The terms tertian and quartan refer to the periodicity of the bouts of fever associates with the disease, with the days counted according to the Roman convention so that tertian fever recurs every 48 hours and quartan every 72 hours. Other plasmodial species are pathogenic to monkeys and birds.

Man becomes infected when he is bitten by a female *Anopheles* mosquito in which the parasites have completed the sexual cycle to be described below. Entering the human blood-stream as a minute spindle-shaped *sporozoites*, the plasmodia pass to the liver where they develop into larger multicellular *schizonts*. Usually about 5 to 10 days after infection (depending upon the plasmodial species) the schizonts disrupt into many *merozoites*. This completes the *pre-erythrocytic* cycle. Some of the merozoites re-enter the liver and the same cycle, now called the *exo-*

erythrocytic cycle, is repeated over and over, except in *P. falciparum* infections. Meanwhile, other merozoites have entered the red cells of the blood and initiated a similar but shorter *erythrocytic cycle*, which ends with the rupture of the infected red cells and the release of further batches of merozoites. The length of the erythrocytic cycle determines the periodicity of the fever, though the patient does not experience symptoms during the first few cycles, which involve relatively small numbers of red cells. *P. falciparum* causes infected red cells to agglutinate, with consequent capillary obstruction and the high incidence of severe cerebral and other complications which have earned for this form of malaria the name 'malignant'.

Instead of developing into schizonts, some of the merozoites which invade red cells become either male or female *gametocytes*. It is on these sexual forms that transmission of malaria depends, for when sucked up by a female *Anopheles* they fuse to form zygotes, which develop into *oöcysts* in the mosquito's stomach wall. Mature oöcysts rupture and release *sporozoites*, which make their way to the insect's salivary glands and are then ready to initiate a fresh human infection.

LABORATORY INVESTIGATION   Plasmodia can be recognized in blood films stained with haemotological stains such as Giemsa's. Since parasites may be few, thick films are used for their detection, but their morphology is more easily studied in thinner films. Species recognition depends upon the appearances of the *trophozoites* (ring-shaped precursors of schizonts), of the schizonts and of the gametocytes, and also upon the presence and colour of pigment granules in infected red cells. *P. ovale* takes its name from the fact that the infected red cells tend to elongate.

TREATMENT AND CONTROL   Quinine, the time-honoured remedy for malaria, has now been joined by an array of synthetic drugs, some of them related to it. Such antimalarial drugs are used for three purposes – to *treat* an acute attack, to *suppress* an infection so that it gives no clinical manifestations, and to *eradicate* the infection. For treatment of an attack chloroquine is the most valuable drug; but in parts of S. America and S.E. Asia *P. falciparum* strains are now encountered which are resistant to chloroquine and related compounds. In such circumstances mepacrine or quinine can be used, or a sulphonamide and pyrimethamine together (see p 342). Chloroquine has also been widely used for suppression of the erythrocytic cycle, and thus of clinical manifestations, in those who visit or live in areas where malarial infection is likely. However, to avoid encouraging the development of chloroquine-resistant strains, proguanil or pyrimethamine should now be used for such suppression. The drugs mentioned so far are active against schizonts and to varying degrees against gametocytes. Since they cannot kill either sporozoites or the exo-erythrocytic stages, they do not prevent infection and they can eradicate it only in the case of *P. falciparum*, which has no exoerythrocytic cycle. Primaquine kills the exo-erythrocytic stages and so in conjunction with one of the other drugs it can eradicate infection by the other species.

Eradication of malaria from a community depends upon a two-pronged attack–treatment of infected human beings so that there is no source of gametocytes, and control of the mosquito vectors. The methods used in achieving the latter vary considerably from place to place because of the varied habits of different *Anopheles* species. They include swamp drainage and other measures to eliminate suitable breeding grounds, oiling the surface of exposed waters to asphyxiate larvae, and spraying houses with long-acting insecticides. Reports of success in the *in vitro* culture of *P. falciparum* suggest the possibility that a vaccine for active immunization against this form of malaria may become available.

THE GENUS TOXOPLASMA
Toxoplasma gondii
First described in 1908, and named after one of its earliest known hosts, an African rodent called the gondi, this species has a world-wide distribution in animals and birds, but its pathogenicity to man was unrecognized until 1939. The probable major source of human infection is suggested by the discovery, reported in 1970, that a sexual phase of the life-cycle of *T. gondii* can occur in the intestine of the domestic cat (which itself could become infected by eating rodents). The majority of human infections are sub-clinical. Of the various clinical manifestations, all of them rare, the following are among the most important:

(1) Transplacental transmission of *T. gondii* from a mother who acquired her primary infection during the pregnancy may result in stillbirth, neonatal death or congenital deformities. Hydrocephalus, microcephaly, intracerebral calcification, chorio-retinitis and psycho-motor retardation are common features of congenital toxoplasmosis.

(2) Infection acquired in early childhood may cause fatal encephalitis.

(3) Infection during later childhood or adult life may cause a benign febrile illness with the clinical and haematological features of infectious mononucleosis; heterophil antibodies are not formed (see p 204).

(4) Chorio-retinitis and other eye lesions may occur as part of one of the above pictures or separately.

LABORATORY INVESTIGATION   The crescent-shaped nucleate protozoa, about 6 μm by 3 μm, can be demonstrated inside and between the cells of affected tissues by staining smears with haematological stains. They may also be found in blood or other body fluids. They can be grown in tissue cultures or in eggs, but intracerebral and intraperitoneal injection into young mice are generally employed for their identification and maintenance.

Antibodies can be detected in the blood of patients, and of many healthy adults who have presumably had subclinical infections. The methods in current use include a fluorescent-antibody procedure similar to the FTA test (see p 263), indirect haemagglutination and complement-fixation procedures and the Sabin–Feldman dye test, which depends upon the fact that after exposure to specific antibodies the parasites resist staining with alkaline methylene blue.

Combined therapy with a sulphonamide and pyrimethamine (see p 342) has given good results in this previously untreatable disease.

MASTIGOPHORA (FLAGELLATES)
THE GENUS TRICHOMONAS
Trichomonas vaginalis

This is a pear-shaped organism, usually 15–20 μm long, with four flagella arising from its blunt end and an undulating membrane down one side. It is found throughout the world, in the genito-urinary tracts of both sexes. In the male, infection is commonly symptomless but there may be a white urethral discharge. In the female *T. vaginalis* may cause vulvo-vaginitis, with a characteristic frothy, yellow or cream-coloured alkaline discharge. It cannot survive at the pH level of the healthy adult vagina, and probably depends upon disturbance of the normal flora for its establishment there. Transmission is commonly but not exclusively by sexual intercourse.

LABORATORY INVESTIGATION   In wet microscopic preparations made as soon as the specimen of discharge is collected *T. vaginalis* is easily recognized by its shape, its ungainly movements and the undulations of its membrane. Identification is considerably more difficult in older specimens or in stained films. In most cases it is possible to grow the organism in artificial culture media.

TREATMENT   Arsenicals and other chemicals have been used for the local treatment of trichomonal vaginitis, with some success but with a high rate of relapse or reinfection because of the difficulty of eradicating the infection from the male or the less accessible parts of the female genito-urinary tract and because no immunity is developed. Metronidazole (p 342), which is given by mouth and reaches all relevant sites, is usually highly effective in treatment; it may need to be given also to the consort to prevent recurrence of the disease.

Other Species
T. hominis and T. tenax
These flagellates, similar to *T. vaginalis* but smaller, appear to be harmless commensals of the intestine and the mouth respectively.

Giardia lamblia
The vegative form of this common inhabitant of the upper part of the human small intestine is similar in size to *T. vaginalis*, and is also pear-shaped if seen 'full-face', though flattened in 'profile'. It has in fact quite a striking resemblance to a human face, with its two symmetrically placed nuclei as 'eyes'. It has eight flagella. The cyst forms are thick-walled ellipsoids, 10–15 μm long. Structural features similar to those of the vegetative forms can be recognized inside these. Heavy intestinal infestation with this species may cause persistent diarrhoea with foul-smelling bulky stools suggestive of impaired fat absorption. In Britain it has for some years been known as a cause of outbreaks of such diarrhoea among children attending day or residential nurseries, but more recently it has been frequently incriminated as the cause of acute diarrhoea in adults, usually those who have just returned from other countries–notably the U.S.S.R. In such circumstances infection is thought usually to be from drinking water, and the incubation of about 2 weeks allows many holiday-makers to return home before they develop symptoms. Mepacrine is usually effective in treatment, as is metronidazole.

THE GENUS TRYPANOSOMA
There are many trypanosomes which are pathogenic to vertebrate animals. Most of them are restricted to Africa or S. America, and all are transmitted by biting insects, in which parts of their life-cycles take place. Only three of them are pathogenic to man. Of these, *T. gambiense*, transmitted by the tsetse fly *Glossina palpalis*, and *T. rhodesiense*, transmitted by *G. morsitans*, cause *African sleeping sickness*, whereas *T. cruzi*, transmitted by reduviid bugs, causes *S. American trypanosomiasis* or *Chagas' disease*. Insects become infected by biting human beings or animals (e.g. cattle and antelopes in Africa, opossums and armadillos in S. America). After appropriate intervals for the completion of the insect stages of their life-cycles, the trypanosomes are to be found in the saliva of the flies and in the faeces of the bugs, and enter the human body through bites contaminated with these materials. In each case an indurated local lesion develops over the course of a few weeks, accompanied by regional

lymphadenitis, blood-stream spread to other parts of the body, and intermittent fever. The African forms multiply while free in the blood, whereas *T. cruzi* does so in the tissues. Meningo-encephalitis with the characteristic lethargy of sleeping sickness takes a month or so to develop in infections with *T. rhodesiense* and longer with *T. gambiense*. Myocarditis is usually more prominent than nervous system involvement in Chagas' disease. Involvement and enlargement of the liver and spleen may occur in any of the three forms, but are most common in Chagas' disease.

When in the human blood-stream the parasites are long sinuous structures, 15–30 μm wide. Each organism has a longitudinal undulating membrane and a single anterior flagellum. In smears stained with haematological stains it can be seen that each has a central macronucleus and a posterior micronucleus. In wet preparations of fresh blood the trypanosomes are actively motile.

LABORATORY INVESTIGATION Diagnosis of African trypano-somiasis is based upon microscopy of blood, lymph node aspirates and cerebrospinal fluid and upon inoculation of such materials into laboratory animals. In Chagas' disease, *xenodiagnosis* is more likely to be positive: this consists of allowing uninfected reduviid bugs to bite the patient and examining their faeces for trypanosomes 7 to 10 days later.

TREATMENT AND CONTROL Intravenous suramin has various toxic side-effects but is highly effective in African trypanosomiasis if given early enough. Pentamine isethionate, given intramuscularly, is less toxic and is highly effective, against *T. gambiense* only, for early treatment or for prophylaxis. For treatment of late cases arsenicals are required, as the other drugs do not penetrate into the brain. There is no effective treatment for Chagas' disease. Prevention of trypanosomiasis depends upon control of animal reservoirs, destruction of insect vectors and protection of human beings against the risk of being bitten.

THE GENUS LEISHMANIA

The three closely similar species of this genus resemble certain stages in the trypanosome life-cycle. All three are pathogenic to man and also have animal hosts, and all three are transmitted by sandflies of the genus *Phlebotomus*. *L. donovani* causes *kala-azar* or *visceral leishmaniasis*, a disease which is patchily distributed throughout the tropical and sub-tropical zones. The liver, spleen, lymph nodes and bone marrow are involved, with resultant fever and emaciation. In the absence of treatment the mortality is high. *L. tropica* causes *cutaneous leishmaniasis*, otherwise known as *oriental sore, Baghdad button* and *Delhi boil*. It is predominantly an Asiatic disease, but also occurs around the Mediterranean Sea and in N. Africa. Local ulcerative lesions occur at the sites of sandfly bites, but there is no visceral involvement and no risk to life. *L. braziliensis* causes *muco-cutaneous leishmaniasis* or *espudia*, which differs from oriental sore in that it occurs in S. America and that it commonly affects the mucous membranes of the nose and pharynx. It is readily transmitted from patient to patient by direct contact as well as by sandflies.

The flagellate stages of leishmaniae occur in the sandfly or in artificial culture, which is possible in a medium consisting largely of defibrinated horse or rabbit blood. (This is also suitable for the culture of trypanosomes.) In human tissues small oval non-flagellate forms called Leishman–Donovan bodies are found. They are of the order of 2—6 μm in diameter, have macro-nuclei and micronuclei as do the trypanosomes, and are found inside endothelial cells. One such cell often contains a tightly packed mass of parasites as a result of their multiplication within it.

LABORATORY INVESTIGATION   The organisms can be recognized in Giemsa-stained smears or sections of scrapings or of biopsy specimens from superficial lesions or of aspirates from lymph nodes or the liver or spleen. Blood or bone marrow smears are also likely to show them in kala-azar. Culture of such materials or inoculation into hamsters or monkeys may also be helpful in diagnosis. So may estimations of the serum proteins, since very high serum globulin levels are common in this disease.

TREATMENT AND CONTROL   Pentavalent antimony compounds, given intravenously, are usually effective in the treatment of kala-azar. They may also be valuable in the superficial conditions when these have failed to respond to simple measures, such as curetting, protective dressings and control of secondary infection by antibiotics. Sandflies are difficult to control. Animal reservoirs can be reduced, dogs and rodents being particularly important in relation to kala-azar and oriental sore respectively. Artificial immunization is of some value in preventing oriental sore.

SARCODINA
THE GENUS ENTAMOEBA
Entamoeba histolytica

This is a common cause of dysentery in the warmer parts of the world. However, in such areas it is also commonly found in the faeces of people who have never had any symptoms, and we do not know whether all of the strains assigned to this species are pathogens.

Infection occurs through taking water or food contaminated with cysts, which usually come from a symptomless excreter. Poor sanitation and food hygiene, assisted by flies, make such contamination possible. In the intestine of the new host the cysts turn into vegetative forms. They may then multiply vigorously in the large intestine and invade its mucosa, producing multiple ulcers. The onset of diarrhoea is less rapid than in bacillary dysentery due to shigellae, and amoebic dysentery is more likely to become chronic. Passage of non-purulent blood-steaked mucus is characteristic of the early stages, though secondary bacterial invasion of the ulcers may cause formation of pus later. In addition to attacking the intestine, amoebae may reach the liver, causing amoebic hepatitis or liver abscesses. The latter may be difficult to diagnose, and may first call attention to themselves by rupturing through the diaphragm into the lung, with consequent expectoration of brown material consisting of altered blood and necrotic liver tissue.

The characteristics of the parasite itself can be conveniently discussed in the next section.

LABORATORY INVESTIGATION   The vegative forms of *Ent. histolytica* are present in the faeces of patients with active dysentery, and are most easily found by examining a specimen as soon as it is passed and by using a warm slide so that the amoebae remain active. A small portion of blood-stained mucus should be mixed with saline on the slide and examined under a cover-slip. It is not sufficient to detect the presence of irregularly shaped organisms, 15–30 μm in diameter, moving by projecting pseudopodia; these may be the common non-pathogenic *Ent. coli* or other commensal amoebae. Full discussion of this differentiation is beyond the scope of this book. It is sufficient to note here that in suitable preparations *Ent. histolytica* moves more rapidly than *Ent. coli* and that its cytoplasm often contains ingested red cells, whereas that of *Ent. coli* contains bacteria and other small particles.

The faeces of patients with chronic amoebic dysentery and of symptomess carriers contain *Ent. histolytica* cysts rather than vegetative forms. These are round structures, 10–20 μm in diameter (or down to 5 μm in the case of small-cyst variants). Their recognition is made easier by using iodine solution (which stains their internal structures) rather than saline when making a wet preparation of faeces for microscopy. Since cysts are non-motile, the freshness of the specimen is less important than when looking for vegetative forms. Once again the chief problem is to distinguish *Ent. histolytica* from *Ent. coli*. Cysts of the latter tend to be larger and to have eight nuclei (well shown in the iodine preparation), whereas those of *Ent. histolytica* have four or less. We would stress the point that the finding of cysts in a patient's faeces and their identification as *Ent. histolytica* do not mean that the patient is suffering from amoebiasis.

The detection of specific antibodies, by immunofluorescence, indirect haemagglutination, gel-diffusion or complement-fixation procedures, may be helpful in the recognition of active amoebic infection, especially when it is in the liver.

TREATMENT   The tetracyclines and some other antibiotics may cause striking improvements in patients with amoebic dysentery, but their effect is mainly upon bacterial secondary invaders of the amoebic ulcers and therefore is as a rule only temporary. Arsenicals, quinine derivatives, emetine and various other drugs have been used against the amoebae themselves, but metranidazole is now probably the best choice for treatment of intestinal and of hepatic amoebiasis.

THE GENERA NAEGLERIA AND HARTMANNELLA

Since 1965 *Naegleria fowleri*, an amoeba found living free in fresh water and soil, has been reported from many countries as causing a rare acute and usually fatal disease, *primary amoebic meningo-encephalitis*. Most of the patients have been adolescents or children who had recently swum or played in fresh water lakes, pools or puddles. Infection is thought to be by inhalation. Amoebae of the genus *Hartmannella* have been shown to cause a more chronic but otherwise similar disease in older patients, not associated with recent swimming or playing in water.

CILIOPHORA (CILIATES)
Balantidium Coli

Man's only ciliate pathogen is also his largest intestinal protozoon, its vegetative form being an oval structure 50 μm or more in length. It is motile by means of short cilia distributed all over its surface. At its anterior end it has a mouth-like recess, the cytostome, and its cytoplasm contains a single large kidney-shaped nucleus, two contractile vacuoles and various ingested particles. The thick-walled cysts are somewhat smaller than the vegetative forms.

This organism is commonly carried by pigs. In man it is a rare cause of severe dysentery which closely resembles that caused by *Ent. histolytica*. It is probable, but not certain, that man usually acquires his infection from pigs. Arsenical treatment is usually successful; surprisingly, tetracycline antibiotics are said to be more effective in some cases. However, metronidazole seems to be the drug of choice.

Suggestion for Further Reading
Section IV of *Bacteriology Illustrated*–see p 159.

PART V

LABORATORY DIAGNOSIS OF MICROBIAL DISEASES

14

Collection and Examination of Specimens
(excluding serology)

We have already dealt quite extensively with diagnostic procedures when discussing particular organisms or groups of organisms. In practice, however, diagnostic microbiology begins not with a known organism but with a patient who is ill, often from an unknown cause. We need, therefore, to rearrange our knowledge so as to provide a coherent scheme for the investigation of patients. It is not possible here to go into much detail about clinical indications for collecting various types of specimen, but we can discuss the collecting and handling of specimens from different parts of the body, and give some idea of the results that they are likely to give in health and disease.

The amount of help that a microbiological laboratory can give to a clinician depends in part upon the following contributions from the clinical end:

(1) Careful and well-informed selection of the right specimens to send to the laboratory.

(2) Proper collection of such specimens. (*Whenever possible, this should be done before antibacterial treatment is given.*)

(3) Rapid transmission of the specimens to the laboratory.

(4) Clear, but preferably concise, indications of the diagnostic problem, the treatment already given, and the purpose for which the specimen is sent.

The importance of these points is illustrated by the following all-too-common situations:

(1) A vaginal swab is often the only specimen sent to the laboratory from a woman with suspected gonorrhoea. Because of the acidity of the adult vagina (see p 29), gonococci do not thrive there and are better sought in the cervix uteri or in urethral discharge.

(2) In the absence of supervision or clear instructions, a patient who has difficulty in producing sputum will often spit out saliva instead. This is, of course, useless as a source of information about his lower respiratory tract. Indeed, if it is examined and reported upon as though it were sputum, the clinician may be totally misled.

(3) Urine is quite a good bacterial culture medium. If it is left to stand at room temperature for some hours after collection, its bacterial content may increase considerably, and since different species multiply at different rates, subsequent culture may give a highly inaccurate picture of what was in the specimen when it left the patient.

(4) The more delicate pathogenic species—e.g. the gonococcus—are liable to die before reaching the laboratory if the specimen is allowed to become dry or is excessively delayed in transit. Their failure to grow on cultures may then give a misleading impression.

(5) The presence of a large number of *Esch. coli* or related organisms in the upper respiratory tract can be interpreted in various ways. In infants it is a common finding, probably a result of regurgitation, and is of no importance. It is also common in patients of all ages who have received antibiotic treatment sufficient to derange their normal flora; in such circumstances the most that is usually called for is modification or cessation of the antibiotic treatment. But in the absence of either of these explanations, such a finding requires further investigation, and the enterobacteria may require specific treatment. The bacteriologist who has not been told anything about the patient's age or treatment is in no position to give intelligent co-operation.

Having received a satisfactory specimen in good condition and with adequate accompanying information, the laboratory staff have to decide what to do with it. Routine procedures in busy laboratories are planned to extract the maximum of useful information from each specimen and yet keep the amount of work within bounds. When the specimen comes from a part of the body that is normally sterile, any organism found is abnormal—though it may have entered the specimen as a contaminant during or after collection. However, it is clearly impossible to apply to each such specimen a routine calculated to detect any known micro-organism; the best that can be done is to look for those which are not excessively rare in such situations and are likely to be relevant to the patient's condition. This is one reason why it is important that the laboratory should be told if any unusual infection is suspected. With specimens from sites that have a normal microbial population it is essential to have clearly defined aims—one of which is usually the discouragement of organisms normally present, in order to increase the chances of detecting those that are abnormal. There can be few hospital bacteriologists who have not at some time received a faecal specimen 'For organisms please'. Isolation and identification of all bacteria, viruses, fungi and protozoa in a single faecal specimen might well take years, whereas the question 'Does this specimen contain known intestinal pathogens?' can usually be answered by a few minutes' work spread over 2 or 3 days.

The presence of a normal microbial population creates problems of reporting. Clearly the report should include the names of any known pathogens found which might be responsible for the patient's illness or which it is undesirable that he should continue to carry. As a rule it will also include information about the sensitivity of such pathogens to appropriate antimicrobial agents. Organisms which are common commensals but also potential pathogens—e.g. pneumococci in the respiratory tract—need to be assessed in the light of circumstances. An unexplained and unusual predominance of one of the normal commensals may be of some significance—e.g. an almost pure growth of viridans streptococci is sometimes obtained from a swab of an inflamed tonsil, and possibly indicates that this organism is in fact causing the tonsillitis. The correct wording of 'negative' reports is a subject of controversy. 'No pathogens isolated' gives the clinician a minimum of information, though it is probably the best formula for faeces and some other specimens for which the range of normal findings is very wide. A list of pathogens which have been sought but not found is sometimes appropriate but is liable to be cumbrous. A report of the predominant organisms in the cultures—e.g. 'viridans streptococci and commensal neisseriae' from a throat swab—does not convey much useful information, and obscures the fact that this predominance was probably determined by the methods of culture. 'Normal flora' is defensible provided that it is taken to mean: 'The varieties and proportions of organisms identified appear to be within normal limits for such specimens when examined by the procedures in routine use in this laboratory.' The last point is important; an abnormality will be detected only if the procedures used are appropriate to its detection.

With these points in mind we will now consider methods of collecting and examining specimens from human beings, first in general terms and then in relation to different parts of the body.

METHODS
Collection of Specimens
Most clinical specimens are collected in one of the following ways:

(1) Materials such as saliva, sputum, faeces, urine, crusts, and scabs and freely discharging pus can be collected *directly into suitable sterile*

containers. (Special containers for faeces are described on p 248.) Because of the labour involved in efficient cleaning and resterilization of screw-capped glass bottles and jars after they have been used for such purposes, they are increasingly being replaced by plastic bottles and jars with watertight caps and by disposable waxed cardboard or plastic cartons with tightly fitting lids.

(2) Sometimes it is convenient to collect small quantities of fluid–e.g. vesicle contents for examination for poxviruses, or exudate from a suspected syphilitic chancre for dark-ground microscopy–into *capillary tubes*, which can then be sealed by heating their ends, so that the fluid does not dry up.

(3) For collection of material from skin and mucous surfaces, and also of exudates and discharges which are too small in amount for direct collection as in (1), a *swab* can be used. This usually consists of a wooden or wire rod about 6 inches long, with a small quantity of cotton wool tightly twisted around one end and the other end inserted into the cork or stopper of the tube in which it is supplied. The swab and the inside of its container are sterile. For use, the swab is withdrawn from the tube, applied to the patient and then replaced in the tube for transmission to the laboratory, or else used for the immediate inoculation of a suitable *transport medium* (i.e. a medium which will keep delicate organisms–notably gonococci or viruses–alive during transit). Modifications of swab design for special purposes are discussed under appropriate headings later in this chapter. Collection of organisms from dry skin is more efficient if the swab is moistened with sterile broth immediately beforehand. Use of serum- or albumin-coated cotton wool swabs increases the chances that relatively delicate bacteria, such as *Str. pyogenes*, will reach the laboratory alive. The efficiency of transfer of organisms from the patient to the culture media by means of a swab is low, particularly if the amount of material on the swab is small, for some of it becomes entangled in the cotton wool. For certain purposes this difficulty can be overcome by using alginate wool; this is soluble in sodium hexametaphosphate solution, so that all of the trapped material is released into the solution and can be concentrated by centrifugation.

It needs to be emphasized that *swabbing is not a satisfactory substitute for the direct collection of such materials as pus*; it should be used only when inadequacy of materials or other factors make direct collection impossible (see p 242).

(4) *Washings* from cavities are used in certain circumstances. Throat washings, sometimes preferred to throat swabs for virus investigations, are obtained by asking the patient to gargle with physiological saline and then expectorate it. Gastric washings for examination for tubercle

bacilli, from patients who cannot produce sputum, are obtained by running saline into the empty stomach and then withdrawing it through a Ryle's gastric tube. Washing out of the maxillary antrum is a therapeutic procedure, but the washings are often sent for bacteriological examination.

(5) *Aspiration*, usually through a needle and often with the assistance of suction from a syringe, is used to collect materials confined within the patient's body, such as blood, cerebrospinal fluid, effusions into body cavities and joints, and closed abscesses. Organ biopsies can be carried out in the same way. Care must be taken to avoid contamination of the specimens, either from the apparatus used or by collecting organisms in the needle as it passes through the skin. (See p 253.) Aspirated materials are either placed in a sterile container or added to suitable media directly from the syringe.

Transmission

In all cases this should be as rapid as possible. Death of some delicate organisms can be delayed by using transport media, or in the case of most viruses by transporting them packed in ice (see p 183). Inoculation of media at the bedside or in the clinic, while necessary in some cases, is unsuitable for general use because of administrative difficulties and the risks of contaminating the cultures. As mentioned on p 234, delay in transmission of some specimens results in unequal multiplication of the contained organisms. If delay is inevitable, virtually all specimens are better kept in a refrigerator than at room temperature.

As well as being rapid for the sake of the organisms, *transmission should be free from risk to all those who handle the specimen on its route from the patient to the laboratory bench*–nurses, doctors, relatives, hospital porters, laboratory staff etc. This means:

(*a*) that a specimen which may contain pathogens (which of course includes virtually any specimen sent to a medical microbiology department) must be securely enclosed in a protective container;

(*b*) that there must be no contamination of the outside of the container during collection;

(*c*) that the container for a fluid specimen must be leak-proof, both in design and in practice–i.e. if it has a cap this must be put on correctly and firmly, etc.;

(*d*) that for any particularly hazardous specimen, such as blood or other body fluid from a patient with possible virus hepatitis or fluid faeces from a patient with enteric fever or cholera, the container itself must be enclosed in a sealed plastic bag. It is of course important that the accompanying request form, which will have to be handled by laboratory clerical and technical staff, should *not* be enclosed in the same bag.

Special regulations govern postal transmission of microbiological specimens and other pathological materials. Those operative in the U.K. are given in *Medical Microbiology* (ed. R. Cruickshank, Churchill Livingstone, Edinburgh, 12th edn, 1973) p 644. An important regulation, relevant also to many specimens not sent through the post, is that when a fluid specimen is sent inside a glass or other breakable container which is itself inside a box, there must be sufficient absorbent packing material in the box to take up all of the fluid if it should leak from the inner container.

Microscopy

WET PREPARATIONS   These are used for counting leucocytes and other cellular elements in such specimens as cerebrospinal fluid and effusions, and are usually more satisfactory than stained smears for the identification of such structures. Wet preparations are also used for the examination of skin scrapings and hairs for fungi and of faeces, vaginal swabs, etc. for protozoa.

GRAM-STAINED SMEARS   These are made from a large proportion of specimens sent for bacteriological examination, and often give valuable leads as to the most appropriate culture procedures. Such smears are of limited value, however, in the study of specimens from the alimentary tract and many of those from the respiratory tract, since even those from healthy subjects are likely to contain bacteria of many different morphological types.

ZIEHL–NEELSEN-STAINED SMEARS   These are made from specimens sent specifically for investigation for tubercle bacilli. Whether they are also made routinely from sputa and other specimens sent for general bacteriological investigation depends on the local prevalence of tuberculosis.

Appropriately stained smears are made from specimens that may contain virus inclusion bodies or elementary bodies (e.g. p 182).

Cultures

A great number of man's parasitic bacteria grow on *blood agar incubated aerobically* at 37°C, and therefore this medium is used for most clinical specimens. *Anaerobic cultures on blood agar* are also put up routinely from most specimens taken from situations to which there is not free access of air. (Anaerobic culture techniques are described below.) *MacConkey's medium* is valuable for all specimens likely to contain enterobacteria

–including, among others, faeces, urine, most pus samples and wound swabs and many ulcerative skin lesions, especially those on the lower half of the body. *Robertson's cooked meat medium* (boiled minced lean meat in peptone water–see p 123) supports the growth of most aerobic and anaerobic bacteria, and is commonly used in addition to the solid media for primary culture of pus and of swabs from many sites. Particularly when there has been delay in transport of the specimen or when the patient has been on antibiotic treatment, growth often occurs in the cooked meat medium when there is none of the primary plate cultures; the cooked meat medium is then subcultured to further blood agar plates for aerobic and anaerobic incubation. Organisms from a patient receiving penicillin treatment will sometimes grow in *broth containing penicillinase* (β-lactamase) when they fail to grow in or on other primary culture media. They too can then be subcultured to blood agar. By careful choice of the right β-lactamase preparation it is possible to extend this neutralizing action to all of the β-lactam (penicillin and cephalosporin) antibiotics. Less straightforward and in general less effective means are available for neutralizing antibiotics of other groups, but *p*-aminobenzoic acid successfully antagonizes sulphonamides (see p 40).

The few media mentioned so far are sufficient for the examination of most clinical specimens except faeces, for which a highly selective approach is necessary (see pp 235 and 249). Specially nutritious media–notably *chocolate agar* (p 106)–must be provided for unusually exacting bacteria. Various media containing selective inhibitors for the isolation of particular groups of bacteria have already been mentioned in discussing the relevant organism, as have those for the growth of viruses and fungi; some of them will be referred to again at appropriate points in the next section of this chapter.

ANAEROBIC CULTURE   The *McIntosh and Fildes jar* is a cylindrical glass or metal container of suitable size to hold a pile of culture plates. It has a heavy metal lid which can be clamped down to give an air-tight joint. When the jar has been loaded with cultures and closed, air is evacuated from it by suction through a tube that passes through the lid, and the jar is refilled with a mixture of nitrogen and hydrogen. The remaining traces of oxygen are removed by combination with some of the hydrogen, a reaction which is catalysed by palladium or platinum in a capsule fixed to the under surface of the lid. When its preparation has been completed, the whole jar can be placed inside an incubator.

Tubes and bottles of media, as well as plates, can be incubated anaerobically in a McIntosh and Fildes jar (they must, of course, have cotton-wool plugs or caps that are not air-tight), but there are a number of other ways in which strict anaerobes can be grown. Anaerobic conditions are to be found in the deeper parts of a tube full of a solid or semi-solid medium, or in a fluid medium which has been boiled and immediately covered with a layer of sterile vaseline. Alternatively, reducing agents, such as a sterile iron nail or strip or a combination of glucose and *sodium thioglycollate*, can be added to the medium. *Robertson's cooked meat medium* is suitable for growing anaerobes because of the reducing activity of the pieces of meat at the bottom of the bottle.

CULTURE IN 5–10% CO_2 Conditions appropriate for the primary isolation of *N. meningitidis* and *Br. abortus* can be produced by placing the cultures, together with a lighted candle, inside any suitable container which can then be closed with an airtight lid. When the candle goes out the CO_2 level is of the desired order. Alternatively, a McIntosh and Fildes jar is evacuated by suction and refilled with a mixture of 10% CO_2 in air.

SPECIMENS FROM DIFFERENT PARTS OF THE BODY
This section has the following aims:

(1) To indicate the *commensal organisms most commonly found* and the *pathogens of greatest importance* in specimens from various situations. The lists are deliberately brief and far from comprehensive, and little reference has been made to pathogens that are rare in Britain.

(2) To indicate *reasonable basic routines* for the collection and initial investigation of specimens. These are by no means the *only* reasonable routines, and they would often need to be supplemented by further investigations. Laboratories differ widely in their choices of methods, and are influenced by many local factors. We indicate appropriate specimens to collect for investigation of virus infections, but say nothing here about laboratory procedures for examining them, which are considered in Chapter Eleven. Nor do we include in this chapter any mention of serological investigation, which is often more important and informative than microscopy and culture, especially in virus infections, but is considered in earlier chapters and in Chapter Fifteen.

Except where otherwise indicated, examination of bacteriological specimens is generally completed within one or two days of receiving them, with the addition of a further day if antibiotic sensitivity determinations are carried out after the organisms have been isolated. A minority of specimens require a few more days for the sorting out of mixed cultures or the identification of unusual organisms, and on rare occasions the latter causes further delay. Culture for tubercle bacilli takes

3 to 6 weeks. Mycological cultures for dermatophytes and some other slow-growing fungi may also take several weeks.

The Skin

COMMON COMMENSALS

Staphylococci (mainly *Staph. epidermidis*) and diphtheroid bacilli. Many other bacteria and some fungi are often present on the skin, but only transiently.

IMPORTANT PATHOGENS

Staph. aureus–pustules, boils, carbuncles, paronychial infections, impetigo, and secondary infections of blisters, bites, burns, ulcers, dermatitis and many other lesions.

Str. pyogenes–much the same except for pustules, boils and carbuncles.

Esch. coli, Proteus species, *Ps. aeruginosa*, enterococci–secondary infection of various lesions, especially on the lower part of the trunk and the lower limbs.

Candida albicans–exudative dermatitis of skin folds (intertrigo) and chronic paronychia.

Dermatophyte fungi–ringworm.

Pox and herpesviruses–appropriate vesicular lesions.

CHOICE AND COLLECTION OF SPECIMENS

Rubbing a dry swab over a dry area of skin is unlikely to provide the laboratory with a useful specimen, but the operation is usually more productive if the lesion is exudative or if the swab is moistened in sterile broth or saline before use. Crusts or scabs, in a sterile bottle, may be even more valuable, especially from suspected virus lesions, from which vesicle fluid in capillaries (see p 236) should also be collected if possible. From possible dermatomycoses, skin scrapings, hairs and nails should be collected as appropriate (p 217).

ROUTINE INITIAL INVESTIGATIONS

For bacteria–Gram-stained smear and aerobic culture on blood agar; also on MacConkey's medium if enterobacteria are suspected or can be seen in the smear.

For *C. albicans*, if suspected clinically or seen in the smear–cultures on mycological media.

For dermatophytes–wet preparation of scrapings, etc., in KOH (see p 217) and cultures on mycological media.

Wounds, Abscesses, Sinuses etc.

COMMON COMMENSALS

Such lesions have no 'normal flora' of their own, but the organisms isolated from them commonly include commensals from any surfaces with which they are in communication.

IMPORTANT PATHOGENS

Staph. aureus–the commonest pathogen in skin wounds and abscesses.

Esch. coli, *Proteus* species, *Ps. aeruginosa*–abdominal wounds, intra-abdominal abscesses.

Cl. welchii and other clostridia–abdominal wounds, contaminated accidental wounds.

Bacteroides species–abscesses, especially in association with the alimentary and female genital tracts; also lung abscesses.

Myco. tuberculosis–'cold' abscesses (i.e. chronic abscesses without the warmth and other features associated with acute inflammation) derived from breakdown of infected lymph-nodes, occurring in many sites but notably in the neck.

Actinomyces israeli–abscesses around the jaw and elsewhere, usually discharging to the surface through multiple sinuses.

CHOICE AND COLLECTION OF SPECIMENS

All too frequently a bacteriology laboratory receives a minute amount of pus on the end of a swab, accompanied by a form that refers to incision and drainage of a large abscess. Whenever pus is present in sufficient amount, it should be collected in a bottle–a syringe and needle being usually the best means of getting it there. A small portion of the wall of an abscess or sinus may also be a good bacteriological specimen. When a sinus suspected of being actino-mycotic has discharged into a dressing, the dressing should be sent to the laboratory, as 'sulphur granules' (p 152) may be found on its contaminated surface.

ROUTINE INITIAL INVESTIGATIONS

Gram-stained smear; culture on blood agar (aerobic and anaerobic) and MacConkey's agar and in cooked meat medium. Anaerobic cultures need to be incubated for at least 2 days for *Bacteroides* and 5 days for *A. israeli*. Gas-liquid chromatography (p 5) may give rapid information about the presence and identity of anaerobes in pus. For *Myco. tuberculosis*–see under Lower Respiratory Tract.

The Conjunctivae and Lid Margins

COMMON COMMENSALS

Bacteria are usually scanty, but they may include staphylococci, diphtheroid bacilli, viridans streptococci, non-pathogenic neisseriae and many others.

IMPORTANT PATHOGENS

N. gonorrhoeae, *Staph. aureus*, *Str. pneumoniae*–neonatal con-junctivitis.

Staph. aureus–styles and blepharitis.

H. influenzae and *H. aegyptius*–conjunctivitis.

TRIC agent–inclusion conjunctivitis (investigations, see p 168).

Adenoviruses and herpesviruses–conjunctivitis, kerato-con-junctivitis.

CHOICE AND COLLECTION OF SPECIMENS

A conjunctival swab is seldom an adequate specimen for bacterio-logy, except when there is visible purulent discharge; even then, the swab should be delivered to the laboratory immediately or sent in a bacteriological transport medium. In most cases it is better to have microscope slides and culture plates to hand in the clinic or ward, or to send the patient to the laboratory, so that smears can be made and cultures inoculated with material taken straight from the con-junctival surface by means of a sterile bacteriological loop (made of platinum, not of nichrome wire, because the latter is liable to abrade the conjunctiva). Conjunctival swabs for virology should be sent in virus transport medium (see p 183), together with a throat swab if adenovirus infection is suspected.

ROUTINE INITIAL INVESTIGATIONS

Gram-stained smear; culture on blood agar and chocolate agar, aerobically and in 5–10% CO_2.

The Ears

COMMON COMMENSALS

External ear: as for skin. Middle ear: normally sterile.

IMPORTANT PATHOGENS

Staph. aureus, Str. pyogenes, Ps. aeruginosa–otitis externa.

Str. pneumoniae, H. influenzae, Str. pyogenes, Staph. aureus–otitis media.

CHOICE AND COLLECTION OF SPECIMENS

A swab can be used to collect material from the external ear–i.e. from an otitis externa or from an otitis media that is discharging through a perforated ear-drum. In the absence of perforation, it is usually possible to aspirate fluid from an infected middle ear by passing a needle through the drum, but this is rarely justified, as treatment can be based on probabilities. Despite the communication between the healthy middle ear and the nasopharynx via the Eustachian tube, swabbing of the nasopharynx is not useful as a means of determining the probable pathogens in otitis media.

ROUTINE INITIAL INVESTIGATIONS

Gram-stained smear and aerobic culture on blood agar and MacConkey's agar and, in the case of otitis media in a child, chocolate agar for the possible *H. influenzae*.

The Upper Respiratory Tract (including the mouth)

COMMON COMMENSALS

Staph. epidermidis and *Staph. aureus* (particularly in the anterior nares), viridans and non-haemolytic streptococci, diphtheroid bacilli, lactobacilli, non-pathogenic neisseriae, haemophili, fusiform bacilli, various spirochaetes; also in young children, *Esch. coli* and related organisms, probably regurgitated from the alimentary tract.

IMPORTANT PATHOGENS

In the mouth:
Borr. vincenti and *F. fusiformis* ('Vincent's organisms').
C. albicans–thrush.

In the throat and nasopharynx:
Str. pyogenes and *Staph. aureus*–tonsillitis.
C. diphtheriae.
H. influenzae (type b)–acute epiglottitis.
Vincent's organisms.
The many viruses that cause respiratory tract infections.
Other pathogens are sometimes to be found in these sites although they produce their main ill effects elsewhere–e.g. *N. meningitidis*, *Bord. pertussis*, polioviruses and the causative organisms of pneumonia (see below).

In the paranasal sinuses:
Staph. aureus, *Str. pyogenes*, *Str. pneumoniae*, *H. influenzae*.

CHOICE AND COLLECTION OF SPECIMENS

Swabbing a mouth lesion is usually a straightforward procedure. So is swabbing of the anterior nares, except that when there is no nasal discharge (e.g. when the purpose is to detect nasal carriage of *Staph. aureus*) the swab should be moistened as for skin swabbing (p 241). Throat swabbing is carried out with the patient's mouth wide open and his tongue depressed, and care must be taken not to touch the swab against anything other than the pharyngeal mucosa. (The results of culture may be vitiated if antiseptics or antibiotics have been applied to the throat in the previous 12 hours or so–a statement which is, of course, equally true about specimens from other sites, but is most commonly forgotten in relation to throat swabs.) The nasopharynx can best be swabbed by passing a pernasal swab, made with fine and fairly flexible wire, along the floor of one nostril; this is the recommended procedure for isolation of *Bord. pertussis*.
Swabbing the epiglottis or even the throat of a child with haemophilus epiglottitis may provoke a fatal supraglottic spasm, and should therefore not be attempted unless steps to maintain the airway have been taken or can be taken immediately. Blood culture,

while it does not provide information soon enough to help in the management of this fulminating condition, is usually positive for *H. influenzae* type b and should be carried out, as the best means of confirming the diagnosis.

Pernasal aspiration of nasopharyngeal fluid through a fine plastic tube provides the best sample for rapid diagnosis of respiratory syncytial and other respiratory virus infections by immunofluorescence. Nose and throat swabs for culture of viruses should be sent in virus transport medium (see p 183).

Investigation of infections in the paranasal sinuses is difficult because of their inaccessibility. If there is a purulent discharge it may contain relevant bacteria. The surgical procedure of washing out the affected sinus provides the best information about what is happening inside it, but clearly is indicated only when the infection has failed to respond to simpler measures.

ROUTINE INITIAL INVESTIGATIONS

Gram-stained smears; smears stained with dilute carbol fuchsin for Vincent's organisms; aerobic cultures on blood agar and on the following media as indicated–Loeffler's serum and a tellurite medium for *C. diphtheriae*, chocolate agar for *H. influenzae* and for *N. meningitidis*, Bordet–Gengou medium for *Bord. pertussis* and mycological media for *C. albicans*.

Information about the diagnosis of diphtheria is available at the following times:

(1) *No information* is available *immediately* after receipt of the specimen; this diagnosis cannot be confirmed or refuted by examination of direct smears made from the specimen.

(2) *Provisional identification* of *C. diphtheriae* may be possible 18 hours or less after receipt of the specimen, on the basis of its characteristic appearances in films made from Loeffler's serum culture at this stage and stained with methylene blue or by Albert's or Neisser's method.

(3) *More definite identification* may be possible 48 hours or more after receipt of the specimen, by examination of colonies on a tellurite medium.

(4) *Confirmation that the strain isolated is C. diphtheriae* usually takes a further day, during which the fermentation reactions of the organisms are tested.

(5) *Confirmation that the strain is toxigenic* takes a few more days. Further details of all these procedures are to be found on pp 111–12.

Bord. pertussis may take 4 days to form visible colonies on Bordet–Gengou medium.

The Lower Respiratory Tract

COMMON COMMENSALS

In the larynx and trachea, much the same as in the nasopharynx. The bronchi are sterile when healthy.

IMPORTANT PATHOGENS

Str. pneumoniae, Staph. aureus, Mycoplasma pneumoniae–pneumonia.

H. influenzae, Str. pneumoniae–chronic bronchitis and bronchiectasis.

Myco. tuberculosis.

Viruses, notably influenza.

(Also *C. diphtheriae* in the larynx and *Bord. pertussis* in the trachea and bronchi, but these organisms are more commonly *isolated* from the upper respiratory tract.)

CHOICE AND COLLECTION OF SPECIMENS

The commonest specimen obtained from the lower respiratory tract is sputum. Ideally this is coughed up from far down the bronchial tree, expectorated immediately with minimal contamination from the throat and mouth, and delivered to the laboratory without delay, since such contaminant bacteria and fungi as have been picked up are likely to multiply in the specimen at room temperature far more rapidly than the pathogens. Even such an ideal specimen (which is rare) may not give straightforward information about the infection that is being investigated. For example, in the early stages of lobar pneumonia (as well as in various other lung infections) the sputum–if there is any–may merely reflect conditions in a bronchus at some distance from the lung lesion; better information may come from blood culture, or from looking for pneumococcal polysaccharide or other relevant bacterial products in the patient's blood or even urine. In acute bronchopneumonia the sputum may well come straight from the 'battlefield' and be highly relevant. Especially in chronic bronchial disease, any one sputum is likely to consist of somewhat diverse contributions from different sources which have stuck together but not mixed, and consecutive sputa may represent different parts of the bronchial tree and give markedly divergent bacteriological results. The problem of contamination from the upper respiratory tract can be minimized by aspirating material direct from the bronchi through a bronchoscope, or from the lumen of the trachea by passing a needle through the skin and anterior wall of the trachea, but such procedures are not suitable for routine use. In children too young to expectorate, the causative organisms of broncho-pulmonary infections can sometimes be found in the nasopharynx; and in patients with pulmonary tuberculosis but no sputum, tubercle bacilli may be found by swabbing the larynx (using a long curved swab) or by obtaining gastric washings. These two procedures both depend upon the fact that ciliary currents carry mucus from the bronchi up the trachea and larynx, after which it is swallowed if its quantity is insufficient to provoke coughing.

For investigation of virus infections of the lower respiratory tract the specimens indicated for upper respiratory tract infections are appropriate.

ROUTINE INITIAL INVESTIGATIONS

Important information may be given by the naked-eye appearance of the sputum–mucoid, mucopurulent, purulent, blood-stained, etc. (In sputum from asthmatics, apparent pus may in fact consist of eosinophils, as can be shown by staining a smear with a suitable haematological stain.) Sometimes the specimen obviously consists mainly or entirely of saliva. Frequently its non-homogeneity is evident. A sample for microscopy or culture which is taken by dipping a loop into an untreated sputum is likely to contain a disproportionately large contribution from the irrelevant surface coating of throat and mouth contamination, together with material taken from only one part (not necessarily a representative part) of the underlying sputum. A better procedure is first to shake up the specimen with a homogenizing agent such as 2% N-acetyl-L-cysteine; any sample from it should then contain a fair representation of all parts of the specimen, and any organism that was present in very large numbers in some part of the original sputum should also be plentiful in the sample. The homogenate can be used for all of the investigations listed below:

Gram-stained smear (which gives further information about purulence, shows the extent of upper respiratory tract and mouth contamination and may give useful indications as to the predominant organisms). Aerobic culture on blood agar and chocolate agar; culture of the homogenate in 1:100 saline dilution as well as neat helps to show which organisms are present in very large numbers and therefore probably important. Anaerobic culture on blood agar when there is a possibility of lung abscess or of bronchial obstruction leading to failure of aeration of part of a lung.

For *Myco. tuberculosis*–Ziehl–Neelsen-stained smear (which must be carefully searched, as the bacilli may be scanty), and aerobic culture on Löwenstein–Jensen or other suitable medium after concentration of the specimen as described on p 146. (Ziehl–Neelsen-stained smears of concentrate may reveal tubercle bacilli when these were not seen in smears of untreated sputum.) Processing of laryngeal swabs is easier and more effective if they are made from alginate wool (see p 236). Gastric washings should be examined and cultured without delay, as the tubercle bacilli may not long survive the action of gastric juice.

The Alimentary Tract

COMMON COMMENSALS

Bacteria of very many varieties are to be found in the alimentary tract, especially in its lower parts, and make a large contribution to the bulk of faeces. The culture procedures used by medical laboratories are selective and give a false impression that enterobacteria are overwhelmingly predominant, but other groups usually present in large numbers and in considerable diversity include lactobacilli, anaerobes of the *Bacteriodes* group, clostridia and streptococci. Commensal protozoa are also common, as are viruses, though the latter are not usually regarded as commensals.

IMPORTANT PATHOGENS

Certain serotypes of *Esch. coli*–gastro-enteritis, mainly of young children.

Shigellae–bacillary dysentery.

Salmonellae–enteric fever and gastro-enteritis (food-poisoning).

Ent. histolytica–amoebic dysentery.

V. cholerae–cholera (see p 136).

Staph. aureus–staphylococcal enteritis (rare).

C. albicans–enteritis.

Rotaviruses.

CHOICE AND COLLECTION OF SPECIMENS

In cases of food poisoning it may be possible and desirable to send vomit to the laboratory, in a suitable water-tight container and with care not to contaminate the outside of the container. The same precaution is essential on the many occasions when it is appropriate to send faeces. All too often a laboratory receives faeces, in unnecessarily large amount, filling and overflowing from an unsuitable container, the outside of which was contaminated during collection and during transport; the hazards of this to nurses, porters, laboratory staff and others are easy to conceive. (See p 237.) It is far better to use a screw-capped, watertight container with, inside it and attached to its cap for convenience of handling, a small plastic spoon that can be used to transfer safely into the container the small amount of material which is all that the laboratory needs. From young children and other patients from whom there is difficulty in obtaining a faecal specimen uncontaminated with urine, a swab inserted into the rectum may be more satisfactory.

ROUTINE INITIAL INVESTIGATION

Naked-eye inspection for consistency and the presence of blood, pus and mucus. Aerobic culture on blood agar for pathogenic serotypes of *Esch. coli* (since these give their most satisfactory slide-agglutination reactions when grown on this medium) and for *Staph. aureus*; on D.C.A. medium for shigellae; and in selenite F broth to be subcultured next day to D.C.A. medium, for salmonellae. Gram-stained smears should be made if either staphylococcal or candida enteritis is suspected, and in either condition usually show the respective pathogens in large numbers. Mycological cultures should be set up when candida enteritis is suspected. Wet microscopic preparations, usually in iodine solutions, are used for the detection of *Ent. histolytica* and other protozoa (as well as worm ova and larvae, which are outside the range of this book).

The Urinary Tract

Apart from skin commensals and transient organisms in the female and the anterior part of the male urethra, the tract is normally sterile.

IMPORTANT PATHOGENS

Esch. coli, *Proteus* species, enterococci, *Myco. tuberculosis*–cystitis, pyelitis, pyelonephritis.

Typhoid and paratyphoid bacilli, while nor primarily pathogens of the urinary tract, may be found in the urine (see pp 127 and 129).

CHOICE AND COLLECTION OF SPECIMENS

For non-tuberculous infections–a mid-stream specimen of urine whenever possible. This is a specimen collected after the patient has passed enough urine to flush out organisms from the urethra. It should also be collected with care to minimize contamination of the urine on its way from the urethra to the sterile collecting vessel. If the patient is male, the foreskin should be retracted and the glans penis cleaned with gauze soaked in sterile saline (not antiseptic, as this may get into the urine). If the patient is female, the vagina should be occluded by a tampon, the vulval area should be cleansed with sterile saline (or, if convenient, by having a bath) and dried, and the labia should be held apart while the specimen is passed. In either case the specimen should be passed directly into a wide-mouthed sterile jar or plastic carton, which must then be closed with a water-tight lid and sent to the laboratory immediately. If delay in transmission is inevitable, addition of boric acid powder (about $1\cdot8\%$) to the urine prevents bacterial growth and gives excellent preservation of cells, but a few enterobacterial strains are reduced in numbers by this procedure. (The use of 'dip-slides' is discussed on p 251.) Since passage of a catheter into the bladder may itself initiate a urinary tract infection in a patient who did not previously have one, catheter specimens of urine should be collected only when it is in any case necessary to pass an instrument into the bladder, or when the patient is unable to co-operate. In the latter case, particularly with young children, it is often better to collect a specimen by supra-pubic aspiration–i.e. by using a syringe and needle to withdraw urine from the full bladder through the abdominal wall. In some circumstances, especially when it is important to find out whether urinary tract infection is limited to one kidney, specimens are collected direct from the ureters, by means of fine catheters inserted via the bladder with the aid of a cystoscope.

For *Myco. tuberculosis*–repeated early morning urine specimens, since these are likely to be the most concentrated and so to offer the best chance of finding the scanty bacilli. If the investigation is solely for tuberculosis, there is no need to take special precautions to avoid contamination of such specimens during collection.

ROUTINE INITIAL INVESTIGATIONS

Cell count–conveniently performed by centrifugation of 10 ml of urine, discarding 9 ml of the supernatant, re-suspending the deposit in the remaining 1 ml, and counting the pus cells and other cells in a counting chamber under the microscope. Two points to remember are: (1) that the pus cell excretion rate per hour is a more informative figure than the number per ml, since the latter is greatly influenced by the patient's level of hydration; and (2) that a significant urinary tract infection, as indicated by the presence of large numbers of pathogenic bacteria in freshly passed specimens, can exist without an appreciable cellular response. Such a condition, which has been given the name *bacteriuria*, may precede the development of a frankly purulent infection of the tract.

Semi-quantitative aerobic culture on blood agar and on MacConkey's agar. Each of these media is inoculated by using a standard loop which transfers approximately 0·002 ml of urine, and this amount is spread as evenly as possible over the surface of the plate. After incubation the bacteria can then be roughly enumerated as well as identified, each colony representing one organism in the inoculum and therefore about 500 organisms per ml in the urine specimen. *If a carefully collected specimen is cultured within 3 hours, contaminant bacteria picked up during collection are unlikely to exceed 10 000 per ml* (i.e. 20 colonies on the blood agar plate) and these are usually a mixture, including staphylococci and diphtheroid bacilli. On the other hand, *a specimen from a patient with a non-tuberculous urinary tract infection is likely to contain 100 000 or more organisms per ml* (200 or more colonies per plate) and these are usually of a single bacterial species which grows well on both the media used and in most cases are Gram-negative bacilli. Delay in examination of the specimen is likely to confuse the distinction between contaminants and pathogens because the former have had time to multiply. Antibacterial treatment also obscures the situation by slowing the multiplication of pathogens in the bladder and therefore lowering their numbers to 'contaminant' levels in fresh urine specimens. A Gram-stained smear of the centrifuged urine deposit may help to unravel the problems: for example, when the deposit from a urine specimen from a female is found to contain many characteristic vaginal epithelial cells with their usual adherent Gram-positive bacilli which have failed to grow on the cultures (lactobacilli), it is clear that the specimen was improperly collected. Use of 'dip-slides' (plastic slides, similar in size to microscope slides, which are coated with culture media and can be dipped into freshly passed urine and then incubated inside closed containers) overcomes some of the problems introduced by delay in transport, since the number of colonies on such a slide depends on the number of bacteria in the urine as passed; but heavy contamination is not easy to distinguish from true infection by such means, and the additional information that comes from cell counts and Gram-stained smears is not available unless a conventional specimen is also available. The main value of dip-slides seems to be as a means of screening large populations of symptomless people in the search for those who may have 'silent' bacteriuria: those whose dip-slides give heavy growths need further investigation. (All that we have said about the importance of heavy growths is inapplicable to chronic renal parenchymatous infection, in which the pathogen may be excreted in the urine intermittently and in small numbers–a difficult condition to detect.)

For *Myco. tuberculosis*–Ziehl–Neelsen-stained smear, and aerobic culture on Löwenstein–Jensen or other suitable medium, of concentrated deposit from a large volume of urine which has been allowed to stand in a refrigerator for a day or two, or of a smaller volume which has been centrifuged. The possibility of tuberculosis should be considered whenever other pathogens are absent from a purulent urine, unless this situation is due to antibacterial treatment.

The Female Genital Tract

COMMON COMMENSALS

A bacterial population similar to that of skin is found in the vulva and lower vagina, and also in the vaginal vault before puberty, late in pregnancy and after the menopause. During the child-bearing period, lactobacilli and micro-aerophilic or anaerobic streptococci usually predominate in the vaginal vault. The cervical canal, uterus and Fallopian tubes are normally sterile.

IMPORTANT PATHOGENS

T. pallidum–syphilitic chancres and condylomata.

N. gonorrhoeae–urethritis, cervicitis, endometritis and salpingitis of adults, vulvo-vaginitis of children.

Trich. vaginalis, C. albicans–vaginitis.

Str. pyogenes, Staph. aureus–puerperal sepsis.

Cl. welchii, Esch. coli, Proteus species etc.–septic abortion.

Micro-aerophilic and anaerobic streptococci–septic abortion, chronic vaginitis and endometritis.

Myco. tuberculosis–endometritis, salpingitis.

CHOICE AND COLLECTION OF SPECIMENS

For *T. pallidum*–exudate collected in capillary tubes from the surfaces of lesions which have first been thoroughly cleaned with gauze and sterile saline.

For *N. gonorrhoeae*–swabs of urethral discharge and of cervical mucopus (*not* a high vaginal swab) placed in transport medium; or preferably, when possible, material collected with a sterile wire loop and used at once to inoculate suitable media; and in either case, smears of discharge suitable for Gram-staining (and, if the technique is available, immunofluorescence for *N. gonorrhoeae*) in the laboratory. When there is no evident discharge but chronic gonococcal infection is suspected, it is important also to send a rectal swab for culture for *N. gonorrhoeae*.

For *Trich. vaginalis*–if immediate microscopic examination of a wet preparation of the discharge is not possible in the ward or clinic, a swab of discharge sent immediately to the laboratory in a suitable transport or culture medium.

For *Myco. tuberculosis* or other causes of chronic endometritis–uterine curettings or other surgical specimens.

For other organisms–swabs of the vaginal vault ('high vaginal' swabs) or of discharges or lesions.

ROUTINE INITIAL INVESTIGATIONS

For *T. pallidum*–immediate dark-ground microscopy of the exudate. The laboratory should be warned in advance, so that the specimen can be given prompt attention.

For *N. gonorrhoeae*–Gram-stained smears (and immunofluorescence); culture on suitable selective medium in 5–10% CO_2.

For *Trich. vaginalis*–immediate microscopy of wet preparation.

For *Myco. tuberculosis*–Ziehl–Neelsen-stained smears or sections, aerobic culture on Löwenstein–Jensen or other suitable medium or guinea-pig inoculation.

For other organisms–Gram-stained smears. Culture on blood agar aerobically (and anaerobically for high vaginal swabs); in cooked meat medium; and on mycological media if *C. albicans* was suspected clinically or seen in the smears.

The Male Genitalia
Exudate from syphilitic chancres and discharge from gonococcal urethritis are collected and examined in the same way as similar specimens from female patients.

The Central Nervous System
When healthy this system is free from micro-organisms.

IMPORTANT PATHOGENS

N. meningitidis, *Str. pneumoniae*, *Myco. tuberculosis*–meningitis at all ages.

H. influenzae (type b)–meningitis, mainly in children aged 2 months to 3 years.

Staph. aureus–abscesses with secondary meningitis at all ages.

Esch. coli, *Listeria monocytogenes*–meningitis in new-born infants.

T. pallidum–the various forms of neurosyphilis (p 154).

Many viruses, notably: polioviruses–poliomyelitis; coxsackie and echoviruses–meningitis; togaviruses–encephalitis.

(*Cryptococcus neoformans*, p 219, and *Naegleria fowleri* and *Hartmannella* species, p 230, are rare causes of meningitis that need to be borne in mind.)

CHOICE AND COLLECTION OF SPECIMENS

Cerebrospinal fluid, by far the commonest microbiological specimen from the central nervous system, is sometimes collected from the ventricles of the brain or elsewhere inside the skull, particularly by neurosurgeons; but far more often by the procedure known as lumbar puncture. In outline, a wide-bored sterile needle is passed between the spines of two lumbar vertebrae and through the dura, and cerebrospinal fluid is allowed to drip from it into a sterile container. From the bacteriological point of view, the most important technical problem is to avoid introducing contaminant organisms either into the subdural space or into the specimen. This calls for rigorous aseptic technique and for antimicrobial treatment of the skin–e.g. by applying povidone-iodine solution or chlorhexidine in 70% alcohol (see p 285).

When a virus infection of the central nervous system is suspected, other specimens besides cerebrospinal fluid should be sent to the laboratory–nose and throat swabs in virus transport medium (see p 183), and also faeces if an enterovirus infection is a possibility.

ROUTINE INITIAL INVESTIGATIONS

The cerebrospinal fluid specimen should be sent to the laboratory and examined without delay. Normal cerebrospinal fluid is crystal clear and colourless; any turbidity indicates either infection or the presence of blood (possibly as a result of trauma during collection of the specimen). In tuberculous meningitis a 'spider web' clot often forms in the fluid shortly after collection. Investigations of a turbid fluid should include a total and differential cell count and esti-mations of its glucose and protein contents. If, as commonly occurs, these are to be carried out elsewhere than in the bacteriological laboratory, two specimens should be collected so that there is no risk of the specimen for culture being contaminated during the removal of material for other purposes. In most cases of acute bacterial meningitis there are thousands of cells per μl, virtually all polymorphonuclear leucocytes (in contrast to the very small number of lymphocytes normally present), glucose is absent or present in much smaller amounts than normal and the protein level is raised. Later, there is commonly a lower total cell count with a larger proportion of lymphocytes, a picture which is also common in tuberculous meningitis. Depression of the chloride level is some-times helpful as an indication of tuberculous meningitis. In virus meningitis, predominance of polymorphonuclear cells, if present at all in the early stages, is usually short-lived and there is little or no alteration of the glucose and chloride levels.

Unless it is very turbid the fluid is centrifuged for bacteriological examination and the deposit is used for making smears and for inoculating cultures.

For *Myco. tuberculosis*–Ziehl–Neelsen-stained smears of deposit, or if a spider web clot is present, part of it should be spread out on a slide, dried, fixed by gentle heating, and stained by the Ziehl-Neelsen method; culture on Löwenstein–Jensen or other suitable medium.

For other bacteria–Gram-stained smear; aerobic culture on blood agar and chocolate agar. (Because the identity of the pathogen may have an important bearing upon the treatment of acute bacterial meningitis, initial investigations applied directly to the cerebro-spinal fluid may include such procedures as attempted identification of the organism itself by capsule-swelling or immunofluorescence, or of its products by cross-over immuno-electrophoresis or co-agglutination.)

The Blood-Stream

Although many oral, intestinal and other bacteria enter the blood in small numbers from time to time, it has no normal microbial flora.

IMPORTANT PATHOGENS

Staph. aureus, *Str. pyogenes* and many other bacteria–acute septicaemia.

N. meningitidis–chronic septicaemia.

Viridans streptococci, enterococci–sub-acute bacterial endocarditis.

Coagulase-negative staphylococci–infections of prosthetic heart valves and other prostheses.

Salmonellae–enteric fever.

Brucellae–undulant fever.

Plasmodia–malaria (see p 223 for investigation).

COLLECTION OF SPECIMENS

Venepuncture should be carried out with the same scrupulous care to avoid contamination as is required for lumbar puncture, using a sterile needle attached to a sterile syringe (or to a sterile evacuated ampoule specially designed for the purpose). The veins in the antecubital fossa or on the forearm are commonly used, and are distended by means of a tourniquet. It may be best to take blood at a time when the patient's temperature is rising, as this is the time at which the number of bacteria in the blood is likely to be greatest. The blood should be transferred as soon as it is taken (before it has time to clot) into two or more bottles containing appropriate broth culture media (see below), as a general rule adding about 3–5 ml of blood to 50 ml of broth. In addition, or as an alternative, to the direct inoculation of broth cultures, blood can be added in a ratio of about 2:1 or 3:1 to broth containing 0·05% Liquoid (sodium polyanethol sulphonate), which both prevents it from clotting and inhibits its bactericidal mechanisms. In the laboratory some of this treated blood can be mixed in a 1:20 ratio with melted nutrient agar, poured into Petri dishes and allowed to set; the rest of the blood can be used to set up broth cultures if this has not already been done at the bedside. All cultures are usually incubated at 37°C. The poured plate technique has two advantages over broth culture: it may provide colonies of bacteria on or beneath the surface of the medium within 18 hours or so of setting up the cultures, in which case identification of the organism is possible sooner than if it is merely growing in broth; and it gives a quantitative estimate of the number of bacteria in the blood–heavy growth indicates that there were many organisms, and contamination during collection is most unlikely to account for more than a very few colonies. Broth culture, on the other hand, is a far more sensitive means of detecting small numbers of bacteria, especially of organisms like brucellae and some of the streptococci that cause endocarditis, which may take several weeks to increase to detectable numbers; but it is also a good means of producing heavy growths from a small number of contaminant organisms. Opinions differ as to whether a broth culture should be subcultured to solid media every few days (thus hastening the detection of any organisms present, but at the risk of introducing contaminants into the bottle and thus confusing the interpretation of subsequent subcultures) or should be left alone until colour change of the blood layer at the bottom of the bottle or turbidity of the supernatant indicates that bacterial growth has occurred. The need for very great care to avoid contamination of the cultures arises from the difficulty of deciding that any organism grown from blood is not a pathogen; bacteria of almost every group have at some time or other been at least suspected, if not convicted, of causing sub-acute endocarditis or low-grade chronic septicaemia.

The following are appropriate broths for various purposes:
For salmonellae–broth containing bile salt (e.g. 0·5% of sodium taurocholate), or even an aqueous dilution of ox bile. Clot culture should also be used (see p 128).
For brucellae–liver infusion broth, incubated in 5–10% CO_2.
For other organisms–a digest broth known to be able to support the growth of fastidious organisms; and a thioglycollate medium if anaerobes are likely to be present. Neutralization of penicillins, cephalosporins, sulphonamides and so far as possible other anti-bacterials that the patient may have been receiving may improve the efficacy of blood culture, as of culture of other types of specimen (see p 239).

Pleural and Peritoneal Cavities, Joints etc.
When fluid from one of these sites is required for microbiological investigation, aspiration should be carried out with the same care to avoid contamination as is required for cerebrospinal fluid or blood. The investigations appropriate to the specimen are determined by clinical indications as to the likely pathogens and by its own nature–e.g. it may be thick pus as from an abscess, it may be a relatively clear fluid on which cell counts and protein determination could be helpful, or it may be virtually pure blood.

Suggestions for Further Reading
Manual of Clinical Microbiology by E. H. Lennette and others, 2nd edn. (American Society for Microbiology, Washington, D.C., 1974).
Also Section III of *Bacteriology Illustrated*–see p 159.

15

Diagnostic Serology and Skin Testing

SEROLOGY

Since microbial infection commonly provokes the host to make specific antibodies, the demonstration of such antibodies in a patient's serum is often of considerable diagnostic value–particularly in conditions in which isolation of the causative organism takes a long time or is difficult or even impossible. However, there are a number of important points which have to be borne in mind when interpreting the results of antibody determinations. They include the following:

(1) Sometimes antibodies are found which react with a particular organism or its products although they were formed in response to infection with a different organism. For example, antibodies that agglutinate various proteus strains are formed as a result of infections with some of the rickettsiae (see p 162, the Weil–Felix test).

(2) The duration of detectable antibody responses to different organisms varies. After infection with some species, antibodies may be detectable for many years, and in such circumstances their presence is evidence only of infection *at some time*, not necessarily of *recent* infection. For example, the finding of rubella antibodies in the serum of a woman a few weeks after she had been exposed to rubella during early pregnancy may mean either that she became infected at that time, with the possibility that her foetus was severely damaged, or that she had her infection some years earlier and was immune at the time of exposure, and so the foetus was not at risk. Two lines of evidence in favour of an infection being recent are the demonstration of a rising titre (see below) and the identification of some of the antibody molecules as IgM (see p 65), since in many infections–notably rubella and brucellosis– antibodies of this class are the first to appear in the serum after a primary antigenic stimulus but may persist for only a few weeks.

In other infections IgM antibodies may persist much longer but their presence can be taken to indicate that the disease is still active. (In still others, however, IgM antibodies may persist long after the infection is, so far as we can tell by any other means, extinct.)

(3) As a corollary of the preceding points about cross-reaction and persistence of antibodies, the significance of a given level of the antibody measured by a particular test cannot be assessed without knowing the levels to be expected in the blood of normal healthy individuals of the same age, habitat and social background as the patient.

(4) In general, antibody responses are not detectable for at least 10 days, and often not for several weeks, after the onset of an infection with an organism of which the host has no previous experience. Thus examination of a serum sample collected during the first few days of an illness cannot be expected to give useful direct information about the cause of the illness. However, in virtually all acute infections for which specific serological tests are available, *it is desirable to collect a serum sample in the acute stage*. This is because demonstration of *a rising level of specific antibodies* is often the best way of identifying a recent infection. If antibodies are found in a serum sample collected 3 weeks or so after the onset of an illness, it may be impossible to say whether they have any connection with that illness and it may be too late to demonstrate a further rise (however, see p 184). But the situation is much clearer if an acute-stage specimen is available to be tested at the same time as the later specimen, and contains a significantly smaller amount of the antibodies in question. It is generally accepted that a 4-fold rise in titre is beyond the range of experimental error of most routine procedures, provided that the two specimens are tested at the same time, and is therefore indicative of a true increase in the amount of antibody in the patient's blood. (The *titre* of a serum is the highest dilution of that serum which gives a clear-cut positive reaction in a given test for antibodies of a given specificity. For example, if in the Widal test described below the *S. typhi* H suspension is agglutinated by the 1:480 and lower final dilutions of a serum but not by the 1:960 dilution, the *S. typhi* H titre of the serum is 1:480–or as some prefer to express it, 480.)

(5) Even a rising titre of specific antibody is not unequivocal evidence that the organism in question was responsible for the illness that is being investigated. Contact with the organism may have occurred coincidentally at about the time of onset of the patient's illness–though this possibility can reasonably be ignored if the patient's condition is strongly suggestive of that which the organism commonly produces. The position may also be obscured by an

anamnestic reaction–i.e. a rise in the level of a previously formed antibody in response to the non-specific stimulus of some quite different infection. This is particularly well recognized in connection with salmonella H agglutinins, which may increase in amount following a wide variety of unrelated febrile illnesses.

(6) When a patient is suspected of suffering from an illness in which detectable antibodies are usually formed, but no appropriate antibodies are found in his blood several weeks after the onset of his illness, considerable doubt is thrown upon the diagnosis–unless there is some derangement of his antibody-forming mechanism.

(7) Detectable antibodies are not necessarily protective antibodies, and therefore the results of serological tests may have nothing to do with the patient's immunity or lack of it.

The principle of tests used for the measurement of antibodies have been outlined in Chapter Eight, and the types of test used to detect infection with particular organisms have been indicated in Chapters Nine to Thirteen, in relation to the following conditions:

> *Str. pyogenes* infections–pp 101–1
> Gonorrhoea–p 109.
> *Enteric fever–p 129 and below (the Widal test).
> *Yersinia* infections–p 133.
> *Brucellosis–p 142 and below.
> *Syphilis–p 155 and below.
> Leptospirosis–p 157.
> *Mycoplasma* infections–p 158.
> Rickettsial infections–p 162.
> Q fever–p 165.
> Chlamydial infections–p 167.
> Most virus infections–pp 184–5.
> Candidiasis, aspergillosis and deep mycoses–p 221.
> Toxoplasmosis–p 225.
> Amoebiasis–p 230.

There are many other infections in which diagnostic serological tests can be used, at any rate by workers with special interest and expertise, and no doubt in some of them such tests will in due course be widely adopted. The serological approach to diagnosis is used far more generally in virology than in bacteriology, but the techniques are more standardized and have been described adequately for our purposes in Chapter Eleven. In this chapter we shall deal with serological tests for the bacterial infections marked * in the list above, since between them these account for the great majority of the serological workload of most diagnostic bacteriology laboratories and since the tests used illustrate many general principles and involve certain theoretical complexities that need to be explained.

The Widal Test

In many cases of fever it is necessary to investigate the possibility of enteric fever or other salmonella infection. The serological part of such an investigation is measurement of the ability of the patient's serum to agglutinate various salmonella suspensions.

THE TEST   Standard bacterial suspensions of known agglutinability are used. The nature of the three types of antigen involved–H, O and Vi–has been discussed on pp 126 and 129. In Britain, H and O suspensions of *S. typhi* and of *S. paratyphi B* are commonly used, and also a 'non-specific salmonella H' suspension which contains antigens common to a wide range of salmonellae. If any other particular salmonella is suspected of being responsible for the patient's illness, H and O suspensions of that type are included in the test.

Serial dilutions of the patient's serum in saline (e.g. 1:15, 1:30, 1:60, 1:120, 1:240, 1:480) are pipetted in small amounts (e.g. 0·5 ml) into special small tubes, one complete set of dilutions being prepared for each bacterial suspension that is to be used in the test. An equal volume of the appropriate bacterial suspension is then added to each tube (the final serum dilutions therefore becoming 1:30, 1:60, etc.). Control tubes are also set up, containing suspensions mixed with saline instead of serum, to ensure that the bacteria do not agglutinate spontaneously.

H and O agglutination tests are incubated in a water-bath at 37 °C (or at 50–55 °C). Floccular agglutination of the H suspensions becomes apparent within 2 hours or so, whereas the more granular agglutination of O suspensions takes from 4 to 24 hours. The results of the tests are expressed as antibody titres, as defined above.

INTERPRETATION   Low levels of antibodies that agglutinate salmonella suspensions are common in the blood of patients with no history of relevant illness or of immunization. In Britain, H titres of 1:30 and O titres of 1:60 for *S. typhi* and *S. paratyphi B* are 'normal'. The picture is greatly confused by previous immunization, for which T.A.B. (killed bacilli of *S. typhi* and *S. paratyphi A* and *B*) or T.A.B.C. (the same + *S. paratyphi C*) are generally used (see p 312), and it is important that all relevant information on this matter should accompany any request for a Widal test. Following such immunization, high levels of H agglutinins for the species used may be present for many years, and rising H agglutinin titres are of doubtful significance because they may represent anamnestic reactions (see p 259). Similarly, after natural infection the H agglutinin level may be high and variable for many years, but in this case it is only the H suspension belonging to the appropriate species which is agglutinated or those which are antigenically related to it. O agglutinin levels, on the other hand, remain high for only a few months after immunization or natural infection, and are less liable to anamnestic rises. Furthermore, O agglutinins are formed more rapidly and more constantly than H agglutinins following typhoid or other salmonella infections, usually being detectable in the serum by about the tenth day of the illness. For these reasons the most reliable serological evidence of a salmonella infection is a 4-fold or greater increase in the O agglutinin level between the first week and the second or later weeks of the illness. However, because there is considerable sharing of O antigens between salmonellae, a rise in the H agglutinin level may give more precise information as to the particular organism causing the patient's illness. Absence of agglutinin response does not exclude the possibility of typhoid, as occasionally patients fail to produce detectable levels of antibodies.

Serological Tests for Brucellosis
Since brucellosis is a possible cause of persistent pyrexia, agglutination tests using suspensions of the appropriate brucella species (in Britain, *Br. abortus* and sometimes *Br. melitensis*) are commonly carried out in conjunction with the Widal test. The technique is essentially that of the Widal test for O agglutinins, and, since the organisms are not flagellate, only a single suspension of each species is required. Neither agglutination tests nor any of the other tests mentioned below can be relied upon to establish firmly the diagnosis of brucellosis, since antibody levels found in the blood of some apparently healthy people, notably of farm workers and others who have long been exposed to risks of brucella infection, may exceed those found in some patients with undoubted brucellosis. If the patient is seen early in the illness, it may be possible to demonstrate that his blood contains IgM antibodies, and such a finding strongly supports the diagnosis of brucellosis. Demonstration of a rising antibody titre may also be possible at this stage, and is a help to diagnosis. But because the onset of this disease is often insidious, the IgM antibodies may have disappeared and the initial IgM antibody rise may be over before the patient presents for investigation. An agglutination titre of 1:1000 or more indicates active brucellosis, but in the chronic infection it is common to find either a low agglutination titre or *zoning* (i.e. failure of the serum to cause agglutination until it is considerably diluted—see p 69), because of which the range of serum dilutions used in the test should extend at least to 1:5000. Both of these findings are attributable to the

blocking action of non-agglutinating IgG antibodies. These can be detected either by a test of the Coombs type (see p 71) or by a complement-fixation test; a titre of 1:32 or more in either of these tests suggests active brucella infection.

Serological Tests in Pyrexia of Unknown Origin (P.U.O.)

The patient with persistent pyrexia and no clear indication as to its cause is a common diagnostic problem. Serological tests may provide vital clues. Tests which it is reasonable to carry out in such circumstances in Britain include the Widal and brucella-antibody tests already described in this chapter and those which we have mentioned in earlier chapters in connection with leptospirosis, toxoplasmosis and Q fever; with the addition, in influenza-like illnesses, of tests for influenza and other viruses capable of producing such illnesses, and of those for psittacosis and mycoplasma infection. Special circumstances or features of the illness may suggest other possibilities.

Serological Tests for Syphilis

REAGINIC TESTS   For over half a century the Wassermann reaction (W.R.) test was the mainstay of the laboratory diagnosis of syphilis, despite the fact that its mechanism is quite different from that conceived by Wassermann and his colleagues. It is a complement-fixation test and therefore conforms to the outline given on pp 70–1. Wassermann's problem was to find a source of a suitable antigen, since the causative organism of syphilis could not be grown in artificial culture. He thought that he had solved the problem by using an aqueous extract of the liver of a dead human syphilitic foetus, since the organ was teeming with syphilitic spirochaetes. The resulting test was highly successful, but it was soon discovered that the liver of a non-syphilitic foetus was equally good, and that alcoholic extracts of various other organs worked even better. Cardiolipin from ox heart was adopted as the standard antigen. The test is·remarkably specific, considering the apparent irrelevance of the antigen. It reacts with an IgG serum component which is called *reagin* (though it is not related to the similarly named IgE antibodies mentioned on p 61). Many other cardiolipin-based serological tests for syphilis have been devised, in which the reaction between the cardiolipin and a positive serum is manifested by formation of a visible floccular precipitate rather than by complement fixation. These too are known as reaginic tests, though the serum component is IgM rather than IgG. Most of them are now obsolete, but the *Venereal Disease Research Laboratory* (V.D.R.L.) test and its variant the *Rapid Plasma Reagin* (R.P.R.) test are widely used, as they are simple and easy to perform and give consistent results. (Another variant, for dealing with very large numbers of sera, is the

Automated Reaginic Test–A.R.T.) They become positive early in a syphilitic infection, before some of the more specific tests mentioned below, and they are valuable screening tests for determining which specimens for syphilis serology need further investigation. However, in view of the basis of the reaginic tests it is not surprising that they give positive reactions in conditions other than syphilis–'biological false positives'. These may occur in many infections, notably in malaria, leprosy, tuberculosis, leptospirosis and infective hepatitis, after smallpox and other vaccinations, and also (by far their commonest cause in Britain) in pregnancy. Such false positives are usually transitory, except in certain chronic diseases such as rheumatoid arthritis and disseminated lupus erythematosus.

TESTS USING TREPONEMAL ANTIGENS   Wassermann's basic problem that the spirochaete of syphilis could not be grown in culture remains unsolved–hence the persistence of the reaginic tests. The *Reiter protein complement-fixation* (R.P.C.F.) test uses as antigen an extract from a culture of the non-pathogenic Reiter treponema strain; it is less sensitive than some of the other tests to be described, and it gives some false positive results, but since its basis is unrelated to that of the reaginic tests the combination of a positive V.D.R.L. or R.P.R. test and a positive R.P.C.F. test is far more likely to be due to a treponemal infection than to coincident false positives in both systems. The more specific tests, which use genuine *T. pallidum* antigens, depend on the fact that this organism can be propagated and produced in fair quantities by serial intratesticular passage in rabbits–though this is a procedure for a specialized reference laboratory only. Where such a preparation of live *T. pallidum* is available, it can be kept alive for several days in a special fluid medium under carefully controlled environmental conditions, and shows itself to be alive by continual flexuous movements that can be observed by dark-ground microscopy. If serum from a syphilitic patient, together with guinea-pig serum, is added to such a suspension of *T. pallidum*, the organisms cease to move. This is the basis of the *Treponema pallidum immobilization* (T.P.I.) test, a highly specific and useful confirmatory test but one which is necessarily limited to reference laboratories. The *fluorescent treponemal antibody* (F.T.A.) test depends on the same source of *T. pallidum*, but they do not have to be alive, and so it can be carried out in a routine laboratory. It is performed by applying dilute serum from a patient to a fixed smear of dead *T. pallidum* on a microscope slide, so that any anti-treponemal antibodies present attach themselves to the treponemes during a period of incubation; the serum is then washed off and antibody-coated treponemes are detected by means of rabbit serum containing fluorescent anti-human-gamma-globulin antibodies (see p

72). (In the improved form of this test known as F.T.A.–ABS the Reiter treponeme appears again, but this time as a means of removing irrelevant antibodies from the serum before it is tested!) The *Treponema pallidum haemagglutination* (T.P.H.A.) test is a passive haemagglutination procedure (see p 69) in which red blood cells (from animals or birds) are coated with a *T. pallidum* extract and are then agglutinable by sera containing appropriate anti-*T. pallidum* antibodies.

THE USE AND INTERPRETATION OF THESE DIFFERENT TESTS   As already indicated, reaginic tests such as the V.D.R.L. or R.P.R. are useful both because they are easily applied in any laboratory to large numbers of sera and because they give positive results during the primary stage of syphilis–i.e. within 2 or 3 weeks of infection. A treponemal-antigen screening test is also desirable because of the problem of false positive results; the R.P.C.F. test has been widely used for this purpose but is being replaced by the T.P.H.A. test, which is more specific and more sensitive (i.e. gives fewer false positive and more true positive results). The F.T.A. test is less appropriate for screening large numbers of sera, as it has to be read under a microscope and so is relatively time-consuming (and difficult to automate, unlike the reaginic tests or the T.P.H.A. test); but it is valuable as a confirmatory test for sera that have given positive results with screening tests, or for the primary examination of patients in whom the probability of positive results is high. Two advantages of the F.T.A. tests are that it becomes positive early in the disease, at about the same time as the reaginic tests and before the other treponemal tests; and that, by use of rabbit serum specific for particular human immuno-globulin classes it is possible to detect IgG and IgM antibodies separately. In an adult, presence of IgM antibodies suggests continued active infection; in an infant, it indicates infection of the infant itself, since maternal IgM (unlike IgG) cannot cross the placenta. The T.P.I. test, for reasons given above, is essentially a reference laboratory test. It fails to detect very early infections, but apart from that it is the most sensitive and most specific serological test for syphilis, with the possible exception of the T.P.H.A. test which is its only close rival. It cannot, however, be carried out on sera that contain antibiotics or other substances which themselves would be toxic to, and immobilize, the treponemes.

Effective treatment very soon after syphilitic infection may prevent development of any serological responses. Treatment some weeks later, during the secondary stage, usually results in disappearance of detectable reagins some 6 months to a year later, but tests using *T. pallidum* are likely to remain positive for years. If treatment is still further delayed, all tests may remain positive for many years, those using *T. pallidum* being the more persistent. This happens despite eradication of the infection by treatment, and subsequent attempts to reverse the positive findings by further antibiotic treatment are of no avail.

The serological tests for syphilis can be applied to cerebrospinal fluid, with positive results in most cases of active neurosyphilis.

The serological responses to T. pallidum infection cannot be distinguished from those to any of the other trepanematoses—yaws, pinta etc. (p 155). Clearly this is most important in parts of the world in which these conditions are endemic, but it needs to be remembered elsewhere. For example, a bacteriologist in Britain is frequently confronted with a set of results which would undoubtedly indicate a past *T. pallidum* infection if they came from the blood of someone who had always lived in this country, and could therefore be used to support a diagnosis of vascular, neurological or other late syphilitic disease; but which in fact came from the blood of an immigrant from the West Indies or some other appropriate area who had had untreated yaws in childhood and had been left with permanent serological memorials of it.

SKIN TESTING

Skin tests used in microbiological diagnosis mostly fall into one of two categories—those for detecting immunity and those for detecting hypersensitivity.

Tests for Immunity

THE SCHICK TEST   If a small amount of diphtheria toxin is injected into the skin of a human being who is not immune to it, local damage results. In such a subject, the minute standard amount used in the Schick test causes a reaction that begins to appear one or two days after injection, reaches a maximum after about four days and persists for a week or two. Its chief component is erythema of the skin in an area a few cm in diameter around the injection site, though there may also be some swelling. However, if the same dose is injected into a subject whose level of diphtheria antitoxin is sufficient to protect him against an attack of the disease, the toxin is neutralized and produces no reaction. The picture is complicated by the fact that diphtheria toxin is prepared from cultures of diphtheria bacilli, and the material used for the test therefore contains other products of the bacilli as well as the toxin. Some patients, probably only those with previous experience of diphtheria bacilli, produce a local erythematous reaction to these other components. However, this 'pseudo-reaction' begins within about 12 hours of injection and lasts only a few days; furthermore, it is produced equally well by an injection of toxin preparation in which the toxin itself has been inactivated by heating.

In a community in which there is very little diphtheria, such as

Britain at present, there is no need to carry out routine Schick tests on small children coming to be immunized for the first time, but they should always be done as a preliminary to immunizing older children or adults, in order to exclude both those who do not need immunization and those in whom it might cause severe reactions.

The Dick test, used in the past to determine the need for immunization against scarlet fever, was essentially similar to the Schick test except that the test material was a preparation of streptococcal erythrogenic toxin and the skin reaction produced was more rapid and transitory.

Tests for Hypersensitivity

THE TUBERCULIN TEST   The theoretical basis of tuberculin testing has been discussed on p 77. It depends on a Type IV hypersensitivity reaction.

It is important to appreciate certain features in which the tuberculin test is fundamentally different from the Schick test:

(a) The test material—old tuberculin (O.T.) or more commonly its Purified Protein Derivative (P.P.D.)—is not itself toxic. Any reaction that follows its injection is due to the host's acquired hypersensitivity, not to the properties of tuberculin itself.

(b) Whereas a positive Schick reaction indicates lack of immunity and a negative reaction indicates immunity, it is the positive tuberculin reaction which is associated with immunity. This association is only an indirect one, however, for there is no clear evidence that tuberculin hypersensitivity is itself part of the mechanism of immunity. All that can be said is that those who have had and overcome tuberculous infections (natural or resulting from B.C.G. vaccination) generally have some degree of immunity to further infection; and, therefore, since tuberculin hypersensitivity indicates past tuberculous infection, it also indicates probable immunity.

(c) The important component of a positive tuberculin reaction is palpable induration, which is maximal two or three days after injection of the tuberculin. Erythema also occurs but is in part non-specific and is difficult to interpret.

Tuberculin testing of human patients can be carried out in various ways. In the *Mantoux* test 0·1 ml of O.T. or P.P.D. solution is injected intradermally by means of a syringe and needle. Since some patients, especially those with active tuberculosis, may give very strong reactions, it is necessary to start with a dilute solution and to repeat the test using stronger solutions if indicated. The *Heaf* test employs a number of very short needles mounted on a spring-loaded device which drives them into the skin through a drop of tuberculin solution placed on the skin in the appropriate site. Although this procedure sounds formidable when described, it is in fact more acceptable to children than is the Mantoux test, and is less liable to produce excessive reactions. Positive reactions range from multiple small papules at the sites of individual punctures to a zone of induration including all of the puncture sites and the surrounding skin.

Purposes for which tuberculin testing of human subjects is useful include:

(*a*) *Diagnosis* of individual patients. The test is positive in all cases of active tuberculous infection except those which are very early or of overwhelming severity. However, its diagnostic value is limited by the fact that it is also positive in a high proportion of older children and adults who are not suffering from active tuberculosis, these being people with healed primary infections (natural or from B.C.G. vaccination). A negative reaction, contraindicating the diagnosis of tuberculosis, is often helpful to the clinician; and a very strong reaction suggests an active tuberculosis infection.

(*b*) *Detection* of foci of infection. In the absence of widespread vaccination, a high incidence of positive reactions in the children of any social unit–e.g. a family or a school–suggests the presence of an active disseminator of the disease.

(*c*) *Surveys* of population groups to determine the frequency of tuberculosis in the communities which they represent. This use also depends upon the situation not having been obscured by widespread vaccination.

(*d*) *Selection* of subjects for B.C.G. vaccination. In the absence of any better criterion of immunity, a negative tuberculin reaction is taken as indicating that vaccination is required.

(*e*) *Assessment* of the efficacy of vaccination. Its use here is controversial (see p 310).

Tuberculin testing of cattle, with elimination of those giving positive reactions, is the basis of the creation of tuberculosis-free herds, which has played an important part in eliminating the risk of human infection with tubercle bacilli of the bovine type.

OTHER TESTS   As we said on p 77, the brucellin test (p 142), the lepromin test (p 148), the Frei test (p 167) and the skin tests used to demonstrate delayed hypersensitivity to fungi (p 221) are essentially similar to the tuberculin test. The usefulness of any such test depends upon the frequency with which positive reactions, due to subclinical infections, are found in healthy members of the community. For example, a positive histoplasmin test is a most unusual and potentially important finding in a patient normally resident in Britain, but far less interesting if the patient comes from an area of the U.S.A. in which histoplasmosis is endemic.

PART VI

PREVENTION AND TREATMENT OF MICROBIAL DISEASES

16

Principles of Prevention

Microbial disease can be prevented by:

(*a*) eliminating sources of the responsible organisms;
(*b*) preventing transmission of the responsible organisms; or
(*c*) raising the resistance of potential hosts so that they are not susceptible to the attacks of the organisms.

The extent to which each of these lines can be followed varies greatly from one disease to another. In many cases it is possible and necessary to advance along two or all three of them at the same time.

ELIMINATION OF SOURCES

The great majority of human microbial infections are acquired from other human beings or from animals. Whether their sources can be eliminated depends upon the ease with which cases and carriers can be found and then treated or destroyed.

In some diseases it is not unrealistic to speak of the possibility of eradicating all sources. Smallpox, for example, appears at present (1977) to have been eradicated from 35 of the 38 countries in which it was endemic 10 years ago. This has been achieved despite the absence of any effective treatment. Relatively rapid eradication has been made possible by the fact that this is a disease of humans only. Furthermore, it is a self-limiting disease, in that patients either die or recover without becoming chronic carriers. Success has been achieved by identifying and isolating all cases (the only sources of infection, though it has to be remembered that virus shed by them into dust can remain infective for many weeks), and by widespread immunization–not merely to protect the immunized but to prevent them from becoming sources of infection.

Tuberculosis provides a somewhat more complicated illustration of the possibility of eradication, since man may be infected from cattle as well as from humans – and indeed there is evidence that cattle may acquire their infections from badgers and other wild animals. In a highly developed community there is no great difficulty in locating all cattle, and those with latent or active tuberculous infection can be identified by tuberculin testing. If all such cattle are destroyed the human population is freed from any risk of tuberculosis of bovine origin. (Alternatively, infected cattle can be segregated from the rest and their milk can be pasteurized, but these measures do not belong to this section of the chapter.) The difficulties of carrying out such a programme are administrative and economic rather than scientific, and have been largely overcome in Britain. Finding human sources of tuberculous infection is a bigger problem, in that human beings are more numerous than cattle and less easy to round up for regular testing. Furthermore, the value of the tuberculin test as a means of detecting latent or active tuberculosis has been considerably reduced by widespread B.C.G. vaccination, which also causes positive tuberculin reactions. However, since infection with the human type of tubercle bacillus usually involves the lungs, it can often be detected on chest X-ray films. Mass-radiography campaigns, involving the collection of such films of as many members of a community as possible, have been widely and effectively used in the search for infected human beings. Unfortunately, as the incidence of tuberculosis decreases as a result of such measures, further routine screening of the apparently healthy population ceases to be either acceptable to the public or cost-effective. As for the active cases that are discovered by one means or another, treatment (with temporary isolation of those that are 'open' – i.e. discharging tubercle bacilli in their sputum or by any other route), must be followed by prolonged surveillance, since it is never safe to regard any tuberculous infection as permanently cured. The contacts of all active cases must also be carefully followed up.

Brucellosis presents a simpler control problem than tuberculosis (in theory, at least!) because domestic animals (cattle in Britain) are the only sources of human infection and elimination of infected farm stock would put an end to the disease (see p 142).

Anthrax is predominantly a disease of domestic animals. As Pasteur demonstrated, the most dangerous source of this disease, at any rate for other animals, is the dead body of one of its victims. Here the problem is not to find the source but to deal with it, since the bacillus is a spore-former and hard to eradicate. Bodies of animals that die from anthrax should either be destroyed by burning or be buried deep in the ground. These are simple procedures when small animals are involved but less simple, when, as in an English zoo some years ago, the victims are elephants! The main sources of anthrax in countries such as Britain are hides, hair and bone-meal imported from countries where anthrax is endemic and where skin and bone are the marketable components of sick or dead animals. The hazards from such materials are reduced by hypochlorite or other appropriate treatment, preferably before shipment but, failing that, on arrival in the receiving country.

It may be difficult or impossible to eliminate the sources of diseases carried by wild animals. A thickly populated island such as Britain has great advantages in this respect, for there are no large tracts of uncontrollable waste land, and land animals cannot enter the country without human help. The rabies virus is not carried by any native wild animals, and has not been endemic among domestic animals since the beginning of the century, although there have been a few localized outbreaks following importation of infected pets. The strict quarantine regulation governing importation of dogs or other potential carriers have been of great value to the country, but are defied – usually for sentimental or commercial reasons – with a frequency which is particularly disturbing at a time when rabies among the fox population is spreading westward across Europe. Control is far more difficult on a continent than on an island, particularly in a country such as Canada, where various wild animal species suffer from rabies – some of them roaming over vast uninhabited areas and others, such as squirrels, coming into close contact with man and his domestic animals.

Persistent hunting for cases and carriers, which is so valuable in controlling chronic widespread diseases as tuberculosis, is less well rewarded in connection with more acute and less common infections. With some of these the best way to locate sources of infection is to co-ordinate information about new cases. This is the purpose of legislation which makes certain diseases notifiable. To search Britain for carriers of typhoid, for example, would be an enormous undertaking with little likelihood of reasonable reward; but as soon as a new case is reported, public health authorities can institute an intensive local detective operation. This may be made easier if there are several new cases due to the same phage-type of typhoid bacillus, since the search for a carrier can then be concentrated in spheres of contact that are common to the people involved. However, finding a typhoid carrier is only part of the problem; eradication of his infection may be a much slower process (see p 127).

There is no possibility of eliminating the sources of some of man's commonest and most important pathogens – e.g. *Staph. aureus* and *Str. pyogenes* – since these are normally carried by a high proportion of healthy people. However, all possible steps must be taken to ensure that people in certain types of employment – e.g. operating theatre staff and food-handlers–are not disseminating strains of such organisms with known propensities for causing trouble (see pp 291 and 306).

PREVENTION OF TRANSMISSION
Control of Migration and Local Movement

We have already touched upon the importance of quarantine regulations in preventing transmission of disease on the international scale. Such regulations require animals or human beings, entering a country in circumstances in which they might be incubating one of certain specified diseases, to be kept in isolation for a period which exceeds the incubation period of that disease. Such an approach is of no use in excluding carriers or those with diseases that have long and unpredictable latent periods. There are other ways of dealing with these, such as insisting that intending immigrants undergo appropriate investigations–e.g. chest radiographs, examinations of their faeces for bacterial and protozoal pathogens, or Wassermann tests of their blood–before leaving their countries of origin, or that they are effectively immunized. This last measure has been widely enforced in relation to smallpox; even efficiently executed vaccination does not exclude the possibility that the immigrant will develop a mild (but transmissible) attack of smallpox several weeks after leaving an infected area, but it does greatly reduce the risk of his doing so.

Unwanted and undocumented animal immigrants can be a serious problem. Hence ships in port have shields on their hawsers which prevent 'hitch-hiking' by plague-carrying rats, and aeroplanes which pass through yellow fever zones are sprayed with insecticides in case they pick up infected mosquitoes.

Quarantine regulations can be imposed on a local basis. It is no longer generally regarded as necessary to restrict the movements of children during the incubation stages of the common infectious fevers of childhood, but similar restrictions can be applied to members of small units, such as families or schools or military camps, who are possibly incubating more serious diseases.

Isolation of infected patients comes under the same heading but is discussed in Chapter Eighteen.

Control of Insect Vectors

Destruction of insect vectors plays a large part in the control of many diseases–notably of rickettsial infections (Chapter Ten), yellow fever (p 190) and malaria (p 224). While it may be difficult or impossible to eradicate an insect species from an area permanently, it is often possible to reduce its numbers to a very low level for a time, and during that time to treat any remaining human cases of the disease and so abolish the reservoir from which the insects might otherwise become infected on their return.

When the relevant insects cannot be destroyed, it may be possible to prevent them from acting as vectors. For example, mosquito nets, fly screens and insect repellants can keep biting insects from attacking prospective hosts, and flies which cannot reach human faeces or human food cannot transmit dysentery bacilli from one to the other.

Communal Hygiene

The spread of disease is made easier when human beings live closely packed together in homes into which little bactericidal sunlight penetrates; in which fleas, lice and bugs abound as vectors; in which accumulated refuse encourages the breeding of disease-carrying vermin; in which lack of water supply discourages personal and domestic cleanliness; and in which there is no adequate provision for sewage disposal. In other words, it is generally true that a well-housed community with a main water supply and proper provision for the disposal of refuse and sewage is also a community relatively free from microbial diseases, and the provision of such conditions must be the aim of those interested in the prevention of such diseases. But transmission of infection is not, of course, limited to the home. In schools, shops, meeting halls, places of amusement, public vehicles, swimming baths and wherever else human beings come together they exchange their microbial parasites. Some of the factors concerned in such transmission are mentioned below under 'Personal hygiene'; public responsibility is generally limited to preventing gross overcrowding and seeing that the individual has the necessary facilities for hygienic behaviour and is encouraged to use them. During serious epidemics, particularly of droplet-borne diseases, it may be wise to prevent people from congregating indoors.

The communal and personal aspects of the proper treatment of food and drink are discussed in Chapter Nineteen.

Personal Hygiene

The individual has a double responsibility in relation to the transmission of disease—to do his best to avoid being either a recipient or a donor. Much of what he has to do about protecting himself relates to the maintenance of his general health and specific immunity, and so is not the concern of this section; but there are some ways in which he can reduce or eliminate his risks of acquiring certain infections—e.g. he can avoid promiscuous sexual intercourse (without which the serious problem of venereal diseases would cease to exist), and if he lives in an area where diseases are transmitted by biting insects he can protect himself from them as indicated above. In many everyday matters it is hard to decide how far hygienic precautions should be taken. Theoretical considerations suggest scrupulous care to keep all potentially infected objects away from the lips and mouth; but since this includes virtually everything except food which has just been cooked or has been kept in a sterile container since being cooked, some compromise with practical reality has to be reached which involves avoiding only those things that are most likely to be contaminated. From a purely microbiological standpoint kissing is a deplorable habit!

Precautions against transmitting pathogens to others are of course most important when one knows that one has an infection to transmit, and at such times it may be one's duty to stay at home or in some other way to reduce one's social contacts to a minimum. However, personal hygiene should also take into consideration the possibility of carrying and disseminating a pathogenic organism without knowing about it. Particular attention needs to be paid to the excretions of the respiratory and alimentary tracts. Airborne droplets, which are the means of transfer of many bacterial and virus infections, can be intercepted to some extent by following the advice of the slogan: 'Coughs and sneezes spread diseases; trap the germs in your handkerchief'. However, the handkerchief itself, replaced in a warm pocket for a period of incubation and then shaken out vigorously before its next use, can make a considerable contribution to the microbial population of the air. There is much to be said for using (and disposing of) disposable tissues. Spitting of sputum on to the ground, where it is allowed to dry, is a potentially dangerous practice at all times and a serious menace if the sputum contains tubercle bacilli. Faeces may contain pathogenic bacteria and viruses, and so good personal hygiene includes proper disposal of faeces and the washing of hands after defaecation. Food-handlers must be particularly careful to avoid transfer of their intestinal bacteria to food – which may prove a good culture medium for pathogens and so an excellent way of transmitting them to large numbers of people!

RAISING HOST RESISTANCE
General Considerations

There is little room for doubt that severe malnutrition, fatigue and lowering of the body temperature by exposure to a cold environment (chilling) all decrease resistance to infection, though there is a surprisingly small amount of clear-cut experimental evidence to support long-established clinical impressions on these points. Fatigue and chilling probably operate more by allowing latent infections to develop into overt diseases than by increasing susceptibility to fresh infection. Potential hosts who are well fed, well rested, well housed and well clothed are therefore relatively resistant to microbial diseases – though excess of food, rest or warmth may be harmful. Treatment of non-microbial diseases – notably of diabetes – may be important in raising resistance to infection.

Prophylactic Medication

While indiscriminate use of antibiotics and chemotherapeutic agents to prevent infection is to be condemned as extravagant and dangerous (see p 323), their use for this purpose is clearly indicated in a few situations. For example, patients who have had rheumatic fever can be protected from *Str. pyogenes* infections (and therefore from further attacks of rheumatic fever and further damage to their hearts) by long-term administration of sulphonamides or penicillins; and human beings who are regularly taking schizonticidal drugs can live and work in malaria-infested regions without developing that disease (see p 223).

Immunization

This very important part of the raising of host resistance has a chapter to itself (Chapter Twenty). Here it is sufficient to stress (*a*) the duty of the individual, for his own sake and that of the community, to see that so far as possible he and his family are immunized against any disease which is a potential menace in his particular environment; (*b*) the responsibility of public health authorities to see that he has the necessary information and facilities to carry out that duty; and (*c*) the responsibility of the employing authorities to ensure that doctors, nurses, ambulance drivers, medical laboratory technicians and others who are specially at risk because of the nature of their work are adequately immunized against such infections as tuberculosis and poliomyelitis.

Suggestions for Further Reading

'International problems of communicable-disease control' by P. Dorolle, *Lancet*, 1972, ii, 525.

Detailed information about the control of a wide range of infectious diseases is to be found in *Control of Communicable Diseases of Man*, ed. A. S. Benenson 12th edn. (American Public Health Association, New York, 1975).

17

Sterilization

This chapter deals with sterilization in relation to both clinical and laboratory practice. As an introduction to it, the section of Chapter Five entitled 'Survival and Death' should be looked at again (pp 36–42).

STERILIZATION BY FILTRATION

Air and liquids can be sterilized by passing them through filters that remove bacteria and larger particles. Free virus particles are small enough to pass through the majority of filters in common use, but for many purposes this is of no importance. Many viruses are arrested by the filters because they are contained in droplets or in cells.

Filtration of Air

The simplest form of air filter is a glass tube tightly plugged with non-absorbent cotton wool. Bacteria and other particles contained in air which passes through such a filter become entangled in the fibres of the cotton wool, which must itself have been sterilized by heating before it is used as a filter, and which must be non-absorbent because motile organisms can swim through it if it becomes wet. Such simple filters are in common use in microbiological laboratories as a means of allowing sterile air to enter tubes and flasks containing cultures. Larger and more elaborate filters are used when it is necessary to provide sterile air to whole rooms used for special work – e.g. the preparation of vaccines – in which it is particularly important to avoid airborne contamination.

Filtration of Liquids

Liquids can be sterilized by passing them through the walls of hollow cylinders of kieselguhr (*Berkefeld* filters) or unglazed porcelain (*Chamberland* filters), through sintered glass filters formed by fusing small particles of glass together, through disks of compressed asbestos fibres (*Seitz* filter pads) or through cellulose membrane filters. Seitz or cellulose membrane filters held in special metal funnels are more convenient than other forms of filter for most purposes in a routine microbiological laboratory. The liquid to be sterilized is drawn through the funnel into a sterile bottle or flask which is connected via an air filter to a vacuum pump. Filtration is more time-consuming than heat-sterilization, the filter and other apparatus have themselves to be heat-sterilized beforehand, and there is always a risk of accidental contamination of the material because of leakage of unsterile air into the apparatus. This process is therefore reserved for materials such as serum and yeast extracts which would be adversely affected by heat. Selective adsorption of certain ingredients on to the filter is another hazard of filtration, but is minimal when sintered glass or a cellulose membrane is used. (Filters–e.g. cellulose membranes–of known pore size can also be used to determine the size of microbial particles or to separate organisms of different sizes.)

STERILIZATION BY HEAT OR RADIATION

The killing of a microbial population, whether by these physical means or by using disinfectants, is a process, not an instantaneous event. The time taken to complete it depends on the size of the population (among other things). Therefore, to use an oversimplified example, if it is found that in specified circumstances and with a particular bacterial strain a sterilizing procedure kills 90% of the bacterial population every minute, 5 minutes of such treatment would be virtually certain to eliminate a population of 100 organisms (failing only once in a thousand times) but would be unreliable against a population of 10 000 (failing once in ten times) and could not be expected to kill all of 1 million organisms. Of course, several hours of such treatment could be relied upon to deal with astronomical numbers of organisms (at least of the strain in question), but unfortunately the sterilizing process often has to be restricted to the minimum that gives a reasonable degree of safety, since anything more than this does excessive damage to the article or material that is being sterilized. Clearly what constitutes 'a reasonable degree of safety' depends on the dimensions of the problem (in terms of bacterial populations and numbers of items to be sterilized) and upon the seriousness of possible consequences of sterilization failure. For example, failure to sterilize 1% of the units processed is of little consequence in the preparation of bottles of culture media for use in a laboratory, but would be potentially disastrous in a factory producing large numbers of bottles of fluids for intravenous administration to patients, or of ampoules of vaccines meant to contain dead pathogenic organisms. Thorough cleaning of instruments and apparatus before submitting them to a sterilization process decreases the risk of sterilization failure by decreasing the number of micro-organisms likely to present (as well as by removing material that might protect them against the process).

When in the following paragraphs about heat sterilization we say that items 'can be sterilized' by the temperature-time combinations named, we mean that these combinations are commonly used because they rarely fail to sterilize the types of item mentioned, yet are not excessively destructive to them.

Dry Heat

INCINERATION   Though it hardly comes within the normal meaning of the word 'sterilization', total destruction by burning in a furnace is a useful means of eliminating the microbial content of such disposable items as dirty dressings, pathological specimens in destructible cartons, some forms of laboratory cultures and the bodies of small dead animals.

FLAMING   Bacteriological wire loops and various other metal instruments can be sterilized by heating them to redness in a flame, but such treatment blunts cutting instruments. A less destructive modification of it, which is not a fully efficient means of sterilization but is sometimes useful as a 'first-aid' measure when proper facilities are not available, is to dip the instruments in methylated spirit (or pour it on to them) and set fire to the spirit–taking care to keep one's fingers out of the resulting conflagration! Bacteriologists use gentle flaming to resterilize the mouths and necks of culture tubes and bottles which they have momentarily opened.

DRY HEAT IN AN OVEN   Glassware, surgical and laboratory apparatus and instruments of many kinds, some forms of dressing and many other solid, heat-resistant items can be sterilized by heating them at 160°C for one hour in a hot-air oven. They are usually packed in bacteria-proof tubes, tins, drums, cartons or paper wrappings so that they remain sterile after removal from the oven. To ensure uniform heating of the contents of the oven, there must be room for free circulation of air between the items (overloading prevents this) and the circulation should be maintained by a fan. Time must be allowed for the entire load to reach 160°C before starting to measure the hour. The measures for ensuring proper use and for monitoring the performance of ovens are much the same as those for autoclaves (see below).

Moist Heat

STEAM UNDER INCREASED PRESSURE   Many materials, instruments and pieces of apparatus which cannot tolerate being heated to 160°C can be sterilized by exposing them to steam at more than atmospheric pressure (and therefore at more than 100°C). Sterilization of suitable items can be achieved, for example, by 15 minutes exposure to steam under 15 lbs/sq in pressure (121 °C). The instrument used to achieve these conditions is the *autoclave*–essentially an enlarged and sophisticated version of the domestic pressure cooker (which itself can be used for the same purpose on a small scale). The efficacy of steam as a means of killing micro-organisms depends on the fact that on reaching the surface of an object that is at a lower temperature than itself the steam condenses, giving up latent heat and rapidly raising the temperature of the object. Its sudden decrease in volume draws in more steam to replace it, and so penetration into porous structure is good. To enable the steam to do its job, air must first be removed. Upward displacement of the air by rising steam, as in the pressure cooker, is an inefficient process because air is heavier than steam. Downward displacement autoclaves, with steam entering at the top and displacing the air downwards and out at the bottom, are adequate for some purposes, provided that the load is not packed in such a way as to retain the air (e.g. in upward-facing bowls). In the most efficient autoclaves the air is evacuated by suction before the steam is allowed in. Then, after the load has been exposed to pure steam for long enough to reach the appropriate temperature and has been at that temperature for the appropriate time, the steam is evacuated and the vacuum is maintained for long enough to dry the load, after which dry air is introduced and the load is allowed to cool.

Clearly an oven or an autoclave (or any other form of sterilizing apparatus) can sterilize its load only if it is correctly loaded and correctly controlled throughout the sterilizing process. Loading necessarily depends on its human attendants, but subsequent control can be made the responsibility of thermometers, thermostats, clocks and other devices. Automatic recorders can show whether these mechanisms are working or have worked correctly, but the human attendants must take due notice of the recordings and decide which loads have been properly processed. As a protection against mechanical and human errors, *indicators* should be incorporated in the load. (It may be thought necessary to do this for every load, or only from time to time.) Chemical indicators which change colour when adequately heated are in common use; they may be in sealed tubes (e.g. Browne's tubes) that can be placed at appropriate points in the oven or autoclave, or they may be incorporated in adhesive tape (e.g. Bowie-Dick tape) that can be wrapped round or strapped across the various packages. These indicate indirectly whether bacteria should have been killed, but a more direct approach is to use bacterial indicators (which can also be used for checking other means of sterilization, such as irradiation or gas sterilization). These consist of standard numbers of viable spores of suitable *Bacillus* species, commonly carried on filter-paper strips or threads, which are placed inside appropriate containers at selected points within the load, and which should fail to grow when placed in culture media after undergoing the sterilization process.

STEAM UNDER ATMOSPHERIC PRESSURE   Many culture media and other aqueous liquids – which cannot, of course, be sterilized in an oven because they would boil – can be sterilized in an autoclave. However, some are damaged if they are raised to temperatures more than a little above 100°C. Twenty minutes at this temperature kills all vegetative micro-organisms. Cotton wool-stoppered bottles or tubes of liquid can be heated in free steam by placing them in a *Koch* or *Arnold steamer*, in which steam is generated by boiling water and is retained under a conical lid which has a small escape vent at the top. Such treatment does not kill spores; but if these are present and the liquid provides a suitable environment, they will germinate after it has been removed from the steamer and allowed to cool. They can then be caught and destroyed in their vegetative state by similar heating on the next day. Further heating on the third day is usually added for extra security. This process of intermittent steaming is called *Tyndallization* after its originator, one of the first British scientists to follow up Pasteur's discoveries.

LOW-PRESSURE STEAM WITH FORMALDEHYDE   A combined physical-chemical method of sterilization, applicable to many heat-sensitive materials but not yet extensively used, is exposure to steam and formaldehyde in a special chamber at sub-atmospheric pressure (temperature about 80°C).

BOILING WATER   Boiling-water-baths have been commonly used in hospital wards and operating theatres for the treatment of bowls, instruments, etc., and were often described as 'sterilizers'. They do not in fact sterilize consistently, since some sporing organisms cannot be killed by boiling. Such pieces of apparatus may have their uses, provided that their limitations are borne in mind and that they are not, for example, expected to sterilize instruments used in wounds with possible clostridial infections.

Radiation

This subject is briefly discussed on p 37. Gamma-rays are now extensively used for sterilization of the many disposable items used in medical practice; but the need for a radiation source and strict safety precautions means that sterilization by ionizing radiations is carried out only in a few special centres. Whereas dry heat (160°C or so) kills organisms by oxidation and moist heat by denaturation of proteins, ionizing radiations kill mainly by damaging nuclear DNA.

THE USE OF DISINFECTANTS

We have not called this section 'Sterilization by chemical means' because chemicals can seldom be relied upon to kill all micro-organisms. For this reason some writers use the term *disinfection* to indicate the less radical operation of destroying all *pathogenic* organisms, and *disinfectant* for a chemical which achieves this. However, such terminology is unsatisfactory for at least three reasons: that it involves a concept which is extremely difficult to define in practical terms so that disinfection can be measured as something other than sterilization; that a minority of pathogens, notably some sporing bacilli, *Myco. tuberculosis* and some viruses, are highly resistant to the action of chemical agents; and that in any case the terms have different meanings when used by other people – e.g. *disinfection* = killing or removal of *non-sporing* organisms. Our own use of the word *disinfectant* is in accordance with the definition given on p 38; we do not use the word *disinfection*.

Disinfectants are widely used in clinical and laboratory medicine for treatment of objects and materials which are potential sources of infection or contamination but for which sterilization by heating is impossible, inconvenient or unnecessary. The properties listed in Table I (p 39) play a large part in determining the suitability of a disinfectant for a particular task. Examples of appropriate uses are:

1 Treatment of Excreta that may contain Pathogens, of Discarded Microbial Cultures and Preparations, etc.

Unusually dangerous specimens should always be sterilized in the autoclave or by some other effective form of heating, but for routine use the clear phenolics are appropriate because of their powerful and rapid action even in the presence of organic matter. However, they are ineffective against most viruses. Formalin is often used for the treatment of faeces in chemical closets, but its usefulness for other purposes is restricted by its pungent smell.

2 Treatment of Surfaces of Dressing Trolleys, Bedside Lockers, Laboratory Benches, etc.

A detergent-hypochlorite mixture has the advantages of physically removing adherent and possibly contaminated matter from the surfaces and of being effective against viruses – including hepatitis viruses, which have to be constantly remembered when blood may have been spilled. However, hypochlorite may cause corrosion of metal. Other disinfectants sometimes appropriate for such purposes include the clear phenolics (when viruses are not a serious hazard) and formalin.

3 Treatment of Instruments and Apparatus that would be damaged by Heat-sterilization

An essential preliminary to any attempt at chemical sterilization of such items is thorough cleaning. This reduces the number of organisms present and deprives them of the protection that might be afforded by blood clot, pus and other extraneous material. Hollow tubular instruments such as cystoscopes and catheters, and more complex devices such as heart-lung machines, are difficult to clean, but prolonged flushing with running water immediately after use often decreases the problem. They can then be exposed to formaldehyde, either as a gas or as a dilute solution (of the order of 5%). Catheters are often treated by sealing them in a container together with paraformaldehyde tablets, which give off formaldehyde gas. Although formaldehyde is effective against sporing organisms, in the concentrations in which it is used it may take many hours to kill them. Glutaraldehyde is less toxic and irritant than formaldehyde and is a more potent antimicrobial agent, but it is expensive and unstable in the pH range at which it is effective. The gas ethylene oxide is a sterilizing agent that penetrates into relatively inaccessible sites in pieces of apparatus, and is also used for sterilizing objects as different as bone grafts and disposable plastic syringes. It has the virtue of not lingering in or on the objects sterilized, as it is rapidly removed by air. But it is toxic, and when mixed with oxygen in a wide range of proportions it is highly explosive.

4 Storage of Frequently Used Instruments

Before the era of disposable instruments it was common practice in busy surgeries, clinics and wards to put scalpels, scissors, forceps and other frequently-used instruments into a 'sterilizing solution' for a short while after each use and then to remove, rinse and re-use them; and to keep syringes and needles in alcohol between uses. Such procedures did not in fact sterilize, and any such practices left over from that time should be abandoned. The safety of the patient requires that when instruments must be re-used (i.e. when no suitable disposable items are available) and are required frequently, a sufficient supply should be held to permit resterilization by heat or some other adequate treatment between uses.

5 Treatment of Skin

Although the term 'skin sterilization' is often used, there is no reliable way of rendering skin sterile without severely damaging it. There are, however, various sets of circumstances in which steps must be taken to reduce its bacterial population, and in particular to eliminate pathogens. (The term *antiseptic* has often been used for a substance that can achieve this purpose, but it has also been used in other meanings–for example, in previous editions of this book, in the meaning that we now give to *disinfectant*.)

(*a*) When there has been known or possible contamination of the skin–usually of the hands–as a result of contact with patients or with laboratory cultures, the organisms in question are on the surface of the skin and can be relatively easily removed with soap and water. For additional safety, the hands can be first immersed for a few minutes in some antiseptic of low toxicity, such as a 5% aqueous or alcoholic solution of chlorhexidine.

(*b*) A more difficult problem is the treatment of the hands of doctors and nurses in order to minimize the chances of their passing on their own resident flora, possibly including pathogens such as *Staph. aureus*, to their patients. Vigorous 'scrubbing up' removes surface organisms but drives others up from the hair follicles and sweat glands; culture of the skin after this procedure may therefore actually yield more bacteria than before. A satisfactory approach to the problem is to wash the hands, wrists and fore-arms carefully with a 'surgical scrub', consisting of a detergent and either chlorhexidine or povidone-iodine (iodine carried on an 'iodophor', which retains the efficacy of the long-established tincture of iodine but does not cause staining or sensitization of the patient's skin, as does the tincture).

(*c*) A patient's skin can be satisfactorily prepared for needle-puncture by rubbing it with a piece of lint soaked in 70% isopropyl alcohol (which is less volatile than ethyl alcohol). For efficacy and also the patient's comfort, the alcohol should be given time to dry before the needle is inserted. For preparation of skin before surgical incision, either povidone-iodine solution or chlorhexidine in 70% isopropyl alcohol is appropriate.

Note that antibiotics have not been mentioned in this chapter. Because of limited ranges of organisms against which they are active and their relative or total inefficiency against those which are not multiplying, they are not to be regarded as sterilizing agents or general disinfectants.

PRESERVATIVES

For many purposes the prevention of microbial growth is an adequate substitute for sterilization. For example, in the laboratory serum can be preserved by adding chloroform (1:400) or 'Merthiolate' (1:10 000), the former having the advantage that it can be driven off by warming when it is no longer required. In the kitchen, sugar, salt, vinegar, alcohol and certain ingredients of smoke have been used as preservatives from very early days. Sodium sulphite, calcium propionate and a small number of other non-toxic chemicals are used in commercially produced foodstuffs. Again, antibiotics are unsuitable for such purposes, for various reasons, including their instability.

Suggestions for Further Reading
See references at the end of the next Chapter.

18

Some Special Problems of Hospitals

The population of a hospital necessarily includes many disseminators of pathogenic organisms and many people whose illnesses or injuries make them particularly susceptible to infection. In the past, before the nature and modes of spread of micro-organisms were understood, hospitals were fearful places into which patients were loathe to go. Highly infectious diseases such as cholera were liable to spread uncontrollably among the overcrowded patients and their attendants; childbirth was commonly followed by puerperal fever which might well be fatal; and wounds all too often became gangrenous and gave rise to septicaemia. 'Let him bear in mind,' wrote the early nineteenth-century surgeon, John Bell, concerning hospital gangrene, 'that this is a hospital disease; that without the circle of the infected walls the men are safe; let him therefore hurry them out of this house of death . . . let him lay them in a schoolroom, a church, on a dunghill or in a stable . . . let him carry them anywhere but to their graves.' This terrible position was transformed by the introduction of Lister's antiseptic techniques (see p 10) and then of aseptic surgery, and by the development of other ways of controlling infection. Antimicrobial drugs have played a part in this control, though early hopes of their dramatic success in this field have been disappointed by the emergence of drug-resistant strains, especially of *Staph. aureus*. But the fact remains that hospitals are by their nature places in which infection is a grave menace that can be reduced to a minimum only by constant care on the part of all concerned.

The term *hospital infection* (or, in American literature, *nosocomial infection*) is used for any infection which a patient acquires in hospital, whether it becomes apparent during his stay there or only after his discharge and whether the organism came from another patient (*cross-infection*), or was one that he himself was formerly carrying in another site (*self-infection* or *auto-infection*). In cross-infection the organism may have been brought into the hospital by the other patient, but commonly it is resident in the hospital or in a particular ward, to be found on the floors, walls, bedding, etc., and maintained by infection of successive generations of patients. Self-infection is illustrated by infection of a wound with a *Staph. aureus* which the patient was carrying in his nose when he was admitted to hospital, or by urinary infection with an *Esch. coli* from his own intestine. While such infection is not due to hospital organisms, it may well have been made possible by operative or other procedures carried out in the hospital and hence be a direct consequence of hospital admission; and in practice it is often impossible to distinguish the two types of hospital infection because the sources of infecting organisms are not known.

Available evidence from this and other countries suggests an actual increase in recent years in the frequency and severity of hospital infections, particularly of those due to antibiotic-resistant enterobacteria, *Staph. aureus* or *Ps. aeruginosa*. The size of the problem is illustrated by a survey of 3354 operation wounds in 38 hospitals in Birmingham, England, during 1967–73. The overall infection rate was over 15%, rising to nearly 50% for wounds liable to faecal or other heavy contamination and with post-operative drains. Enterobacteria, *Staph. aureus* and *Ps. aeruginosa* were isolated from 43%, 24% and 7% of infected wounds respectively. (Cultures were aerobic only, so *Bacteroides* species –now known to be of great importance in such situations, see p 143 –were not detected.) Wound sepsis and other forms of hospital infection cause the death of some patients, and prolong the stay in hospital of many others. Such prolongation may be a serious matter for the patient and for his family; his maintenance in hospital and treatment are expensive; and meanwhile a bed is occupied which might otherwise be used for another patient.

Of course, problems similar to those encountered in hospital arise in connection with patients nursed at home, and much of what is said in this chapter applies also to them. But they are less liable to cross-infection, and any bacteria that they do acquire are more likely to be sensitive to antibiotics. Multiple drug-resistance is a feature of 'sophisticated' organisms bred in the highly selective environment of a hospital (see p 334). However, antibiotic-resistant strains of *Staph. aureus* and other bacteria are increasing in frequency among the general population, presumably derived from patients who were discharged from hospital carrying them.

PATIENTS REQUIRING ISOLATION

It is obvious that patients with easily transmissible and serious diseases such as smallpox, Lassa fever, diphtheria, typhoid or even open tuberculosis should not be nursed in open wards among patients suffering from other diseases. In accordance with the circumstances prevailing, they should be isolated either in special hospitals, in special wards for patients with the same condition or in separate rooms or cubicles. Similarly, children with such conditions as measles or whooping cough should not be nursed in general children's wards, though in many cases there is no reason why they should not be nursed at home. The desirability of isolating patients with *Staph. aureus* infections is less widely recognized. In most hospitals these are so numerous and the number of suitable cubicles is so small that there would be no possibility of isolating them all, and in most cases this is not necessary. But some, such as those with staphylococcal pneumonia or with large infected areas of dermatitis or burns, liberate very large numbers of staphylococci into their environment and certainly require to be isolated if possible. This is particularly important if the *Staph. aureus* in question is resistant to a number of antibiotics and belongs to one of the phage-types known to be able to cause serious epidemics of hospital sepsis—e.g. types 80/81 and 75/77. If such a patient is in a ward, the staphylococci become freely distributed throughout the ward, colonize and multiply in the noses of other patients, invade wounds and respiratory tracts, and may make it necessary for the ward to be closed; attempts, not always successful, must then be made to rid the ward of its staphylococci by extensive washing with disinfectants. *Staph. aureus* can be particularly troublesome in the nursery of an obstetric unit, and babies with even minor lesions should be isolated. Isolation is also desirable for babies with *Esch. coli* gastro-enteritis, and indeed for patients of all ages with diarrhoeal diseases; and for many patients with *Ps. aeruginosa* infections.

An isolation cubicle should be so designed, equipped and managed that so far as possible no micro-organisms can pass from it to a ward. Since for administrative reasons it is usually close to a ward and the patient is usually cared for by the ward staff, the success of isolation depends on the thoughtfulness and scrupulous carefulness of *everyone* concerned. The ventilation of the cubicle must be so designed that all air from it passes to the outside of the building, not into the ward or corridors. Washing facilities for the patient and attendants must be provided inside the cubicle. Attendants should put on gowns on entering the cubicle and remove them on leaving, remembering that this is not a mystic rite but an attempt to prevent contamination of themselves or their clothes and consequent carriage of pathogens out of the cubicle. Everything inside the cubicle should be regarded as contaminated, dressings should be discarded into paper bags in which they can be removed to an incinerator, bedding and clothing should be placed in disinfectant solution before being sent to the laundry, excreta should also be treated with appropriate disinfectants, and cutlery or crockery should not be allowed to return to a kitchen without sterilization. When the patient finally leaves the cubicle, it should be thoroughly washed with a disinfectant and all equipment should be sterilized so far as possible.

When isolation is necessary but no cubicle is available, '*barrier nursing*' of patients in open wards is commonly used. The patient's bed is surrounded by screens and a routine similar to that for true isolation is applied to the area inside the screens. While this procedure serves as a reminder to the patient's attendants to use special care, it is not a satisfactory alternative to the use of cubicles, particularly as airborne micro-organisms are not impressed by the 'barrier'.

'*Reverse isolation*' is used for patients who particularly need to be protected against infection – e.g. those with extensive burns or severe bone-marrow disease, those on immunosuppressive drugs to prevent graft-rejection, and those receiving heavy X-ray dosage for malignant disease. The procedure is much the same as that described above, except that the object is to prevent introduction of organisms *into* the cubicle. This is helped by a constant supply of sterile air into the cubicle at a pressure which ensures that all air-currents around doors and windows are outward.

GENERAL WARD HYGIENE

Even the patients who do not require isolation must always be regarded as potential sources or recipients of infection with pathogenic organisms. Overcrowding increases the ease with which organisms can pass from one bed to another, and lack of ventilation allows a high concentration of micro-organisms to be built up in the ward air. Bedding, particularly blankets, can become heavily loaded with bacteria, which are thrown off into the air by vigorous bed-making. For this reason it is bacteriologically desirable, though not always administratively convenient, that dressings which have to be changed in the ward should be dealt with before beds are made, and indeed as early in the day as possible since any movement of a patient in bed adds to the bacterial content of the air. Blankets should be laundered regularly, and those made of wool, which cannot be boiled, should be washed in a detergent which will kill vegetative bacteria; treatment with oil at the end of the laundering process reduces the dissemination of bacteria into the air during subsequent use of the blankets. Ward dust is often rich in pathogenic organisms and should be removed by a vacuum cleaner rather than a brush; and the vacuum cleaner must be fitted with a suitable filter so that it does not fill the ward air with bacteria collected from the floor. Appropriate steps should be taken to prevent transmission of pathogens by bed-pans and other common utensils, and each patient should have his own thermometer or disposable thermometers should be used.

HOSPITAL STAFF AS CARRIERS OF PATHOGENS

Nurses or medical staff or students can easily act as vectors of organisms from one patient to the next by allowing their clothes to be contaminated or by failing to wash their hands after attending to or examining a patient. This, however, is probably of little importance by comparison with the possibility of their being true carriers–i.e. those in or on whose bodies pathogenic organisms are multiplying. There are many microbial species which can be carried and disseminated around a hospital in such a way–*Str. pyogenes*, salmonellae and shigellae and the viruses of respiratory infections, for example–but once again *Staph. aureus* is by far the most important species in this context in present-day Britain. There is little point in routine swabbing of hospital staff aimed purely at detecting carriage of this species, since it is very common (see p 95) and there is little that can be done about it or indeed needs to be done about it in most cases. There is some point in such routine swabbing of the staff of special units if the phage-types and antibiotic sensitivities of carried strains can be determined. In this way it may be possible to pick out an occasional member of the staff who is carrying an organism which could be really troublesome. Frequently, however, the search for carriers of such strains is carried out not as a routine but in an attempt to find the cause of an outbreak of staphylococcal sepsis. It may be that the number of cases of staphylococcal infection in a ward or unit has been abnormally high and that at least a proportion of them were due to strains of the same phage-type. Swabbing of the staff and of all other regular visitors to the ward may reveal one or more carriers of the appropriate phage-type. It does not follow that these were the source of infection for the patients–they may in fact have acquired their staphylococci from the patients or from a common source–but as carriers of organisms which have shown themselves capable of causing an outbreak of sepsis these people must be excluded from contact with patients, and may be allowed to return only when such carriage ceases. This may occur spontaneously after a few weeks, or may be assisted by application of antiseptic or antibiotic creams or sprays to the nose. The use of systemic antibiotics for such a purpose is seldom justified. Medical or nursing staff or others who have staphylococcal lesions such as boils must be removed from duties in which they may infect patients, since the nature of their lesions proves the pathogenicity of their staphylococci. Similarly, members of staff who develop diarrhoea must be removed from such duties until it can be established that they are not excreting pathogens.

SOME VARIETIES OF HOSPITAL INFECTION AND THEIR PREVENTION

Wounds and Burns

Any breach of the skin surface, whether accidental or surgical, provides an open door for bacterial infection. Bacteria can establish themselves more easily in damaged than in healthy tissue, and it therefore important to remove all tissue debris from accidental wounds and burns and to reduce to a minimum the amount of tissue crushed, bruised or otherwise harmed during operations. Aseptic surgical technique is aimed at preventing entry of bacteria from any source into wounds during operations, and dressings should be so designed and applied that they fulful the protective function of the missing skin barrier. A drain in a wound makes it more difficult to exclude air-borne organisms and also is liable to predispose to infection by damaging the tissues. When dressings are changed, great care must be taken to protect the wound or burn from infection and to dispose of dressings from already infected wounds in such a way that organisms from them are not transferred to other patients. While there are considerable advantages in changing dressings in special side-rooms rather than in open wards, careless technique which allows contamination of the air and equipment of such dressing rooms can be the means of extensive cross-infection.

The Urinary Tract

The passage of a catheter or other instrument into the bladder is liable to cause infection of the urinary tract, usually with *Esch. coli* or other Gram-negative bacilli. Such instrumentation should therefore be carried out only when it is essential, and with full aseptic technique. Used catheters are difficult to sterilize, but this possible source of cross-infection is eliminated by using presterilized disposable catheters. When it is necessary to drain the bladder continuously through an indwelling catheter, the receptacle must not be open to the ward air (otherwise organisms can enter the urine, multiply in it and ascend to the bladder) and should preferably be a disposable plastic bag.

The Respiratory Tract

Patients who lie still for long periods as a result of unconsciousness, major operations, paralysis or other causes, and some who have respiratory tract virus infections or other predisposing conditions, are liable to acquire pneumococcal, staphylococcal or other infections of their respiratory tracts. Apart from general hygienic measures there is little that can be done to prevent this. Attempts at antibiotic prophylaxis often do more harm than good (see p 326); antibiotic treatment of an established infection is quite a different matter.

The Alimentary Tract

Outbreaks of *Esch. coli* gastro-enteritis among babies and of *Sh. sonnei* dysentery occur from time to time in hospitals. They can be prevented or controlled by measures already outlined in this chapter—isolation, general hygienic precautions and exclusion of carriers.

Infection Due to Injection or Transfusion

Introduction of a needle and extraneous fluids into a patient's sub-cutaneous or muscular tissues or his blood stream may involve the introduction of pathogens. This can be avoided by adequate skin preparation (see p 285), aseptic technique including particular care not to contaminate the prepared skin with organisms from the operator's respiratory tract or hands, and use of properly sterilized syringes, needles, blood-giving sets and fluids. Since there is little that can be done about sterilization of blood, donors must be chosen with care to avoid any likelihood of their blood containing pathogens—in other words, they must be in good health and give no serological evidence of hepatitis B or syphilitic infection. Unsterilized tatooing instruments can transmit pathogens collected from the skin or blood of previous customers.

Baths as Means of Cross-Infection

Baths are difficult to sterilize and in general should not be used by patients who may contaminate them with pathogens. There is a strong case for the more general use of showers rather than baths for ambulant patients. Bathing of a series of babies in the same bath or sink can result in dispersal of *Staph. aureus* and other pathogens through a nursery; if newborn babies need to be bathed at all, this should be done in stainless-steel bowls which can be autoclaved after the bathing of each child.

INVESTIGATION OF OUTBREAKS OF HOSPITAL INFECTION

We can deal only very briefly with this large and complex subject. Investigation of such an outbreak is a detective operation, and begins with the accumulation of evidence—the number of patients involved; their distribution in the hospital or ward; the times of onset of their symptoms and the probable times at which they were infected; whether all or the majority of cases followed operation and, if so, whether they were operated on in the same theatre or by the same team; and any other clues as to the way in which they became infected. If their infections are all due to apparently identical bacteria, a human carrier or other source of the appropriate organism must be sought, whereas an outbreak of infection due to various organisms suggests a breakdown in theatre or ward ventilation, in aseptic technique or in the sterilization of dressings or instruments. In many hospitals today a member of the medical staff (a clinician or a bacteriologist) is appointed Control of Infection Officer, and is assisted by a Control of Infection Nurse in the task of keeping a record of all cases of sepsis and continually reviewing the cross-infection situation. Such work can be valuable provided that there is some mechanism for ensuring that appropriate administrative action is taken when there is evidence of trouble. A small committee–including, for example, a surgeon and a bacteriologist, the Control of Infection Officer (if he is not one of the first two), the Control of Infection Nurse (who must be of adequate seniority to speak for the nursing administration) and a hospital administrator, with other members co-opted as the occasion demands–can be a suitable body for dealing with such episodes, and can also be responsible for defining the hospital's policies for preventing cross-infection. (It is, of course, easier to define policies than to ensure that they are carried out by all concerned!)

Suggestions for Further Reading

Hospital Hygiene by Isobel Maurer (Arnold, London, 1974)–an excellent small book, full of good practical advice.

Control of Hospital Hygiene: A Practical Handbook, ed. E. J. L. Lowbury and others (Chapman & Hall, London, 1975).

19

The Bacteriology of Water, Milk and Food

WATER

Factors which determine the total bacterial content of a water supply include the following:

(1) Rivers fed by surface drainage contain many bacteria, some collected from the air by the water as it fell in the form of rain or snow and many collected from the soil or other surfaces on to which it fell or over which it passed.

(2) Water from deep wells or springs usually has a low bacterial content because it has undergone filtration as it percolated through the soil to reach underground lakes or rivers.

(3) Bacterial multiplication may occur in running water if it contains suitable organic nutrients and if the temperature and other conditions are appropriate.

(4) When water comes to rest in large lakes and reservoirs, its bacterial content is as a rule greatly reduced as a result of sedimentation and other factors.

(5) Supplies to most developed human communities are usually first stored, then further purified by filtration through sand-beds (which owe their efficiency as filters to a surface layer of protozoa and algae), and finally chlorinated. Chlorine, in a concentration as low as 1:5 000 000, rapidly kills nearly all vegetative bacteria provided that there is very little organic matter present.

It is not the total bacterial content, however, which is important in assessing the suitability of a water supply for human consumption. What matters is the possibility that it contains organisms capable of causing disease in those who drink the water. Important among these organisms are the bacilli of typhoid, paratyphoid, dysentery and cholera; some pathogenic viruses can also be water-borne–notably those of polio-myelitis and hepatitis A. Presence of such organisms result from contamination with human excreta, or in some cases with animal or bird droppings. There are a number of obvious precautions which can be taken to reduce the risk of such contamination–e.g. drawing supplies only from relatively uninhabited catchment areas, seeing that one community is not discharging its untreated sewage into a river upstream from the point at which another is drawing off its supply, or, in places where there is no main water supply or main drainage, seeing that wells are so situated and protected that there cannot be any leakage into them from pit-latrines and the like. There are few occasions, however, when it is safe to assume that a water supply has not been contaminated–though a dangerous level of contamination is highly improbable in the case of water taken from a fast-running stream in a hill or mountain area above the level of human habitation. With this exception it is virtually always unwise to drink unboiled water derived from a source that has not been subjected to thorough and repeated testing, as described below, or to filtration and chlorination with adequate bacteriological control.

Although most non-chlorinated water supplies contain Gram-negative bacilli, including enterobacteria such as *K. aerogenes*, the presence of 'faecal coliforms'* such as *Esch. coli* indicates contamination with human or animal faeces, and their presence in more than very small numbers indicates that the water is not safe for human consumption. *Str. faecalis* and *Cl. welchii* have a similar significance, though the latter, being a sporing organism, survives longer than other faecal organisms, and its presence without them suggests that contamination was not recent. There is seldom any point in examining a water supply directly for the presence of pathogens, for if contamination has occurred other faecal organisms are likely to be far more numerous and easier to detect, and the presence of these organisms in a supply that does not at present contain detectable pathogens implies that it may well do so on other occasions. Since contamination may be intermittent, a single satisfactory bacteriological examination does not guarantee the safety of a water supply. Regular testing of any supply to be used for drinking is essential, and in the case of a non-chlorinated supply any deviation from the pattern of results obtained over the course of previous years must be taken as indicating that there has been a change in the source of the supply and that it must be regarded with suspicion.

Almost all piped drinking water in Britain is chlorinated. The presence of any coliform bacilli at all in a 100 ml sample of chlorinated

---

*The terms *coliforms* and *coliform bacilli* continue to be used in connection with the bacteriology of water and milk, as collective terms for lactose-fermenting enterobacteria (see p 122).

water collected at its point of entry into a public supply (i.e. before there is any chance of mixing with unchlorinated water) indicates that the chlorination procedure was defective.

BACTERIOLOGICAL EXAMINATION   As we have indicated, the most important part of the bacteriological examination of water is the detection and enumeration of coliform bacilli, and in particular of those that are of faecal origin. This can be done by adding portions of the water sample–e.g. one of 50 ml, 5 of 10 ml and 5 of 1 ml–to bottles or tubes containing a suitable liquid lactose-containing medium and incubating overnight at 37°C. Production of acid and gas in a bottle or tube indicates the presence of 'presumptive coliforms'. Because organisms may be irregularly distributed in the water, it may well happen that, for example, growth of 'coliforms' occurs from some of the 1 ml samples but fails to occur from some of the 10 ml samples. However, by comparing the results obtained with McCrady's probability table worked out for this purpose, it is possible to arrive at a figure for the most likely number of 'coliforms' per 100 ml of the water.

Not all bacteria that produce acid and gas under the conditions of the presumptive coliform count are in fact faecal organisms. If any such bacteria are detected, they are further tested for ability to grow and to produce gas in the same or a modified fluid medium incubated at 44°C. With rare exceptions, the ability to do this is confined to true 'faecal coliforms'. The finding of any such indicates that the water is not fit for human consumption.

An alternative procedure for the bacteriological sampling of water is to pass a known volume of water under pressure through a special porous cellulose acetate membrane which holds back all bacteria. The membrane can then be placed in a Petri dish on top of a pad of filter paper or other suitable absorbent material which is saturated with a fluid culture medium. On incubation, colonies form on the surface of the membrane. By using appropriate media and incubation temperatures it is possible to carry out total counts, counts of lactose-fermenting organisms that will grow on bile-salt lactose medium and counts of those which will do so at 44°C. However, gas production cannot be detected and the results are therefore not strictly parallel with those of the tests in liquid media.

MILK

Human milk taken by the baby straight from the mother is seldom a vector of pathogens. Only minor bacteriological problems are associated with the collection and storage of expressed human milk. Cow's milk, on the other hand, presents many important problems. It may contain pathogens derived from the cow; the circumstances of its collection, unless carefully controlled, permit it to become heavily contaminated with a wide variety of micro-organisms; it is a good culture medium for many of these; it may spend hours or days at temperatures suitable for bacterial multiplication before it is consumed; and, as the result of pooling, milk from a single cow may be distributed to a large number of human beings.

Organisms which may be present in cow's milk include the following:

(1) *Pathogens excreted in the milk or derived from the animal's udders.* The most important of these are *Myco. tuberculosis* and *Br. abortus* (*Br. melitensis* being transmitted similarly in goat's milk in some countries). Other pathogens which occasionally come under this heading are *Staph. aureus*, *Str. pyogenes* (including scarlet fever strains), salmonellae and *Coxiella burnetii*.

(2) *Pathogens derived from the hands or respiratory tracts of dairy workers during or after milking; from utensils or bottles washed inadequately or with water from a contaminated supply; or from airborne or other contamination.* These include *Staph. aureus*, *Str. pyogenes*, *C. diphtheriae*, salmonellae and shigellae, and possibly viruses such as those of poliomyelitis and infectious hepatitis.

(3) *Non-pathogens* of many varieties and from many sources, which may multiply in the milk and cause souring or other changes in it. Souring, which is due to the production of lactic acid from lactose by such organisms as *Str. lactis* and lactobacilli, is deliberately encouraged for such purposes as the production of butter and cheese, but is otherwise undesirable.

Regular tuberculin-testing of cattle, tests for brucella agglutinins in milk (see p 261) and scrupulous attention to the general health of the cattle and to any local lesions of the udders are important steps towards eliminating pathogens of the first category. Subsequent contamination can be reduced by a high standard of hygiene in cow-sheds and by efficient washing and sterilization of all utensils and containers. Multiplication of organisms can be kept to a minimum by cooling the milk as soon as it is collected, keeping it cool during transmission, and delivering it to the consumer early in the day while the atmospheric temperature is still low. But even a combination of all these measures does not guarantee that the milk will be safe to drink. This can be achieved only by heating it, as described below.

Pasteurization

A process which Louis Pasteur devised to deal with a problem of the wine industry has been generally adopted as the most satisfactory treatment for milk. If milk is heated to 63–66°C and kept at this temperature for 30 minutes (the *Holder process*) or is heated to 71°C for at least 15 seconds (the *High Temperature Short Time process*), all vegetative pathogens are killed; spore-forming pathogens are of no importance in this context. The milk must then be rapidly cooled to 10°C or less, so that surviving organisms do not multiply. The adequacy of the treatment which a specimen of milk has received can be tested by a simple procedure–the *phosphatase test*. This depends upon the fact that the enzyme phosphatase is constantly present in fresh milk and is destroyed by heat treatment that just conforms with the above standard. Inability of treated milk to liberate phenol from disodium phenylphosphate is therefore evidence that it has been effectively pasteurized.

Pasteurization does not impair the taste of milk, and there is no evidence that it appreciably lowers its nutritional value. It does make the milk entirely safe to drink, provided that it is delivered into sterile bottles immediately after treatment and is kept sealed until it is consumed.

Sterilization

More vigorous heat treatment is required in order to destroy all bacteria in milk and so prevent it from being soured or otherwise spoiled by bacterial multiplication. Such treatment inevitably causes a change in the taste of the milk, due to caramelization. True sterilization by steam under pressure is necessary for such products as condensed milk, which must be able to survive prolonged storage in tins at room temperature, but heating at or around boiling point, which destroys all but the most resistant spores, is adequate for less long-term purposes. Such treatment causes coagulation and precipitation of proteins and therefore *the turbidity test* can be used to check that it has been carried out efficiently. In this test ammonium sulphate is added to the milk, which is filtered five minutes later and then boiled for five minutes and cooled. 'Sterilized' milk should show no sign of turbidity at the end of this procedure.

'Ultra Heat' Treatment (U.H.T.)

A 1965 regulation permits the sale in this country of milk, designated 'ultra heat treated', which has been treated to 132°C for 1 second under specified conditions, has been delivered aseptically into sterile containers which are then sealed so as to be air-tight, and has a very low bacterial count as determined by specified tests. Such milk has a shelf life of several months.

Bacteriological Examination

Milk can be examined for its content of coliforms and other bacteria by tests similar to those used for water. Its total bacterial content can also be assessed by microscopic examination of stained films (since the number of bacteria is likely to be very much higher than in samples from water supplies) or by the *methylene blue reduction test*. This is a non-specific test for the presence of organisms producing enzymes that reduce and thereby decolorize methylene blue. Milk collected with reasonable care to avoid contamination, and therefore suitable for distribution or pasteurization, should not have a bacterial population that is able under standard conditions to decolorize methylene blue in less than 30 minutes. Examination for individual pathogenic species such as *Myco. tuberculosis* or *Br. abortus* is carried out by culture on suitable media and, in the case of those two species and some others, by guinea-pig inoculation. Milk from cows with brucellosis may contain brucella agglutinins. When such milk has been mixed with a large volume of milk from healthy cows, it may be easier to detect the agglutinins, by the sensitive *brucella ring test*, than to isolate brucellae. In this test, haematoxylin-stained dead brucellae are added to a sample of the milk; if they are agglutinated, they rise up in the fat globules and form a blue ring in the cream layer.

Milk products, such as butter and cheese, and milk-containing foods, such as ice-cream and custards, are of course liable to contain pathogens similar to those found in milk, and are exposed to greater risks of contamination by handlers. It is, however, very much more difficult to devise bacteriological standards and tests for these products, apart from cultures to exclude the presence of named pathogens.

FOOD

Many foods make good microbial culture media and 'go bad' unless protected from the deleterious effects of multiplying bacteria and fungi. This protection can take the form of cooking, refrigeration, drying or the addition of sugar, salt or other preservatives (see pp 285–6).

The role of food as a vector of pathogenic organisms is not closely associated with obvious deterioration. Food which has been made unpalatable by the activities of multiplying organisms is not necessarily harmful to eat, and on the other hand food may contain large numbers of pathogens and yet be normal in appearance and pleasant to eat; if this were not so, there would be few outbreaks of food-poisoning.

What we said above about the difficulties of devising bacteriological standards and tests for milk products applies even more strongly to other food substances, because of their great diversity.

Of the important food pathogens the salmonellae, *Cl. welchii*, *Cl. botulinum* and *B. cereus* are discussed separately below, and *V. para-haemolyticus* and the campylobacters were mentioned on pp 135–6. The organisms of dysentery–both bacillary and amoebic–may be carried by food, especially in communities in which human excreta are used as fertilizers for lettuce and other vegetables which are eaten raw. Some outbreaks of gastro-enteritis are caused by food in which there are no recognized pathogens to be found but large numbers of various other bacteria, usually including *Esch. coli* and *Proteus* species. It seems probable that the gastro-enteritis in such cases is due to products of bacterial metabolism which are present in the food. These may be results of food breakdown rather than true bacterial toxins.

Treatment of food-poisoning is mainly symptomatic. Antibiotics are liable to do more harm than good in cases of salmonella food-poisoning (see p 130) and are irrelevant to forms of food-poisoning due to preformed bacterial toxins. The use of *Cl. botulinum* antitoxin is discussed on p 118.

Salmonella Food-Poisoning

AETIOLOGY   Contamination of food with salmonellae can arise in many different ways and can come from a wide range of natural sources.

Salmonella infections are common among chickens, ducks and turkeys, and the organisms may be found in their eggs. Occasional cases of food-poisoning result from eating lightly-cooked individual eggs, but far more serious trouble arises from the mixing and spray-drying or freezing of large batches of eggs for use in the catering trade. Eggs often travel from one country to another in these forms, and can carry large numbers of salmonellae with them. The danger of such egg preparations is increased by the fact that they are often used in preparing food items that undergo little cooking. The carcasses of the birds themselves, especially of those reared in the crowded conditions of modern intensive production, are often heavily contaminated with salmonellae by the time that they reach the kitchen.

Pigs and cattle may have salmonella infections, and some human infections are due to eating inadequately cooked meat. In connection with this and all forms of food-poisoning it is important to appreciate that heat penetrates very slowly to the centre of large joints of meat or other large volumes of solid or semisolid food during cooking, so that even vegetative organisms may still be alive at the centre long after the periphery is well cooked.

Oysters grow particularly well near sewage outlets, and readily become contaminated with faecal bacteria. Since they are eaten raw, it is important that they should be kept for long periods in fresh water before they are marketed.

Rats and mice are commonly carriers of salmonellae and must therefore be kept away from food stores.

Finally, human carriers may contaminate food with salmonellae, of the food-poisoning or the enteric varieties. Transmission can easily occur via a substance such as ice-cream, which is readily contaminated during manufacture, is a good culture medium and is not cooked before it is eaten. Sometimes the route from man to man is long and complex. For example, salmonellae have been known to travel from Ceylon to Britain in desiccated coconut.

Although typhoid is not strictly 'salmonella food-poisoning', international transmission of salmonellae is well illustrated by the 1964 Aberdeen typhoid outbreak, which was the largest of several that occurred in Britain within a few years in association with the distribution of corned beef imported in large cans from South America. These cans were in effect cultures of typhoid bacilli, which they had presumably acquired from river water, contaminated with human excreta, that had been used to cool the cans after sterilization and had been sucked into them through faulty joints, as described below in connection with an outbreak of staphylococcal food-poisoning. The large scale of the Aberdeen outbreak–507 cases–was a result of contamination of a slicing machine and other utensils in the shop in which the corned beef was sold, and consequent transfer of typhoid bacilli to various other foods sold in the same shop. A fortunate feature of this series of outbreaks was the very low frequency of secondary cases–i.e. of patients who had not themselves eaten the contaminated food but had acquired their infection from those who had.

Salmonellae usually produce gastro-enteritis only when ingested in large doses. Their multiplication, which is encouraged if infected foods of appropriate composition are allowed to stand for some hours in a warm room, is even further stimulated by 'warming up' the food for too short a time to kill the bacteria and then allowing it to cool slowly through the temperature range that suits their growth.

CLINICAL PICTURE   The presenting symptoms are headache, fever, abdominal pain and diarrhoea. They usually come on 12 to 36 hours after eating the offending food. Vomiting may occur but is not commonly a prominent feature. Recovery may take a week or two, and convalescents may remain carriers for long periods. A small proportion of cases are fatal.

Staphylococcal Food-Poisoning

AETIOLOGY   In contrast to the 'infection' type of food-poisoning caused by salmonellae, this is a 'toxin' type–i.e. it is due to the ingestion of preformed toxin, not to any action of the organisms themselves upon the patient. Milk may be contaminated with *Staph. aureus* from cows (rarely in Britain today) or from human beings, so cream-filled cakes and other foods containing uncooked milk products are prominent in the literature of this disease. Cooks with staphylococcal finger infections may infect various other 'culture media' which are left to stand in a warm room or are 'warmed up'. Multiplication may also occur inside tins of food. For example, one outbreak was traced to the following sequence of events: In a certain factory tins of vegetables were placed in cold water immediately after they were sealed, in order to cool them down before labelling; the cooling process produced a partial vacuum in the tins, and one of them had a small leak, through which it sucked in some of the water; the worker responsible for lifting the tins out of the water had boils on her arms and had contaminated the water with *Staph. aureus*; labelling sealed the small leak, and the staphylococci were left to multiply in an apparently normal sealed tin. Once formed, the staphylococcal enterotoxin is more heat-resistant than the organism itself, and will even withstand boiling for a short while. Many of the *Staph. aureus* strains that have been shown to cause food-poisoning belong to a small number of types in phage-group III (see p 97).

CLINICAL PICTURE   Vomiting, which may be violent, comes on within 2 to 6 hours of eating the food. Diarrhoea often follows. The patient may be prostrated and usually has abdominal pain. Complete recovery takes place by the next day.

Clostridium welchii (Cl. perfringens) Food-Poisoning

AETIOLOGY   As indicated on p 121, many of the *Cl. welchii* strains responsible for this condition differ from other members of type A in being able to survive prolonged boiling. They are also antigenically distinct. They are found in the intestines of man and animals, and meat is often contaminated with them either in the slaughter-house or at some other stage before it reaches the consumer. A characteristic story of an outbreak of this type of food-poisoning begins with a large quantity of meat or stew being boiled for some hours and then left to cool. The clostridia find themselves in an excellent anaerobic culture medium, similar to Robertson's cooked meat medium which is used for growing just such organism in the laboratory. Cooling in the centre of a large mass of food is slow, especially if it is not immediately refrigerated. Multiplication of the clostridia begins when the temperature falls below 50°C, continues until it reaches 20°C or lower, and is resumed if the food is gently heated on the next or subsequent days before being served. The bacilli are commonly found in very large numbers in food which has caused outbreaks of this form of poisoning. They are there in the vegetative form, but on ingestion they sporulate in the intestine. The final stage of sporulation involve lysis of the remainder of the vegetative cell, with liberation of an enterotoxin that was formed during the earlier stages and is the cause of the clinical manifestations.

CLINICAL PICTURE   Abdominal pain and diarrhoea, which is often violent, come on within 8 to 24 hours of eating the food. Prostration is common, but there is no fever and seldom any vomiting. In most cases recovery is complete by the next day, but occasional fatalities occur among the old and infirm.

Botulism

AETIOLOGY   *Cl. botulinum* is another organism that can survive prolonged boiling and can multiply in the anaerobic environment provided by food that has been treated in this way. Unlike *Cl. welchii* it is not found in the intestines of animals but is a soil saprophyte in many parts of the world, notably in the U.S.A., and may contaminate vegetable foods as well as fish and meat. Home-preserved vegetables, particularly beans, have figured in a number of incidents; careful supervision of commercial canning of such items ensures that they are raised to temperatures that are lethal to clostridia. The very severe human illness that results from eating food in which this organism has multiplied is described on p 117. It is far less common than the other forms of food-poisoning described in the present chapter. It is due entirely to the exotoxin, the organisms themselves being harmless; and can be prevented by quite gentle cooking immediately before the food is eaten, as the toxin is destroyed in 10 minutes at 100°C.

Bacillus cereus Food-Poisoning

AETIOLOGY   *B. cereus* is a common soil organism, found on many sorts of vegetable matter destined for human consumption (notably rice), and is a spore-former and consequently resistant to drying and heating. Episodes of food-poisoning associated with its presence in food have been reported from as far back as 1906, and have been more frequently recognized since 1950, but since 1971 a special association with Chinese fried rice has been noted in many countries. The typical story behind an outbreak of this kind is that the rice has been boiled (which does not destroy *B. cereus*) and then allowed to remain warm for many hours before being lightly fried. The organism multiplies briskly in the warm rice if it is in the range 30–37°C, and produces one or more enterotoxins, which are not destroyed by the final frying.

CLINICAL PICTURES   Two distinct pictures can be recognized, and are due to differences between strains of *B. cereus* in the number and proportions of toxins that they produce. Most of the rice-associated outbreaks are characterized by nausea and vomiting coming on 1 to 5 hours after eating the rice. In contrast, vomiting was uncommon in most of the outbreaks of the kind recognized in earlier years, which were characterized by abdominal pain and diarrhoea coming on 8 to 16 hours after eating the food responsible.

LABORATORY INVESTIGATION OF FOOD-POISONING

The nature of the organism responsible for a food-poisoning outbreak is often suggested by the pattern of the outbreak – whether it is confined to a household or involves large numbers of people, the time relationships, the nature and severity and duration of the symptoms, and so on. Except in salmonellosis the investigation of an outbreak has little bearing upon treatment and is principally concerned with finding out what went wrong and preventing further outbreaks. The laboratory's contribution is to try to isolate the responsible organism, by culture of faeces and vomit (if available) from a manageable proportion of the patients and by microscopy and culture of the offending food if it can be identified and if some of it is still available. Sometimes the history of the outbreak clearly incriminates a particular item or at least a meal, but in other cases detailed detective work is necessary. If the food is available and either a salmonella, a heat-resistant *Cl. welchii*, or a *B. cereus* is involved, there is not usually much difficulty in growing the organisms from the food and from at least some of the patients, and in showing that they are identical. *Cl. botulinum* is also likely to be recoverable from the food, and although it is unlikely to be recovered from the patients it produces a highly characteristic clinical picture. The case against a staphylococcus, however, may be difficult or impossible to prove. These organisms, being less heat-resistant than their enterotoxin, may have been killed during cooking, and there is no simple and satisfactory procedure for demonstrating the presence of the enterotoxin, though it can be detected by tests used in specialized food-hygiene laboratories.

PREVENTION OF FOOD-POISONING

The responsibility for preventing food-poisoning is shared by many people, including public health authorities, wholesale and retail food distributers, caterers and their staffs, and housewives. The following are among the more obvious precautions:

(1) All animals should be inspected before being slaughtered for human consumption, and their meat should be inspected afterwards, for evidence of relevant disease.

(2) All consignments of potentially dangerous food ingredients such

as spray-dried or frozen eggs should be tested bacteriologically.

(3) All food should be protected from flies, rodents and other possible vectors of pathogens at all times—during distribution and storage and after being cooked.

(4) All food in or on which bacteria could multiply should be kept in a refrigerator, or at least cool, at all stages. This applies particularly to such excellent culture media as ice-cream mixtures and synthetic cream.

(5) Cooking, especially of meat, should be thorough, and food which is not to be eaten immediately after cooking should be cooled rapidly. If reheating is necessary, temperatures of more than 60°C should be attained with a minimum of delay. These precautions are particularly important with large quantities, especially of meat. Cooling of large joints is accelerated if they are cut into several pieces immediately after cooking.

(6) If there is any ground for doubting the effective sterilization of home-preserved foods in a part of the world in which botulism occurs, they should be raised to 100°C for more than 10 minutes immediately before consumption. This destroys *Cl. botulinum* toxin, and even if the organism itself is still alive, it can be eaten with impunity if it is given no time to make more toxin.

(7) Known carriers of salmonellae, shigellae or *Ent. histolytica* and people with known staphylococcal lesions, especially of the hands, should be excluded from work involving the handling of foods. Appropriate laboratory tests for the intestinal pathogens should be carried out on all those about to be engaged in the kitchens of institutions, restaurants, etc., or in the food-distribution trade at points at which contamination of the food could have serious consequences.

(8) A high standard of personal hygiene, especially the careful washing of hands after defaecation, should be observed by all food handlers (and indeed by all!).

Suggestions for Further Reading
Food Poisoning and Food Hygiene by Betty C. Hobbs, 3rd edn. (Arnold, London, 1974).

20

Immunization

Immunological theory has been considered in Chapter Eight. Here we are concerned with its practical application to the artificial enhancement of immunity–i.e. immunization. This chapter includes an outline of commonly used procedures for immunization against particular diseases, and then a discussion of immunization programmes, but it is necessary first to enlarge upon the distinction made on p 56 between active and passive immunization and to make some general remarks about vaccines.

ACTIVE IMMUNIZATION

This involves administering antigens which stimulate the recipient's own immunological mechanisms. In many cases he responds by producing measurable circulating antibodies; sometimes the only measurable result is an alteration in his subsequent reaction to the same antigen–e.g. an increase in his resistance to infection by the organisms from which the antigen was derived. When we speak of immunization, we are usually referring to the use of microbial preparations, but the term can also reasonably include such procedures as the desensitization of atopic patients (see p 75). The types of antigenic preparation commonly used in active immunization against microbial diseases are discussed on pp 309–10.

Since active immunization of a subject who has no previous experience of the antigen takes several weeks to produce effective protection (see p 64) it is of prophylactic but not of therapeutic value. Boosting of existing immunity, however, may be of immediate therapeutic value. Immunity following adequate active immunization may last for many years.

PASSIVE IMMUNIZATION

This involves the giving of ready-made antibodies formed by another host in response to artificial immunization or to natural infection. For the production of antitoxic sera (i.e. sera containing toxin-neutralizing antibodies) used in the treatment of diphtheria and tetanus, the horse has been generally employed because it is a good producer of such antibodies, has a large blood volume, and is easy to inject, bleed and maintain. However, human beings are liable to develop horse-globulin sensitivity if they are repeatedly exposed to such sera, and some do so even as a result of frequent contact with horses. The antitoxin antibodies are themselves horse-globulins, and although before use they are purified and are treated with enzymes and gentle heat to reduce their antigenicity, it is impossible to eliminate the risk that they will cause anaphylactic reactions (see p 75) or serum sickness (see p 76) in such sensitive people. Alternatively, the recipient may have developed a different form of antibody to horse-globulin, which produces no hypersensitivity reaction but combines with the horse antitoxin and makes it ineffective; this is detectable only by the fact that the antitoxin fails to protect the patient. Similar problems arise when animals other than the horse are used to produce the antisera. Immunoglobulin from human volunteers immunized with tetanus toxoid is relatively safe to use but supplies are limited. Immunoglobulin from human convalescents is used to protect infants and other specially susceptible patients against measles and other virus infections, and to prevent cases and control outbreaks of hepatitis A (see p 210).

Passive immunization begins to be effective as soon as the antiserum enters the recipient's circulation, but its effect lasts at most for only a few months. This is because the antibody molecules, like all protein molecules in the body, have only a short life, and they are not replaced as are those produced in response to active immunization. Consequently passive immunization is of use only for short-term prophylaxis or for treatment of existing infection.

The main differences between active and passive immunization can be summarized as follows:

	Active	Passive
Immunizing agents	Live or dead organisms, toxoids	Sera from immunized animals or humans
Rapidity of protection	2 to 3 weeks' delay if no previous immunity	Immediate
Duration	Usually several years	At most a few months
Complications	Various (see later) but rarely serious	Anaphylaxis, serum sickness
Uses	Long-term prophylaxis	Short-term prophylaxis
	Treatment only if previously immunized	Treatment

VACCINES
The words *vaccine* and *vaccination*, derived originally from the use of

material from the cow (Latin *vacca*) for immunization against smallpox, have gradually extended in meaning to include all immunizing preparations of living or dead organisms or of materials derived from organisms. Vaccines can be classified as follows:

(a) *Live organisms of limited virulence* – usually attenuated derivatives of pathogens, but sometimes naturally occurring organisms closely related to pathogens (e.g. cowpox virus, or the vole tubercle bacillus which has been used for immunizing humans against tuberculosis). Because live cultures are used, it is important to ensure that they do not contain contaminant pathogenic organisms (see p 310 – the Lübeck disaster). A particular hazard of virus vaccines that have to be grown in primary tissue cultures – i.e. in cell populations directly derived from animal embryos or organs – is that they may contain wild viruses that were already in the tissues. Provided that a live vaccine 'takes' and multiplies in the recipient's tissues, a single dose usually gives a satisfactory degree of immunity, since it provides a prolonged antigenic stimulus.

(b) *Dead (or inactivated) organisms.* Suspensions of dead bacteria have on the whole been disappointing as inducers of immunity, though some are misleadingly successful in stimulating the production of measurable antibodies. The position may be improved by research aimed at finding for each organism the culture conditions and method of killing which give the best yield, not just of organisms but of those antigenic components which stimulate protective responses. Inactivated virus vaccines have been somewhat more successful, but disasters have resulted from failures of the inactivation processes and consequent inadvertent administration of live virulent viruses. Because a dead or inactivated organism does not multiply in the recipient's tissues, several suitably spaced and relatively large doses have to be given, usually by injection.

(c) *Purified microbial products.* The classical examples of these are *toxoids*, which are bacterial toxins – e.g. of diphtheria or tetanus – that have been made harmless by heat or formalin treatment, but are still effective as antigens and stimulate the production of antibodies which neutralize the corresponding toxins. Also in this category of products are the *B. anthracis* protein antigen mentioned on p 116 and the pneumococcal and meningococcal capsular polysaccharides. The ultimate aim in active immunization must be the maximum of protective response with the minimum risk of unpleasant or harmful reactions. Administration of whole organisms, alive or dead, is a somewhat crude approach to this aim as compared with administration of refined preparations of 'protective' antigens, from which virtually all irrelevant and potentially 'reactogenic' material has been removed.

IMMUNIZATION AGAINST PARTICULAR DISEASES DUE TO BACTERIA
Tuberculosis

Immunization against tuberculosis, using the living attenuated bovine-type tubercle bacillus of Calmette and Guerin (B.C.G.), has been in use since 1922, but its widespread adoption was greatly delayed by the Lübeck disaster of 1930, in which 72 out of 251 infants vaccinated died of tuberculosis soon afterwards. There is little doubt that this was due to contamination of one batch of vaccine with virulent tubercle bacilli. In recent years B.C.G. has been given to many millions of people with few complications; a very small number of generalized and fatal infections have been attributable to unsuspected hypogammaglobulinaemia.

The vaccine is given as a small intradermal injection of a suspension of the live bacilli–usually a reconstituted freeze-dried culture. For a variety of reasons the upper arm is the most satisfactory site for this and most other forms of vaccination. B.C.G. vaccination in Britain (and in many other countries) is preceded by tuberculin testing, and is confined to those giving negative results. This is partly because a positive result is presumptive (though not conclusive) evidence that the subject is already protected against tuberculosis; but mainly because B.C.G. vaccination in the presence of tuberculin hypersensitivity results in a destructive Koch phenomenon (p 77). The omission of preliminary tuberculin testing in large-scale B.C.G. immunization programmes in developing countries speeds up the programmes, and hypersensitivity reactions have not been found to be a serious problem. In the absence of pre-existing hyper-sensitivity, a small tuberculous ulcer develops a few weeks after vaccination and persists for several months before it heals, leaving a small scar. The recipient usually gives a positive tuberculin reaction from the sixth week after vaccination.

While B.C.G. vaccination does not give complete protection against tuberculosis, there is clear evidence from trials in Britain and many other countries that it greatly decreases the chance of contracting the disease and virtually eliminates the danger of developing it in its more virulent primary form (see p 144). How long this protection lasts is not so clear. Reversion to tuberculin negativity after 3 or 4 years or less is quite common, and may be regarded as an indication for revaccination, but there is in fact no certainty that protective immunity has also waned at the same time as the hypersensitivity. Some American trials have failed to show any protective effect following B.C.G. vaccination. A possible explanation of this failure is that the populations concerned were already enjoying, as a result of natural infection with non-tuberculous mycobacteria, a degree of protection against tuberculosis comparable to that conferred in less fortunate communities by B.C.G. vaccination.

Whooping Cough

This disease can be serious, even lethal, in the first year or so of life, and responds poorly to antibiotic treatment. Effective prophylaxis is therefore clearly desirable, and ideally would give protection even in the first months of life, since there is little transfer of maternal immunity to this disease. Vaccines consisting of killed suspensions of *B. pertussis* have been available since the 1930s, and are given by intramuscular or subcutaneous injection. Early trials showed that they were effective, and some (though by no means all) of those in use in Britain and elsewhere in the 1950s were shown (in excellent Medical Research Council trials) to give good levels of protection. However, subsequent British surveys from about 1963 onwards have shown whooping cough incidences among vaccinated children that were disturbingly similar to those among otherwise comparable unvaccinated children. This has been attributed by some to the emergence of antigenic variants of *B. pertussis* against which the previously successful vaccines failed to protect, and by others to changes in methods of preparing and standardizing the vaccines. Among the factors that have complicated the situation is the lack of any satisfactory test for the potency of a batch of vaccine (other than using it and studying the consequences). There is also a lack of evidence as to whether the decreased incidence of whooping cough and the wider spacing of outbreaks that have undoubtedly occurred since the introduction of vaccination were due to it, or would have happened in any case for other reasons. Also there has been fierce controversy about the true frequency of brain damage attributable to *B. pertussis* vaccination. While there seems to be no doubt that this does occasionally cause encephalopathy, not every case of brain damage detected in a child who had received *B. pertussis* vaccine at some earlier time should be attributed to the vaccine. There is a shortage of good control data about the incidence of such brain damage in the unvaccinated. Unfortunately but understandably, public discussion of all these doubts about whooping cough vaccination has caused many parents to doubt the wisdom of having their children vaccinated at all—against any disease, not merely against whooping cough.

Typhoid and Paratyphoid

Immunization against enteric fever by injecting killed suspensions of the causative bacilli was introduced at the end of the last century and has been very widely used, especially in war-time, ever since then; but for many years there was surprisingly little definite evidence that it gave any protection. This was in part because army units and other groups of people with high vaccination rates have usually also had high standards of general hygiene which could equally well have been responsible for their low incidence of enteric fever; and in part because the effectiveness of such a vaccine varies with its method of preparation. However, carefully controlled large-scale trials in Yugoslavia in 1954–55 established that recipients of a heat-killed phenol-preserved *S. typhi* vaccine developed typhoid significantly less often than did those who received either a *Sh. flexneri* vaccine (presumably irrelevant) or an alcohol-killed *S. typhi* vaccine (which, on the evidence of this trial, was of little or no value).

It has been customary to use heat-killed suspensions of *S. typhi* in mixed vaccines containing heat-killed *S. paratyphi* A and B (T.A.B.) or A, B and C (T.A.B.C.) and sometimes other antigens (notably tetanus toxoid – see below); and to give two initial injections, with an interval of 10 days to 4 weeks between them, followed by booster doses at intervals of a year or two years to those liable to continuing exposure to risk of infection. Subcutaneous injection of these vaccines commonly produces painful local swelling, often accompanied by a general febrile reaction. These reactions are reduced in frequency and severity by giving the vaccines intradermally. It now seems doubtful whether the paratyphoid components should be included, since there is little evidence that they give useful protection and they certainly increase the adverse reactions. Acetone-killed *S. typhi* vaccines have now been shown in a number of trials to give more complete and more lasting protection than heat-killed phenolized vaccines, and seem likely to replace them.

All of these vaccines, even those that are not protective, stimulate vigorous antibody responses which greatly reduce the diagnostic value of subsequent Widal tests (see p 260).

Diphtheria and Tetanus

Both active and passive immunization against these diseases date from the pioneer work of von Behring and Kitasato at the end of the last century (see p 11), and from the time of their discovery there has never been any room for doubt about the efficacy of these procedures. In both diseases the damage is done by toxins and immunization is aimed at neutralizing these.

ACTIVE IMMUNIZATION   In each case toxoid for active immunization is made by heat- and formalin-inactivation of toxin obtained from a culture of the relevant organism. Elaborate steps are taken to purify this *formol toxoid* so as to eliminate unnecessary ingredients which might act as antigens and give rise to hypersensitivity reactions, or else might be directly toxic.

Diphtheria formol toxoid is an inadequate antigen when given on its own, but whooping cough vaccine given with it acts as an adjuvant (see p 65). Of various other means used to enhance the efficacy of the formol toxoid, adsorption onto aluminium phosphate or hydroxide is the most successful. Two intramuscular or deep subcutaneous injections of such an adsorbed vaccine, given 4–6 weeks apart, constitute an adequate primary course, and adverse reactions are uncommon and virtually never serious in children up to 10 years old. Older children and adults are more likely to have trouble from it. It is therefore best to carry out Schick tests (see p 265) on such subjects, so as to discover those for whom diphtheria immunization would be unnecessary or unwise, and to immunize the rest with the preparation known as toxoid antitoxin floccules (T.A.F.), to which they are much less likely to react adversely. However, this preparation consists of formol toxoid that has reacted with antitoxin from an immunized horse, and therefore must not be given to anyone who is allergic to horse protein; and it is a less potent antigen than the adsorbed vaccines, so that 3 doses are required.

'Provocation poliomyelitis' is a possible complication of diphtheria immunization in a community in which polioviruses are circulating–as in Britain in the 1950s, before vaccination against poliomyelitis had been carried out here on a large scale. At that time it was found that paralysis of the injected limb occurred with a frequency of about 1 per 37 000 injections of diphtheria toxoid, and that it could follow use of formol toxoid with whooping cough vaccine or of alum-precipitated or aluminium-phosphate-adsorbed toxoid without whooping cough vaccine. It apparently depended on local tissue damage converting a non-paralytic poliovirus infection into a localized paralytic form of the disease.

Tetanus formol toxoid is itself a potent antigen, but an adsorbed vaccine is also available. For either the recommended primary course consists of 3 intramuscular or subcutaneous injections, with 6 to 12 weeks between the first two and 6 to 12 months between the second and third.

As we shall see later, diphtheria and tetanus vaccines are commonly used in combination with one another and with other vaccines, and the timing of doses is therefore a matter of finding the best compromise between the optimal schedules for individual components of the mixture.

PASSIVE IMMUNIZATION   The danger to life in *diphtheria* depends largely upon circulating toxin, and there is a good chance of neutralizing this by giving intravenous diphtheria antitoxin (usually horse serum) as soon as the diagnosis is made or suspected. Since this is the only effective treatment, it must be given with the minimum of delay, but it must be preceded by a small subcutaneous dose of the serum to ensure that the patient is not sensitive to horse protein. If the test does cause any systemic reaction, desensitization must be attempted (see p 75). There is virtually never any call for the prophylactic use of diphtheria antiserum.

The position regarding *tetanus* is more complex. *Prophylactic* intramuscular or subcutaneous injection of anti-tetanus serum (A.T.S.) was long considered an essential part of the routine treatment of all lacerating or penetrating injuries. However, the widespread administration of horse serum is attended by serious risks of hypersensitivity reactions and even of fatal anaphylaxis. These risks are increased if such treatment is given on several occasions to the same patient or if there is any history of atopy (see p 75), and are not entirely eliminated by the time-consuming preliminary use of test doses as described above. Antitoxin in the form of immunoglobulin from hyperimmunized humans is much safer, but more difficult to produce in adequate amounts and far more expensive. Lesions potentially infected with tetanus spores are common, and their treatment would be simpler and safer if everyone was actively immunized in infancy and received regular booster injections. An injured patient could then be safely and efficiently protected by giving him a further dose of toxoid. As it is, all too often the patient either does not know or is incapable of telling the doctor that he has been actively immunized. Branding or the wearing of marked disks have been suggested as ways of overcoming this problem. When the immunization status of a potentially infected patient is not known, or when he is known not to have been recently immunized, it is now widely agreed that A.T.S. should not be given, and that it is better to rely on preventing multiplication of the bacilli by careful surgical toilet of wounds including removal of damaged and avascular tissue and by use of antibiotics, until active immunity has been established.

Therapeutic use of A.T.S. in cases of tetanus is also highly unsatisfactory, and here the problems are not overcome by substituting human immunoglobulin. In contrast to the position in diphtheria, it is toxin already fixed in the nervous system which endangers the patient's life. It seems probable that this cannot be neutralized even by very large amounts of intravenous antitoxin, and that the best to be expected of such treatment is the neutralization of any further toxin released by the bacilli. If this is so, the same end can be achieved by using antibiotics to inhibit or kill the bacilli.

IMMUNIZATION AGAINST PARTICULAR DISEASES DUE TO VIRUSES
Smallpox
When nearly 200 years ago Jenner introduced a safe means of immunization against smallpox (see p 11), he began the first (by many years) and one of the greatest of medicine's success stories; but it was not until the

last few years that we reached what may well be the last chapter of that story. With the prospect that smallpox may soon be an extinct disease (see p 205) and that many of our readers will never have to carry out this formerly common procedure which has achieved so much, we have abbreviated the account of the technicalities of smallpox vaccination which we gave in previous editions.

The relationship between the vaccinia and smallpox viruses and the preparation of vaccines for smallpox vaccination are discussed on p 206.

Vaccination is carried out by placing a drop of vaccine on the skin (preferably of the upper arm, where the risk of bacterial infection of the vaccinial lesion is minimal) and using a sterile needle either to scratch the underlying skin lightly or to make a number of small pricks in it by the special procedure known as 'multiple pressure'. In a previously non-immune subject a papule develops at the site of the vaccination after 3–4 days. This turns into a vesicle, which becomes a pustule by about 10 days and then develops a scab that separates during the third week, leaving a scar. This lesion is due to the activities of the live vaccinia virus, and results in prolonged immunity without the need of a second dose, since the virus has been continuously present in increasing amounts as a persistent stimulus while the lesion was present. For purposes of international travel certificates smallpox vaccination has been regarded as providing protection for up to 3 years, but in most cases it lasts much longer – even for life in some. In those already immune the vaccinial lesion is aborted and heals sooner, but the interpretation of results of re-vaccination is often complicated by the development of cell-mediated hypersensitivity to ingredients of the vaccine.

Complications of smallpox vaccination – all extremely rare but serious enough to constitute a strong case against widespread vaccination when there is no longer a significant risk of smallpox infection – include *generalized vaccinia* (a systemic illness with a widespread vesicular eruption), *encephalitis* and, in eczematous children, *eczema vaccinatum*.

Poliomyelitis

Immunization against this disease, as introduced by Salk in 1953, involved repeated injections of formalin-inactivated suspensions of all 3 poliovirus types. Salk-type vaccines made a great contribution to the control of poliomyelitis, but Sabin-type vaccines, consisting of live attenuated viruses, are now in general use. These are cheaper to prepare, are taken by mouth, and have other advantages. The live viruses establish themselves in the recipient's intestinal wall, and in addition to providing him with an antigenic stimulus they are for some weeks excreted in his faeces and may be transmitted to other people around him. Immunity develops sooner and lasts longer after Sabin-type than after Salk-type vaccination, and it includes resistance to propagation of wild polioviruses in the intestine, whereas after Salk-type vaccination such viruses are prevented from reaching the nervous system but are permitted to propagate in the intestine and so can be disseminated through the community. If live-virus vaccination is attempted in a community in which certain other enteroviruses are prevalent, it may be unsuccessful in some cases because of interference (see p 174). Similarly, when vaccine strains of all 3 poliovirus types are administered simultaneously, that of one type (commonly type 2) may establish itself in the intestine to the exclusion of the other two, and the resultant immunity is against only the one type. However, the strain that 'takes' on the first occasion is in consequence unable to do so if a further dose of the trivalent vaccine is given after a suitable interval, and immunization against all 3 types can be achieved by giving 3 doses of the trivalent vaccine at monthly intervals. Alternatively, monovalent vaccines can be used, each being given once only and the intervals being sufficient to prevent interference.

When, as in Britain at present, the circulation of polioviruses within the community is insufficient to maintain herd immunity (the importance of which is outlined on p 58), it is essential that it should be maintained instead by a high level of vaccination–otherwise imported viruses can cause havoc. Furthermore, the community may need protection against the vaccine strains themselves. There has been no confirmation of early fears that the virulence of these might be rapidly enhanced by a few passages through human contacts of those who had been given the vaccine. However, it now appears that a slower change is going on; some of the polioviruses circulating in Britain today, and capable of causing clinical illness with neurological symptoms, have genetic characters suggesting their derivation from vaccine strains that have been able to adapt to life in the community. A falling level of herd immunity might permit such strains to cause more serious trouble. Vaccination is clearly indicated for previously unvaccinated individuals going from a country with a low prevalence of polioviruses to one where they are common.

Measles

Measles may be a severe infection, complicated by otitis media, broncho-pneumonia and even in a few cases by encephalitis. Active immunization, by means of a single injection of a chick-embryo culture of a live attenuated virus, is commonly followed by fever and rash and sometimes by bacterial infection of the respiratory tract, but these complications are far less serious than those of the natural measles which virtually every unvaccinated child acquires. Vaccination in the early months of life commonly fails to prevent subsequent development of measles, probably because maternal antibodies neutralize the vaccine. The beginning of the second year of life seems to be the best time for routine vaccination. As the vaccine did not become available until 1963, information about the duration of protection is still incomplete, but it seems to last for 10 years or so in most cases; a small proportion of children, however, prove to be still susceptible after vaccination. Eradication by mass immunization has proved difficult to achieve except in small closed communities, as transmission of the virus continues unless nearly 100% of the population is immune.

Rubella
Immunization against this disease is discussed on pp 192–3.

IMMUNIZATION PROGRAMMES
Active immunization of a large proportion of a population can be used either to bring a disease under control or to prevent its return to a community from which it has been eradicated. Such use of any immunizing procedure must be governed by the answers to the following questions:

(1) *Is it effective?* Smallpox vaccination was made compulsory in Britain in the middle of the last century, and the disease, formerly common, was virtually eradicated from the country by the end of the century. However, there was still no *proof* of the efficacy of vaccination. The improvement could have been due to other factors, though more recent evidence has shown that vaccination does in fact prevent smallpox. Today such prophylactic procedures are tested in carefully controlled trials, such as that of typhoid vaccines mentioned on p 312, or those described in the papers included in the suggestions for further reading at the end of this chapter.

(2) *Is it safe?* No form of vaccination is entirely free from risk – there are very few things in life which are! Safety in vaccination has to be assessed by comparison with the risks of being unvaccinated. The death-rate from variolation (see p 11) was on a scale that would be called disastrous today; but it was safer to undergo this procedure than to run the risks of natural smallpox infection. The fatality rate from Jennerian vaccination is probably less than 1/10 000 of that from variolation, but even this is too high a risk to permit the continuation of routine vaccination today in countries that are free of smallpox. (Allowing herd immunity to fall is thought not to be dangerous, as immediate vaccination of first-line contacts of anyone who brings smallpox into the country can be relied upon to prevent spread.)

(3) *How great is the need?* Normal adults can develop whooping

cough, but they do not need to be protected against it, since it carries no serious risks for them. On the other hand it is potentially lethal for small children, who need to be protected. In this disease the need for protection and the hazards of immunization (as some estimate them) are sufficiently in balance to provoke vigorous controversy (see p 311). In general, the need for immunization against a disease depends on the risk of acquiring it, the likelihood that the illness will be serious, and the effectiveness of available means of treating it.

(4) *Is it practicable?* This depends on many social and economic factors. Repeated small outbreaks of diphtheria, with quite high death rates, have occurred in some countries which could, in theory, have prevented them, but which could not in fact afford to divert their available medical, administrative and financial resources from larger and more urgent problems.

(5) *Can it be made acceptable?* No programme of mass-immunization can succeed without popular support. This depends largely upon successful propaganda, and is much easier to secure when the disease is still prevalent and its dire effects are known. 'Diphtheria is deadly', an effective slogan in Britain of the early 1940s, is today liable to produce the reply, 'What is diphtheria? Surely it doesn't happen any more.' Popular support also depends upon absence of disfigurement (such as large vaccination scars) and absence of unpleasant (even if harmless) reactions. One reason for never immunizing anyone who is at all unwell is that any illness which he may be incubating will be attributed to the injection. A single death *following* (not caused by) immunization outweighs much expensive propaganda. Finally, immunization is made more acceptable by minimizing the number of visits to the clinic or surgery which are necessary. This means using potent and, where possible, combined vaccines.

Syringe-and-needle injections require a skilled operator, particularly when vaccines that have undesirable effects when placed too deeply, such as B.C.G. and T.A.B., are being given. To inject a large number of people using a fresh syringe and needle for each one takes a long time; but to use the same needle, or even the same syringe with different needles, for several people is to risk cross-infection, particularly with hepatitis viruses (see p 207). Intradermal injections can now be given in the form of a high-pressure jet from an instrument that does not touch the patient's skin. This technique increases the safety, practicability and acceptability of mass-immunization programmes: the safety because it eliminates the risk of cross-infection, the practicability because a relatively unskilled operator can carry out immunizations rapidly, and the acceptability because the patient does not have to be pricked with a needle.

Combined Vaccines

In Britain it is currently recommended that young children should be immunized against diphtheria, tetanus, whooping cough, poliomyelitis and measles. If immunization against each of these diseases was carried out separately, the primary courses alone would require at least 12 administrations of vaccine. However, three doses of *triple vaccine* (diphtheria and tetanus toxoids and a killed suspension of *Bord. pertussis*) constitutes an effective primary course for the first three diseases, the whooping-cough vaccine acting as an adjuvant to enhance the efficacy of the toxoids as well as fulfilling its primary function. Three doses of oral live poliovirus vaccine can be given at the same times as the injections, so that after three visits to the doctor the child needs only to be immunized against measles (one visit). One point to remember is that if a person receives an injection of a combined vaccine of which he has previously encountered only one component, his antibody response may be concentrated entirely on that component to the exclusion of the others. For example, if a child has received one dose of whooping-cough vaccine, he should be given two more doses of that vaccine and then a separate course of diphtheria–tetanus vaccine, as his response to triple vaccine may be inadequate as regards diphtheria and tetanus.

Time-Table for Immunization of Children

Attempts at immunization of a new-born baby are generally unsuccessful both because of the immaturity of its antibody-forming mechanisms and because maternal antibodies in the baby's circulation may neutralize the antigens. (B.C.G. vaccination is an exception to this.) If advantage is to be taken of the triple vaccine, there is a problem about when to use it. *Whooping cough* immunization should start as early as possible if it is to protect the infant during the dangerous period, but *diphtheria* and *tetanus* immunization are more efficient if started when the child is at least 6 months old. In the schedule published by the Department of Health in 1972 for use in this country, the first doses of triple vaccine and of oral *poliovirus* vaccine are given together at some time between the ages of 3 and 6 months, the second doses are given 6–8 weeks later and the third doses 4–6 months after that. *Measles* vaccination is given in the second year, at least 3 weeks after the last dose of poliovirus vaccine. Booster doses for diphtheria, tetanus and poliomyelitis are then given at the time of starting school, and further booster doses for the last two around the time of leaving school. *Rubella* vaccine is recommended for all girls between the ages of 11 and 13 years, even those with histories of rubella-like illness. In countries where infants run a high risk of tuberculous infection they should be given B.C.G. soon after birth, but in Britain such vaccination is carried out in infancy only when there has been known or probable exposure to a source of tuberculous infection; otherwise it is reserved for those aged 10 to 14 years, who are entering a period of special susceptibility, and for nurses, medical students and other young adults who are particularly at risk.

Vaccination for International Travel

To pass from one country to another a traveller may need to produce certificates of recent vaccination against one or more diseases. The details depend on his country of origin and his route, and vary from country to country and from time to time in accordance with the distribution of foci of active disease and the current anxieties of health authorities. The prospective traveller should make sure of the prevailing regulations by asking travel agents or official representatives of the countries to which he is going. Vaccination against smallpox, still (in 1977) required for some journeys, or against cholera can be carried out by his own doctor, but yellow fever vaccination can be carried out only at designated centres. If time is short it may be important to remember that an interval of at least 3 weeks should be allowed between primary smallpox vaccination and yellow fever vaccination carried out in that order, but 4 days is sufficient if the order is reversed. Certificates of vaccination against any of the 3 diseases mentioned so far are acceptable only if they are on international certificate forms obtainable from travel agents or health authorities. Poliomyelitis, typhoid or other vaccinations may be recommended, or in special circumstances required, but there are no international certificates for them.

Suggestions for Further Reading

Symposium on immunization in *The Practitioner*, 1975, vol. 215, pp 285–326.

Good examples of carefully controlled trials of immunizing agents are: to be found in the following Medical Research Council reports: 'Vaccination against whooping cough', *Brit. med. J.*, 1959, i. 994; and 'B.C.G. and vole bacillus vaccines in the prevention of tuberculosis in adolescents', *Brit. med. J.*, 1959, ii. 379.

A comprehensive survey of mishaps and disasters associated with immunizing procedures is to be found in *The Hazards of Immunization* by Sir Graham Wilson (Athlone Press, London, 1967).

21

Antibacterial Drugs*

PERSPECTIVE

Up until 1935 no drugs were available for the treatment of systemic bacterial infections other than syphilis. Doctors could do no more than treat symptoms and, with the invaluable help of nurses, look after the patient's general condition while he overcame the infection himself, or failed to do so. Then came the sulphonamides and other drugs for systemic treatment of bacterial infections, notably the antibiotics. The situation was rapidly transformed, and the morbidity and mortality of bacterial infections were dramatically reduced (see p 12). It is hardly possible to overestimate the importance of antibacterial drugs.

However, this is far from meaning that today the correct answer to a bacterial infection is simply to give the right antibacterial drug. In many cases, as we shall see, choosing the right drug is by no means a simple matter. Furthermore, choosing the right drug is only part of the right management of the patient. The doctor who treats pneumonia merely by giving a suitable antibiotic, and forgets the principles of general medical and nursing care and the importance, for example, of giving oxygen for anoxia, may lose his patient even though he cures the infection. Similarly, the surgeon who ignores the rules of aseptic surgery and relies on antibiotics to prevent or cure wound sepsis is on the way to disaster. Antibacterial drugs must be seen in proper perspective. To use them is to intervene in the struggle between the host's defences and the invading organisms. If the weapons are rightly chosen and rightly used, such intervention is likely to be decisive; but at no time can we afford to neglect the defenders' morale or supplies, or to allow the invaders to build up massive reinforcements.

* Information about drugs for use against viruses, fungi or protozoa is to be found in Chapters Eleven to Thirteen.

Hazards

Neither can we afford to forget that antibacterial drugs are foreign substances so far as the patient's body is concerned, and are potentially harmful to him. They vary in the frequency and severity of their adverse effects, but none of them is perfectly safe, and almost all of them have on occasions killed patients. Most of the troubles for which they are responsible fall into the following three categories:

(1) *Direct toxicity to host cells.* These drugs depend for their effectiveness upon their toxicity to bacterial cells. They may interfere with folic acid metabolism (sulphonamides, trimethoprim), with building of cell walls (penicillins, cephalosporins), with protein synthesis (aminoglycosides, chloramphenicol, tetracyclines, macrolides, clindamycin), with nucleic acid synthesis (metronidazole, rifamycins) or with the integrity of the cytoplasmic membrane (polymyxins). These mechanisms of action are discussed on pp 39–41 and 342–3, but are mentioned here to emphasize the point that a successful antibacterial agent must attack bacterial cell mechanisms or structures, but to be of clinical use it must not do comparable damage to host cells. If it attacks a process peculiar to bacterial cells–their mechanism for cell-wall construction, for example–it is likely not to be harmful to human cells except when given in very large doses (e.g. benzyl penicillin) or by some unrelated mechanism (e.g. the nephrotoxicity of cephaloridine). If it attacks a metabolic process similar to one carried on by some or all host cells, then there may be only a narrow margin between the concentration that is effective against bacteria and the toxic concentration. Indeed, for every antibacterial drug that has been developed for clinical use there are many that have been tested and rejected because this margin was too small or non-existent. (This problem is even more serious in relation to antiviral drugs–see p 180–since the metabolic processes of virus replication are in fact host-cell processes.)

(2) *Hypersensitivity reactions.* Patients may become hypersensitive to almost any antibacterial (and indeed, almost any other) drug, but the antibacterial drugs with which this type of problem is most commonly encountered are the penicillins, otherwise the least harmful of antibiotics. Penicillin hypersensitivity may take the form of rashes, of Type III 'serum sickness' reactions (see p 76) or even of severe, sometimes rapidly fatal Type I anaphylactic reactions (see p 75). Hypersensitivity is not merely unpleasant or dangerous in itself; it also means that the patient is in future deprived of the possibility of being treated with the drugs to which he has become hypersensitive–and in practice this all too often means that the use of an antibiotic for a

condition for which it was unnecessary or inappropriate debars its subsequent use in a more serious situation in which it might have been extremely valuable.

(3) *Alteration of the host's bacterial flora.* The doctor who prescribes an antibacterial drug is aiming it at a known or suspected pathogen, but the drug itself is by no means so selective! As we have indicated in earlier chapters, man's normal bacterial population is of great value to him, and any major interference with it can have unpleasant and sometimes serious consequences (see pp 25, 95 and 125–6). The availability of powerful antibiotics has made such interference possible, and indeed easy to achieve. Freed from the restraining influence of their more numerous but antibiotic-sensitive neighbours, more resistant organisms that are normally present only in small numbers–e.g. *C. albicans*, *Ps. aeruginosa* and some of the enterobacteria–may be able to proliferate vigorously and may become 'opportunist' pathogens, particularly if the patient is debilitated or immunologically deficient. Furthermore, antibiotic-resistant variants of the pathogen for which the patient is being treated, or of any other pathogen that he may be carrying, may be present as a result of mutation or plasmid-transfer (see pp 32 and 34); and if so, the selective advantage conferred on them by the antibiotic treatment may enable them to multiply and so both to cause serious trouble to the patient and to be transmitted to other patients or potential patients in his vicinity. We shall return later in the chapter to the problem of bacterial resistance to drugs; here we would simply point out that a large part of the problem has been created by their use (wise or unwise).

USE AND ABUSE OF ANTIBACTERIAL DRUGS

As far back as 1956 Professor Jawetz, one of America's leading authorities on this subject, hazarded a guess that not more than 5 to 10% of the vast output of antibiotics was employed on proper clinical indications. He went on to give a vivid description of the various pressures, notably from the manufacturers and from patients and their relatives, which cause doctors to misuse such drugs. The number of new antibacterial drugs introduced since 1956 has increased our capacity both for effective treatment and for misunderstanding and mistakes, and it may well be that Jawetz's estimate is not far from the truth today. To provide his patients with optimal antibacterial therapy the doctor needs to answer a number of questions, which we can group under three headings: *Why?*, *Which?*, and *How?*.

WHY does this patient need antibacterial treatment?

This is the most important of the questions. Unless there is a valid reason–scientific, not just social or emotional–for giving an antibacterial drug, the patient would probably be better off without it. (For a placebo effect it is usually possible to choose something safer and cheaper.) Valid reasons include the following:

(1) *Treatment of a known or suspected bacterial infection* that is unlikely to undergo rapid and satisfactory spontaneous resolution, and that can be expected, on the available evidence, to respond to the drug given.

Patients in the early stages of acute upper respiratory tract infections are commonly given oral penicillin or some other antibiotic. This is often a clear example of the misuse of such drugs, since the infection is usually caused by a virus and is likely to be rapidly self-limiting; the antibiotics cannot therefore be expected to do good but may well do harm. However, if the patient has tonsillitis or pharyngitis and there are clinical, epidemiological or bacteriological reasons for suspecting that it is due to *Str. pyogenes*, penicillin treatment is indicated.

Sometimes a patient is known to have a bacterial infection due to an organism which is sensitive to antibiotics *in vitro*, but their clinical use is contra-indicated by existing knowledge. For example, attempted antibiotic treatment of enteritis due to the 'food-poisoning' salmonellae commonly results merely in prolonged carriage and excretion of the offending organism (see p 130).

On many occasions, however, use of antibacterial drugs is clearly indicated. Patients with lobar pneumonia, purulent meningitis, serious post-operative wound infections, or specific bacterial infections such as typhoid, tuberculosis, syphilis or gonorrhoea–to name but a few of many possible examples–must receive prompt and effective antibacterial treatment. In many other cases the indications are less clear, but one or more antibacterial drugs should be given because of the probability that the patient has a bacterial infection, or of the less strong possibility that he has such an infection which, if present, could be serious unless treated promptly. However, as we shall see more clearly when we come to our next question, if there is any doubt about the presence or nature of a bacterial infection it is the doctor's duty to ensure that so far as possible all necessary specimens for precise bacteriological diagnosis are collected before antibacterial treatment is given.

(2) *Prevention of bacterial infection.* There are a few definite indications for prophylactic administration of antibacterial drugs, such as the following:

(a) Patients who have had rheumatic fever need to be protected from *Str. pyogenes* infections which might precipitate further attacks. Fortunately this species is always highly susceptible to penicillin and nearly always to the sulphonamides, and either of these can safely be given in prolonged low dosage for prophylaxis.

(b) During such procedures as dental extraction, other major dental treatment or tonsillectomy, bacteria from the mouth or pharynx enter the blood stream. In such circumstances patients with congenital or rheumatic heart abnormalities may develop sub-acute bacterial endocarditis due to viridians streptococci (see p 103). This can be prevented by ensuring that at the time of, and for a short while after, operation they have in their blood concentrations of antibiotic that can kill the streptococci before they have a chance to establish themselves in the fibrinous vegetations in the heart. It has been customary to give for this purpose an injection of penicillin immediately before the operation, but there is evidence that a more rapid and more reliable bactericidal effect can be achieved by giving streptomycin or gentamicin as well.

Starting the antibiotic treatment a day or two before operation is a serious mistake, as this allows antibiotic-resistant streptococci to proliferate in the mouth and pharynx and to be the organisms that enter the blood stream and possibly cause endocarditis, which in such circumstances is likely to be very difficult to treat.

(c) Operations involving the intestine, particularly the appendix, colon and rectum, almost inevitably result in some contamination of the peritoneal cavity and incised tissues with mixed intestinal flora. Various procedures for pre-operative 'gut sterilization' have been tried, without convincing evidence of success; but 'peri-operative prophylaxis', starting just before operation and continued for a few days, can reduce the frequency of wound infections and other types of post-operative sepsis. In particular, metronidazole (given by mouth, by rectal suppository or intravenously, as appro-priate) has proved highly effective in preventing infections due to anaerobes.

(d) Cl. welchii and other clostidia are predictably sensitive to penicillin (and to metronidazole, but the value of this drug in the situations that we are about to describe has not yet been assessed). Patients at special risk of developing gas-gangrene (clostridial myositis) include: those who have suffered major trauma with soil contamination; those who have lower limb amputations for vascular disease; and those who have operations on their hip-joints or femoral heads. These 3 classes of patient have in common the presence of devitalized muscle or bone fragments and the likelihood of clostridial contamination of these—due, in the last two classes, to the frequency with which the patient's intestinal clostridia are to be found on the skin of the thigh and the difficulty of eradicating these sporing organisms by pre-operative skin preparation. For all such patients penicillin prophylaxis is indicated.

Antibacterial prophylaxis can be justified in a few more conditions—e.g. extensive burns, open heart surgery, leukaemic patients with severe marrow depression, and some patients with recurrent urinary tract infections—but in most others it is likely to do more harm than good. Antibiotics are frequently given to patients with virus infections, in order to prevent superinfection by bacteria. This is nearly always unwise; its most likely result is to ensure that the superinfection is by antibiotic-resistant bacteria and therefore more difficult to treat. Attempted prophylaxis against pneumonia in paralysed, unconscious or debilitated patients has much the same effect. In general it is better to wait until bacterial infection occurs and then treat it with an appropriate drug.

WHICH drug or drugs should this patient receive?
This question breaks down into a number of subsidiary questions:

(1) *What is the pathogen, and to what drugs is it sensitive?*
Right use of antibacterial drugs requires that the problem be defined as closely as possible, so that the best tool or tools for dealing with it can be selected. Sometimes the patient's clinical condition is characteristic of the activities of a particular pathogen—e.g. a typical staphylococcal abscess, typhoid or syphilis—and the drug sensitivities of that organism are predictable enough for a suitable drug to be chosen without laboratory help. Sometimes an illness could be due to any of a number of organisms but stained smears of pathological material give all the information that is needed—pneumococci may be recognized micro-scopically, for example, in pus from otitis media or in cerebrospinal fluid from meningitis, and can be relied upon to be sensitive to penicillin (in most countries). But in many cases in which immediate drug treatment is necessary, it has at first to be based on informed guesses as to the organism and its sensitivities. Except in an emergency or when no laboratory facilities are available, *all specimens necessary for the isolation of the causative organism should be collected before treatment is started*. If this is not done, treatment may obscure the diagnosis without being adequate to effect a cure. For example, a patient may have a streptococcal endocarditis which has not yet been diagnosed. If he is given tetracyclines before blood cultures have been set up, it may then be impossible to isolate the organism. His clinical picture may be temporarily improved, but it is highly unlikely that cure will result (see p 353). When tetracycline treatment stops, he is likely to relapse, and

his proper investigation and treatment will have been delayed by some weeks. Whenever intial treatment has been based on guesses, it needs to be reviewed in the light of subsequent laboratory reports about the nature and sensitivities of the organism isolated. However, the ultimate test of a drug's suitability is its therapeutic effect; laboratory sensitivity reports are at best only an indication of probabilities, and if the patient is responding well to the initial treatment, it is usually unwise to act upon a report which suggests that he ought not to be doing so! In many cases there is no urgent need to start treatment until the laboratory report is available.

(2) *Narrow or broad spectrum?*

The ultimate in precision tools for dealing with identified pathogens – a dream in Ehrlich's time and still no more than a dream – would be an array of drugs, each one of which would with antibody-like precision attack one pathogenic species, leaving other micro-organisms and the host intact. At the other extreme would be a drug which would deal with all bacterial (and preferably other) pathogens. This might be a pharmaceutical manufacturer's dream, as he might hope that all doctors would give it to most of their patients; but to a bacteriologist it is more like a nightmare, because of its inevitable complex side-effects. Real-life antibacterial drugs come between these hypothetical extremes. Cloxacillin, benzyl penicillin, the macrolides and the polymyxins have useful levels of activity against only some parts of the 'spectrum' of bacterial genera, whereas some of the other penicillins, the aminoglycosides, chloramphenicol, the tetracyclines and others are effective against at least some members of most genera, and are often referred to as 'broad spectrum' antibiotics (particularly by manufacturers, who are naturally concerned to promote their wide-spread use). In practice, when the identity of the infecting organism is known or virtually certain the doctor's primary question about any particular antibiotic is not about the width of its spectrum but whether it is the most suitable means of dealing with this pathogen; though when there is a choice between drugs that are equally appropriate in other respects, narrowness of spectrum is at least in theory an asset. On the other hand, when the pathogen has not been identified or when there is more than one pathogen to be treated, it may be best to use a drug with a spectrum wide enough to cover all the probable or known organisms. The alternative approach is to use more than one drug – see below.

(3) *Cidal or static?*

It appears to be true of the treatment of most bacterial infections that there is no need to use drugs that can kill the invading organisms; if they are prevented from multiplying, the patient's own defence mechanisms can eliminate them. However, there are exceptions to this general statement. It is probably best to use bactericidal therapy when the patient's immunological defences are seriously impaired, or when the infection is overwhelming. Chronic bronchitics may have longer spells free of bronchial suppuration if the offending organisms, in the bronchial lumen and so apparently beyond the reach of the host's defences, are eradicated by treatment rather than merely suppressed (see p 000). But the classic, and in some ways the most surprising, example of a disease in which bactericidal treatment is required is bacterial endocarditis. It might seem that organisms in fibrinous vegetations in the heart and major blood vessels were well within the reach of blood cells and antibodies, but in fact all available evidence indicates that in such a site they are unusually well protected against both of these. Bacteriostatic treatment, so long as it is continued, may bring about apparent cure; but the organisms persist inside the vegetations, ready to resume activity when the treatment stops. They require treatment with drugs that can kill them (see p 353).

(4) One drug or drugs?

It is possible to demonstrate *in vitro* four types of results when antimicrobial drugs are mixed: *indifference*, the combined effect being indistinguishable from that of the more powerful drug used alone; *addition*, the combined effect being the sum of the individual effects; *synergy*, the combined effect being greater than can be explained by simple addition; and *antagonism*, the combined effect being less than that of the more powerful drug used alone. The type of result depends upon drug concentrations, the microbial strain used and many other factors, and it is therefore meaningless to describe a drug combination as synergic or antagonistic without specifying the circumstances of such interaction. In general, synergy is likely to be observed only in a mixture of two bactericidal drugs (e.g. penicillin + streptomycin) and antagonism only in a mixture of one bactericidal and one bacteriostatic drug (e.g. penicillin + tetracycline). In at least some instances the mechanism of antagonism appears to be that the bacteriostatic drug prevents the organisms from multiplying and so from entering the phase of growth in which they are susceptible to the bactericidal drug.

These various types of result also occur *in vivo*. Antagonism was clearly illustrated as far back as 1951 in one series of cases of pneumococcal meningitis, in which the mortality of patients treated with penicillin + tetracycline considerably exceeded that of comparable patients treated with penicillin alone. The possibility of such an interaction is a strong warning against the use of drug-combinations without definite reasons. Furthermore, use of more than one drug increases the likelihood of adverse reactions; and when these occur in such circumstances it may be difficult or impossible to decide which drug is responsible, and should therefore be discontinued and not given to this patient on future occasions. Drug incompatibilities are also possible (see below), and the expense is of course increased–a factor which we have not mentioned so far in this chapter, but which needs to be considered in many decisions about antibacterial therapy. However, there are situations in which it is justifiable and may even be essential to use combinations of antibacterial drugs, including the following:

(a) When the patient is suffering from infection with two or more organisms and no single drug is likely to be effective against both or all.

(b) As a temporary measure in a severe acute illness which might be due to any of several organisms and when again no single drug is likely to be effective against them all–see p 354 (meningitis).

(c) To prevent the emergence of resistant strains–see p 334 (drug resistance), p 352 (*Staph. aureus* infections) and p 356 (tuberculosis).

(d) When synergy can be expected–see p 342 (co-trimoxazole), p 353 (bacterial endocarditis).

(e) When there is empirical evidence that a particular combination gives the best results–see p 142 (treatment of brucellosis).

(5) *Is it compatible with other medication?*

Even when an antibacterial drug is appropriate in all other respects for treating an infection, it may be contraindicated or may have to be given with special precautions because of its possible interactions with other drugs that the patient is receiving. Some combinations of drugs are physically or chemically incompatible when mixed in high concentrations. Thus when a doctor prescribes two or more antibiotics which are to be mixed before injection or are to be given together in an intravenous infusion, he needs to be sure that they do not precipitate or inactivate one another. Similarly, when giving any antibiotic by slow intravenous infusion he must be sure that it is not adversely affected by other components of the infusion fluid (e.g. the aminoglycosides are incompatible with heparin, and ampicillin is fairly rapidly inactivated in the presence of 5% dextrose). This is clearly of great practical importance, since incompatibility may result in a patient never having an effective blood level of an antibiotic which is being given in apparently adequate doses. Also very important, and in general even more serious in their consequences, are the pharmacological incompatibilities of some drug combinations at the levels achieved in the patient. Renal damage may follow the giving of gentamicin with cephaloridine, for example, or of one of these with either of the diuretics frusemide or ethacrynic acid; and either nalidixic acid or co-trimoxazole may enhance the effects of anticoagulant drugs and lead to severe bleeding. As more new drugs are introduced, and more undesirable interactions between older ones are recognized, this subject becomes increasingly complex and worrying. Information about known incompatibilities involving antibacterial drugs is to be found in tables in the two books *Antibiotic and Chemotherapy* and *Antibiotics in Clinical Practice* mentioned at the end of this chapter.

HOW should the drug or drugs be given?

This question overlaps with the previous one at many points. For example, however appropriate a drug may be for dealing with a particular pathogen, it is not the right one for the patient if it can be given only in a form inappropriate to his situation – e.g. orally to a patient who is vomiting, intramuscularly to one with a severe bleeding tendency, or intravenously to an out-patient. Nor is it sufficient to be able to give the drug to the patient; having been given, it must be capable of arriving at the site of the infection in adequate concentration. We therefore have to think about the route by which a drug can be delivered, not merely into the patient but to the place where it is needed; and also about dosage.

(1) **Route**

For a superficial infection of the skin or an accessible mucous surface it may be possible to apply the drug in high concentration directly to the lesion; but unfortunately such topical application, notably of the penicillins, is particularly liable to provoke a hypersensitivity reaction and so to deprive the patient of subsequent systemic use of the group of antibiotics in question. A different form of local application that gives less trouble and is sometimes indicated is direct injection into a body cavity – intrapleural, intraperitoneal, intrathecal or intra-ocular, for example.

Oral administration is possible only if the drug can be produced in a palatable form; if it survives the action of the gastric secretions (or can be protected from it in capsules that dissolve in the small intestine); if it does not provoke significant gastro-intestinal upset; and above all if it is reliably absorbed into the blood (unless its site of action is to be the bowel lumen) and passes through the liver without being inactivated. Sometimes an ester or other derivative, itself not an effective antibacterial drug, meets all of these requirements and is converted into the active form after absorption. Oral preparations have, in addition to their unsuitability for patients who are vomiting or cannot swallow, the disadvantage that their absorption may be unreliable in very ill patients, in whom it is particularly important to achieve good levels rapidly and consistently. Some antibacterials, notably metronidazole, are well absorbed when given as rectal suppositories, provided that the patient does not have diarrhoea.

Parenteral (i.e. non-alimentary) administration is usually intramuscular or intravenous. For intramuscular injection it is necessary to produce a strong solution (so that the volume is tolerable) which is of physiological pH and which does not cause excessive pain, or damage the injected muscle; this is not possible for some antibiotics. Also, having been injected, the drug must be rapidly and reliably absorbed into the blood (unless it is deliberately given as a slow-release depot preparation, as is sometimes done with penicillin). Intravenous injection or infusion is in some ways the ideal way of getting a drug into the blood, but it is seldom the most practicable or convenient. Furthermore, some drugs are difficult to give repeatedly by this route because they cause local phlebitis and thrombosis and a consequent shortage of accessible veins.

Once in the blood-stream, drugs vary in their distribution to tissues and body fluids and in their renal handling, and therefore a high blood level is no guarantee of good tissue levels. Indeed, a high and sustained blood level could well be due to the drug's inability to get out of the blood! Part (but it is not clear whether it is an important part) of this variability in tissue penetration is related to differences in binding to plasma proteins. Virtually all antibacterials are bound to some degree, but some very much more than others–even others in the same group. Bound drug is in general no longer active against bacteria, so two drugs may give comparable total blood levels but with one mostly bound and inactive and the other mostly free and active. There is a reversible equilibrium between bound and unbound drug, but it may be only the unbound portion that is free to diffuse out of the circulation–and even then its troubles are by no means over, as it may bind to tissue proteins.

Rapid excretion of an antibacterial drug by the kidneys may make it highly suitable for dealing with urinary tract infections (see p 355), provided that it is not, like chloramphenicol, excreted mainly in an inactive form (see p 349). Such rapid excretion also necessarily means that blood and tissue levels are not well sustained–which may be an advantage, as we shall see below, under (2) (a). Conversely, persistent high levels will be achieved if a drug that is not excreted in bile or metabolized in the liver or elsewhere is only slowly excreted by the kidneys–either because of its nature or because of renal failure.

Antibacterial drugs also vary widely in their ability to pass into body fluids other than urine. For example, sulphadiazine or chloramphenicol levels in cerebrospinal fluid are usually 40–80% of the prevailing blood levels. On the other hand, only traces of the penicillins or of streptomycin reach the cerebrospinal fluid from the blood if the meninges are healthy, though much larger amounts go through and much higher cerebrospinal fluid levels are achieved when the meninges are inflamed. Similarly, when ampicillin is used in treatment of suppurative chronic bronchitis it may pass fairly readily into the sputum at first, but as the infection is brought under control and the sputum ceases to be purulent its ampicillin content falls sharply. However, penetration of the closely related drug amoxycillin into sputum is far less dependent upon local inflammation. Penicillin given to pregnant women may reach much higher concentrations in the liquor amnii than in the maternal blood; yet streptomycin, the tetracyclines and chloramphenicol hardly penetrate to the liquor at all. These examples indicate something of the complexity of a subject which is of great clinical importance but is far from being thoroughly understood.

(2) **Dosage**

Nowhere in this chapter do we go into details about dosage schedules for individual drugs; these are to be found in the books mentioned at the end of the chapter, as well as in the manufacturers' literature and in many other places. However, we do need to consider some general principles.

'Give enough, for long enough, and then stop'. This facile generalization embodies three important points:

(*a*) *'Enough'* The aim of antibacterial treatment must be to ensure a drug level at the site or sites of infection which is sufficient to kill or inhibit the pathogen. The patient must therefore be given his drug in doses adequate to achieve this, with due allowance for his size and other factors that may affect the distribution of the drug. To give him less than this is to deny him the help of the antibiotic without necessarily sparing him the hazards; it may well encourage development of drug-resistance by the pathogen or by other potential pathogens; and it is a waste of the drug and of the money spent on it. When bacteriostasis is the aim, theoretical considerations suggest that an effective concentration should be maintained all the time. The same is not necessarily true for a bactericidal effect. For example, since the action of penicillins is on cell wall formation, they can do nothing to a bacterium which is inhibited and not trying to make cell wall; and it is still debatable, after all the years for which we have had penicillins to use, whether the best mode of attack is by a sustained high level or by a transitory high level ('peak'), followed by a period ('trough') during which the level is low enough to allow any survivors to resume multiplication and so to be susceptible to the next peak. Sometimes toxicity also has to be considered. For example, with gentamicin it is possible to produce toxic effects (mainly on the 8th nerve) by maintaining a blood level that is never high enough to be cidal to any but the most susceptible pathogens; it is therefore essential to achieve bactericidal peak levels but to ensure that for most of the time between doses there is a trough that is below the toxic level. With this and related drugs, laboratory monitoring of both peak and trough levels can be an important aid to treatment. This is particularly so when impaired renal function makes it difficult to predict the rate at which the drug will be excreted, and therefore the interval between peaks which is necessary to ensure adequate troughs.

(b) 'For long enough'. The length of treatment necessary to eradicate a bacterial infection depends, obviously enough, on the nature and location of the pathogen. The tubercle bacillus, with its very long generation time by comparison with most bacteria, needs months or even years of treatment. A pathogen that is well 'dug in' in a fibrotic chronic lesion may call for considerably longer treatment than one that has just arrived and is causing an acute infection. But so far as any generalization is permissible, it seems to be true that for many acute bacterial infections it is appropriate to give an antibacterial drug for 5–7 days. By then it will probably have done its job – or failed to do it, in which case a change of treatment is indicated and may well have taken place already. Unfortunately patients who are not closely supervised, including doctors themselves, commonly give up or forget their drugs as soon as symptoms are abating; relapse of infection following inadequate treatment is therefore all too common. Perhaps we need to learn more from the veterinary profession about the value of a single very large dose of an antibacterial. Venereologists, with their special problems of patient supervision, have made some progress in this direction (see pp 109 and 155).

(c) 'And then stop'. No good purpose is likely to be served, and harm can be done, by continuing to give an antibacterial drug after it has had a proper chance to do its job. 'Tailing off' – i.e. continuing for a while with reduced doses – is even more deplorable, unless it is done for some clearly defined prophylactic purpose.

DRUG RESISTANCE

An antibacterial drug kills or inhibits a bacterium by interfering with some vital process. Any one drug is effective against only some bacterial groups and species, and usually against only some (though often nearly all) strains of any given species. The remaining bacteria owe their resistance to:

(1) impenetrability of their outer layers to the drug;

(2) lack of any important metabolic process to which the drug has any relevance–e.g. sulphonamide resistance due to possession of a dihydrofolic acid reductase which does not 'confuse' sulphonamides with PABA (see p 40);

(3) ability to destroy the drug or convert it into an inactive form–e.g. penicillinases (β-lactamases), which open up the β-lactam rings of penicillins and to variable extents also of cephalosporins; or the acetyltransferases by means of which some bacteria can acetylate chloramphenicol. Since the bacteria that produce such enzymes are as a rule intrinsically sensitive to the drug, their resistance may not be manifested when small numbers of them are exposed to an adequate concentration of the drug without being given time to produce enzyme; this is particularly the case when the enzyme is inducible rather than constitutive (see pp 33–4).

Even when an antibacterial drug is first introduced, the existence of naturally resistant bacterial species and strains places limits on its usefulness. However, there can have been few pathogenic bacteria in circulation 30 years ago which could have survived the onslaught of our present-day armoury of drugs if these had all become available at once. Many of our modern therapeutic problems are due to the fact that in most cases the introduction of a new drug has been followed by proliferation of bacterial strains resistant to it. *Staph. aureus* has been notably successful in keeping pace with new discoveries. In relation to penicillin it is thought that evolution of new strains has played a relatively small part, the increase in frequency of penicillin-resistant *Staph. aureus* and other species being largely due to a 'take-over' by existing resistant strains as their more sensitive colleagues were eliminated. But with most other drugs sensitive strains give rise to rare resistant mutants; these normally have no particular survival value, but in the presence of an appropriate concentration of the drug in question they alone are able to multiply, giving rise to a new strain with increased drug resistance (see p 33). In most cases each mutation involves only a small increase in resistance, and therefore such selection depends upon the drug concentration being not much above the minimum to which the original strain is sensitive; but with streptomycin in particular a marked increase in resistance may develop by a single mutational jump rather than by a series of short steps.

Prevention of the emergence of resistant strains is one of the main indications for the clinical use of combinations of drugs (see p 329). As a result of spontaneous mutation, one cell in every thousand million (10^9) might be resistant to drug A and one in 10^{12} might be resistant to drug B. 10^9 and 10^{12} are not very large populations by bacteriological standards. But provided that the mechanisms of action of the two drugs are unrelated, the incidence of cells resistant to both should be one in $10^9 \times 10^{12}$, which is a very large population. Therefore if both drugs are given in adequate dosage, the risk of the emergence of a resistant strain is very much less than if either is used alone.

Resistance to one or more antibiotics can be transmitted from one bacterial strain to a related but previously sensitive strain by bacteriophage transduction (see p 33). It is not clear yet whether this mechanism is an important source of therapeutic difficulties. But since 1965 it has been clear that *transferable* or *infective resistance* presents a serious threat to antibiotic control of infectious diseases. The mechanism of such resistance-transfer is described on p 34. It is important for the following reasons:

(1) The transferable plasmids commonly determine resistance to several unrelated drugs, and organisms possessing them have a selective advantage in the presence of any one of these drugs. Thus for example the reduction in numbers of streptomycin-sensitive organisms in the intestines of a streptomycin-treated patient or animal may favour the growth of an enterobacterial strain resistant to streptomycin and also (incidentally) to tetracyclines, chloramphenicol and sulphonamides, substances which the patient or animal has never received.

(2) Such plasmids are transferable not merely to related strains of the same species but to strains of other species and genera. Thus a patient under treatment with streptomycin for tuberculosis or a urinary tract infection might have a large population of multiple-resistant but harmless *Esch. coli* in his intestine as a result of the mechanism described in the last paragraph; he might then ingest some shigellae or salmonellae to which the plasmids determining the multiple resistance could be transferred in his intestine; and these pathogens might then be unresponsive to treatment with any of the drugs concerned. Strains of *Sh. flexneri* resistant to chloramphenicol and various other antibiotics were current in Mexico before 1972, but in that year *S. typhi* strains with the same resistance pattern appeared there and were isolated in Britain and other countries from patients who had acquired them in Mexico. These *S. typhi* strains were resistant by virtue of plasmids which they had presumably acquired from the *Sh. flexneri* strains.

(3) It is possible for multiple-resistant enterobacteria to develop in farm animals and be transmitted to man. Some antibiotics are widely used as food supplements for young animals, since partial suppression of intestinal flora can accelerate their weight gain. Antibiotic treatment of sick farm animals is also widespread, and often economically important, but it is uncoordinated. Resistant organisms that have

proliferated as a result of such antibiotic usage have excellent opportunities for dissemination because of the prevailing conditions for maintenance and marketing of stock and because of the transfer of young animals from farm to farm. The dangers of such a situation were clearly illustrated when Anderson and his colleagues reported a disturbing increase in frequency of isolation of *S. typhimurium* from calves in Britain in 1964–66. Nearly all of the strains isolated during this period, from many parts of the country, showed multiple resistance and belonged to a single phage-type (29); and during the same period many similar strains of the same phage-type were isolated from sick humans, many of whom worked on farms. A few of these patients died–an outcome to which the drug resistance of their salmonellae may have contributed.

(4) There is no reason to suppose that what happens among farm animals following widespread use of antibiotics does not also happen, in some measure at least, in human populations similarly treated. For some years development of resistance by man's bacterial flora was mainly a problem of hospitals, where antibacterial drugs are most heavily used and where they can be detected in the dust and even in the air! However, it now seems that widespread use of antibacterials in general practice encourages the spread through the community of multiple-resistant strains brought home by patients returning from hospital, and may even be responsible for the appearance of others that are 'home-grown'.

Although the progressive sophistication of man's bacterial flora, including his pathogens, appears to be an inevitable consequence of the use of antibacterial drugs, we cannot afford to have a complacent or defeatist attitude to this growing problem of drug resistance. There are ways in which we can slow down or arrest its growth. As we have indicated repeatedly, antibacterial drugs should not be prescribed–to men or to animals–without valid indications for doing so. We have also indicated other precautions that should be observed so as to minimize the proliferation of resistant strains–such as isolating patients who are distributing these strains into their environments; always giving antibacterial drugs in adequate doses; and using drug combinations when appropriate. Another approach to the problem that has had some successes is to introduce an *antibiotic policy* for a hospital or area. This usually involves designating certain antibiotics as available for general use but withdrawing others from circulation or permitting their use only on rare and special occasions. If all goes well (and in particular, if all relevant clinicians abide by the policy), the incidence of strains resistant to the reserved antibiotics falls considerably in the months following institution of the policy, and in due course it may be judged right to reintroduce these drugs for general use and to withdraw others.

LABORATORY PROCEDURES
Sensitivity tests

We said on p 326 that the right use of antibacterial drugs requires that the problem be defined as closely as possible. Frequently an important part of that definition is to determine the antibacterial sensitivities of the pathogen. We described on p 5 one of the rapid methods for doing this which may before long be in routine use, but at present most routine diagnostic laboratories use some form of disk-plate method. In essence, this involves inoculating the whole surface of a plate of suitable culture medium with the organism under test, and then placing at appropriate intervals on the surface of the plate a number of filter-paper disks impregnated with different antibacterials. The plate is then incubated, usually overnight. The antibacterials diffuse out of their disks into the medium, and bacterial growth is inhibited in a circular zone around any disk that contains a drug to which the organism is sensitive. 'Sensitive' is of course not an absolute term. The object of this type of test is to distinguish between strains susceptible to drug concentrations that are attainable in patients (and therefore designated *sensitive*) and significantly less susceptible strains (designated *resistant*) – with the option, thought by some authorities to be a useful one, of dividing the latter into those which might be treatable by achieving unusually high concentrations (designated *moderately resistant*) and those whose resistance cannot be qualified in that way. For each drug the disk content should be such that a sensitive strain (as just defined) will give an inhibition zone large enough for any significant decrease to be readily detectable but not so large as to interfere with the zones around neighbouring disks. The amount that achieves this depends on the diffusibility of the drug through the culture medium and also on the levels of it that can be attained in the patient. (For most purposes this means attainable blood levels, but for tests on urinary tract pathogens it usually means the higher levels attainable in urine.) Zone sizes are at the mercy of many factors besides the amount of drug; these include the heaviness of the bacterial inoculum, the medium composition and pH, and the temperature and atmospheric conditions of incubation. Reproducibility of results depends on careful control of all of these factors. One method of standardization depends on faithful reproduction of precisely the right conditions and then the comparison of the inhibition-zone measurements with a table of the results to be expected from sensitive, moderately resistant and fully resistant strains of the species in question. The other approach is to compare the zone sizes given by the test organism with those given by a control sensitive strain tested at the same time and under the same conditions.

Like any *in vitro* method, the disk-plate method can at best only give an indication of what might happen in the very different circumstances prevailing inside the patient's body. In its basic form it does not distinguish between bactericidal and bacteriostatic action. This distinction can be made by the further procedure of transferring to fresh culture plates the bacteria that were originally inoculated on to the zones in which growth was inhibited, and so giving them a chance to show whether they are still alive. One anomaly of the disk-plate method is that resistance dependent on inducible enzyme (notably that of *Staph. aureus* to penicillin) is manifested not so much by a reduction in size of the zone of inhibition as by vigorous growth around the edge of the zone; bacteria near to the disk were overcome before they could produce enzyme, but those further out had time to defend themselves against the advancing drug, and then had the benefit of the additional nutrients diffusing from the nearby depopulated zone.

It is possible to use the disk-plate technique for *direct sensitivity determinations*—i.e. disks can be applied to plates inoculated with pus, sputum or other pathological material and inhibition can be observed in this primary culture. In such circumstances there is virtually no control of inoculum size, and difficulties of interpretation may arise if the specimen contains a mixture of bacteria; for example, it is impossible to assess the penicillin sensitivity of other strains in the presence of one which produces penicillinase. However, this method has the compensatory advantage of speed, since it may be able to provide a rough guide to appropriate therapy as soon as any visible growth is present— sometimes in as little as 6 hours from the time of the collection of the specimen, well before it would be possible to pick single colonies from the primary culture and set up a properly standardized test.

Sometimes it is desirable not just to classify an organism as sensitive or resistant but to determine more precisely the smallest drug concentration that will inhibit it—the *minimal inhibitory concentration* (*M.I.C.*). This is done by testing its ability to grow in the presence of the drug in a series of concentrations, either in tubes of broth or incorporated in solid media in plates. By appropriate subculture from such a series of tubes or plates it is possible to determine also the *minimal bactericidal concentration* (*M.B.C.*). Since M.I.C. and M.B.C. values are expressed in numbers (e.g. 0.5 μg/ml or mg/l) they appear more accurate than they are; with some organisms and some antibiotics in particular, they are markedly dependent on inoculum size and the precise techniques used.

Assays of Drug Levels in Body Fluids

Chemical methods are available for the assay of some antibacterial drugs, but may give misleading results through failure to distinguish between biologically active drug and inactive derivatives. Biological methods (bio-assays) are more commonly used. A simple bio-assay method is similar in general design to the disk-plate sensitivity test method. A plate is inoculated with an appropriate standard bacterial strain sensitive to the drug to be assayed. In place of the disks of the sensitivity test method small cylindrical wells are cut in the medium; some of these are filled with various dilutions of the fluid under test, and others with fluid containing known concentrations of the drug in question. By comparison of the diameters of the zones of inhibition around the standard solutions after incubation and those around the dilutions of the fluid under test, the drug concentration in the latter can be calculated. More rapid results can be obtained by means of sensitive systems for early detection of either metabolic inhibition or enzyme production; these are used to compare the effects of dilutions of the test fluid and of standard solutions of the drug on a test organism.

Most antibacterial treatment can be carried out satisfactorily without any monitoring of the levels achieved in blood and other body fluids. This is because, by the time that an antibacterial drug is on the market, the ranges of levels to be expected following recommended dosage schedules have been reliably established. Monitoring may be required, however, when there is wide individual variation in the levels resulting from a standard dose, so that some patients need unusually high dosage in order to have levels within the therapeutic range. This is true, for example, of gentamicin and related drugs, and for them there is the additional complication of a narrow margin between dosage which is adequate and that which may give toxic levels (see pp 333 and 347). For these and many other antibacterial drugs, impaired renal function is one of the most important factors that may invalidate deductions based on results obtained in healthy volunteers, so that it is necessary to check the levels actually achieved in the patient (see p 357). Other reasons for monitoring include attempts to deal with a moderately resistant organism, for which unusually high concentrations of the drug are required; determining whether oral administration, the least reliable means of administration for most drugs but in some cases the most convenient or most acceptable, is giving adequate levels in a particular patient; and the need to discover whether a drug is penetrating in adequate amounts into some body fluid other than blood. In general, assays as part of patient management are aimed at determining either that the patient is having enough of the drug for a therapeutic effect to be likely, or that he is not having too much and therefore exposed to unnecessary hazard. They may also be undertaken, of course, for research purposes.

As an alternative to assay of a drug by use of a standard bacterial strain, it is sometimes more satisfactory to carry out a direct test of the effectiveness of the patient's serum or other body fluid against a culture of his own pathogen, isolated before he started the treatment. This approach is particularly useful when the patient is receiving more than one drug, since assay of one in the presence of others may be difficult. It is common practice in the management of bacterial endocarditis (see p 353) to expose a culture of the offending streptococcus to serial dilutions of the patient's serum in nutrient broth, and to test for cidal action by subculturing these serum dilutions after overnight incubation. Treatment may well fail unless for at least part of each day the concentration of drugs in the serum is such that a 1:8 dilution of the serum is cidal to the streptococcus (under defined test conditions).

THE DRUGS THEMSELVES
The contents of this section are subject to the following limitations:

(1) *Dosages* are not given. They are not necessary for a discussion of the principles of antibacterial therapy, and for its practice they would have to be considered in far greater detail than our present space permits.

(2) *Trade names* are also omitted. It is understandable that each manufacturer should want to promote the sales of his own product rather than those of identical or similar materials produced by other firms, but much confusion results from the consequent multiplicity of names. The marketing of antibiotic or sulphonamide-antibiotic mixtures under names which suggest that they are single new compounds is another source of bewilderment. The wisest policy is to ignore trade names and to think entirely in terms of official names.

(3) *Antibacterial ranges* of drugs are impossible to define briefly in other than general terms. Strains of the same species may differ widely in their sensitivities, and strains resistant to a particular drug are likely to become far more common in any community in which that drug is widely used, as we have already noted. In this section we have merely indicated the important groups of organisms commonly sensitive to each drug or class of drugs.

(4) The drugs described here as bactericidal are those of which it is possible to achieve in the body concentrations that are lethal to susceptible organisms. They may have only a bacteriostatic action when used in lower concentrations or against less susceptible organisms. Some of the drugs described as bacteriostatic are in fact bactericidal *in vitro* but not in concentrations that have any relevance to their therapeutic use.

The meanings of the terms *chemotherapeutic agents* and *antibiotics* are given on pp 39–40.

(a) CHEMOTHERAPEUTIC AGENTS
Sulphonamides (see also pp 39–40)
These compounds have the general formula NH_2 ⬡ SO_2NHR, the simplest of them being sulphanilamide in which $R = H$. There are about twenty such compounds which are of therapeutic value. All have much the same wide bacteriostatic range, including Gram-positive and Gram-negative cocci and bacilli, but there is some variation in their relative potency against individual species, and resistant strains are common in all groups–especially in those countries where sulphonamides have been heavily used. A strain that becomes resistant to one sulphonamide is resistant to the others, as is to be expected from their common mode of action. All can be given by mouth, and a few by injection, though these parenteral preparations are highly alkaline and usually need to be given intravenously with care to avoid leakage from the vein. Sulphonamides vary widely in their absorption and subsequent behaviour after oral administration. Of those that are rapidly absorbed, *sulphadiazine* is excreted slowly enough by the kidneys to give high blood levels, is not much protein-bound, and hence diffuses well into tissues and into cerebrospinal fluid. Others which are not rapidly excreted are protein-bound, and the consequent depot effect means that high levels can be maintained by giving only one dose a day, or even in one case one dose a week; but it is not clear that such preparations have any merits other than convenience. Those which are rapidly absorbed and rapidly excreted by the kidneys are of particular relevance to the treatment of urinary tract infections. Some are very little absorbed, and therefore useful only when given with other antibacterials for the purpose of suppressing bowel flora. *Sulphacetimide*, one of the earliest of the sulphonamides and no longer used systemically, is highly soluble and is used in eye drops and eye ointments.

Toxic reactions to sulphonamides include hypersensitivity of the serum sickness type, bone marrow depression and renal tubular obstruction. Either of the last two may be fatal. Bone marrow depression, usually manifested as agranulocytosis, is of abrupt onset and so is difficult to anticipate by repeated examinations of the blood. It has been most commonly reported following long courses of treatment. Renal tubular obstruction results from concentration of the drugs and their acetyl derivatives in the urine, with crystal formation since they are of low solubility in acid or neutral urine. This complication can be avoided by oral administration of citrates to keep the urine alkaline and of plentiful fluids to keep it dilute; and also by using a relatively soluble sulphonamide such as *sulphadimidine* or a mixture of several sulphonamides which have additive antibacterial actions but retain their individual solubilities.

Trimethoprim, Co-Trimoxazole

Sulphonamides are bacteriostatic because they block conversion of *p*-aminobenzoic acid to folic acid (see p 40). Much of their original value in therapy has been lost because of the emergence of increasing numbers of streptococcal, pneumococcal, gonococcal and meningococcal strains that are not susceptible to this action. Trimethoprim is one of a series of compounds that inhibit enzymes responsible for the next stage in the same metabolic chain–the conversion of folic acid to folinic acid. The extent of the inhibition varies with the compound and with the species involved. Trimethoprim is the most effective in blocking bacterial enzymes and has no significant effect on mammalian metabolism; it is therefore itself a potentially valuable chemotherapeutic agent, though not yet used extensively on its own. When it is used together with a sulphonamide, the two may be synergic (see p 328) against bacteria and are effective against many that are relatively resistant to sulphonamides on their own. Furthermore, such a combination is bactericidal (in some circumstances, at least), although each of its components when used alone is only bacteriostatic. *Sulphamethoxazole* is the sulphonamide currently used with trimethoprim for clinical purposes, since its absorption and excretion rates are appropriate. This mixture, which has been given the name *co-trimoxazole*, has proved to be a valuable addition to our range of antibacterial weapons. However, the 5:1 sulphonamide:trimethoprim ratio in commercially available preparations appears not to be the best for some purposes, because of different rates of penetration of the two components to various sites, and preparations with different ratios may be desirable.

(Similarly, *pyrimethamine*–a compound related to trimethoprim–is used together with a sulphonamide in treatment of the protozoal diseases malaria and toxoplasmosis, as mentioned on pp 223 and 225).

Metronidazole

This substance has been in use since 1959, in the form of oral tablets, for the treatment of trichomonas infections (see p 225). Later it was discovered also to be effective in giardiasis and in amoebiasis (see pp 226 and 230). Some years passed, however, before clinical use was made of its inhibitory action on anaerobic bacteria. Metronidazole itself is inactive against micro-organisms, but on entering the cell of an anaerobic organism–protozoal or bacterial–it is reduced to a form that inhibits nucleic acid synthesis. It seems probable that all strictly anaerobic bacteria are affected in this way, though it remains to be seen whether its widespread use will be followed by the emergence of resistant strains. It is of particular value against strains of *Bacteroides fragilis*, which are highly susceptible to it and are often resistant to most of the commonly used antibiotics. Patients who cannot take it by mouth can have it in the form of rectal suppositories or intravenously. It has rapidly acquired an important place in prophylaxis for intestinal surgery (see p 325), and in treatment of wound infections, septicaemia and other conditions for which anaerobes might be responsible. Apart from an unpleasant metallic taste it rarely produces immediate side-effects, but its otherwise great promise has been called into question by animal experiments that suggest the possibility of a carcinogenic activity. As yet the evidence that it may be harmful is not sufficient to stop the use of a drug which is undoubtedly of great benefit to many patients.

Nitrofurantoin and Nalidixic Acid

These two unrelated substances have in common that when given by mouth they are rapidly absorbed and are excreted in high concentration in the urine. They are of use only in treatment of urinary tract infections. Nitrofurantoin achieves urinary concentrations that are bactericidal to some members of most bacterial groups, especially if the urine is acid–a condition not likely to be fulfilled if the infecting organism is a *Proteus* or other urease-positive strain, converting urea into ammonia. Nalidixic acid is bacteriostatic, and effective only against Gram-negative bacteria. Its range does not include *Ps. aeruginosa*, and therefore its usefulness is restricted to enterobacterial infections of the urinary tract. Resistance to it develops readily. Thus although both of these drugs have been widely used in treatment of urinary tract infections they are not reliable for this purpose without laboratory evidence of a suitably sensitive pathogen, and in the case of nalidixic acid in particular the sensitivity may not last long.

Chemotherapeutic Agents for Treatment of Mycobacterial Infections

Information about these is to be found on pp 149 and 356–7.

(b) ANTIBIOTICS (For modes of action see p 41)

Penicillins (see also pp 40–1)

The name 'penicillin', used on its own, refers to the first-discovered member of the group, *benzyl penicillin* (penicillin G). This remains one of our most valuable antibacterial drugs. It is bactericidal to a range of bacteria that includes many streptococci, the neisseriae, most Gram-positive bacilli, some Gram-negative bacilli (especially when it is in high concentration), spirochaetes and actinomycetes. Most staphylococci were sensitive to it when it was first introduced, but penicillinase-producing and therefore resistant strains are now common, especially in hospitals. It is a remarkable drug in that it is tolerated by the body in almost unlimited quantities; such adverse reactions as do occur are due to hypersensitivity and are virtually independent of dosage (apart from the toxic encephalopathy occasionally produced by giving very large doses to patients with poor renal function, in whom exceptionally high blood levels can be achieved, or by giving a large excess intrathecally). Two of its unsatisfactory features are that it has to be given parenterally because it is acid-labile and destroyed to an unpredictable degree in the stomach, and that high blood levels are hard to maintain because it is rapidly excreted in the urine. The latter feature is occasionally beneficial, since high urinary concentrations can be achieved; more often it is merely wasteful of a relatively inexpensive compound; but sometimes, when persistent high blood levels are required, it is necessary to give *probenecid* which blocks renal tubular excretion of penicillin.

It is still an open question whether the most effective way of using penicillin is to maintain continuous high blood levels. It is possible that as good or better results can be obtained in most cases by intermittent high levels (see p 332). These can be achieved by suitably spaced intra-muscular or intravenous injections. A steady blood level can be main-tained by continuous intravenous administration, provided that incom-patibilities are avoided (see pp 329 – 30). However, it is often sufficient and more convenient to give a daily intramuscular injection of a slowly absorbed compound which will maintain an adequate blood level through-out the day, and in some cases there is a considerable advantage in being able to give a single dose which will maintain a moderate blood level for many days (see for example p 155, treatment of syphilis). *Procaine penicillin, benethamide penicillin* and *benzathine penicillin* are slowly absorbed compounds of benzyl penicillin which respectively give useful blood levels for many hours, several days and several weeks after a single injection.

By varying the substrate for growth of the moulds, the acid-resistant *phenoxymethyl penicillin* (penicillin V) can be produced. When given by mouth, salts of this compound are sufficiently well absorbed to give reliably useful blood levels.

In 1959 it was discovered that the 'nucleus' of all penicillin molecules, 6-aminopenicillanic acid, could be made by substrate varia-tion or by enzymic removal of side-chains from benzyl penicillin or other existing penicillins. By attaching various side-chains to this nucleus it has been possible to make a vast range of new semi-synthetic penicillins, some of which have special properties that make them useful therapeutic agents. These include:

(a) *phenethicillin* and *propicillin*, acid-resistant and absorbed more efficiently than phenoxymethyl penicillin, but correspondingly less potent and therefore comparable with it in effectiveness.

(b) *methicillin*, *cloxacillin* and *flucloxacillin*, penicillinase-resistant and therefore active against penicillinase-producing staphylococci. The cloxacillins are also acid-resistant and effective when given by mouth, flucloxacillin being the better absorbed of the two.

(c) *ampicillin*, which can also be given parenterally or by mouth, and its orally administered and better absorbed esters *talampicillin* and *pivampicillin*; somewhat less potent than benzyl penicillin against many Gram-positive bacteria, but markedly more effective against some of the enterobacteria (including salmonellae and shigellae) and against *H. influenzae*; liable to provoke rashes (distinct from those due to hypersensitivity to all penicillins), especially in patients with infectious mononucleosis. Ampicillin itself commonly causes intestinal disturbances, due to the action of the unabsorbed portion of the drug in the bowel lumen.

(d) *amoxycillin*, structurally related and similar in range to ampicillin; better absorbed (comparable to the esters); more effective in eradicating some infections (see p 129, treatment of typhoid, and p 355, chronic bronchitis); a better oral drug than ampicillin, and recently made available in a form suitable for parenteral use.

(e) *mecillinam* and its ester *pivmecillinam*, also structurally related to ampicillin; highly active against some enterobacteria that are ampicillin-resistant, apparently by a different mode of action; only recently made available.

(f) *carbenicillin*, the only penicillin yet available that is effective against *Ps. aeruginosa*. It is also active against *Proteus* species and some of the enterobacteria, but is relatively ineffective against Gram-positive organisms. It has to be given by injection. The doses needed for treatment of some *Ps. aeruginosa* infections are very large and can be given only by the intravenous route. An indanyl ester and a phenol ester (*carfecillin*) can be given by mouth for treatment of urinary tract infections, but do not achieve blood levels that are of any value for systemic infections.

Apart from the adverse effects mentioned under (c) above, the penicillins all share the lack of toxicity of benzyl penicillin, but also share its liability to provoke hypersensitivity reactions (see p 322). When hypersentivity occurs, it applies to all members of the group, so that none of them can be given to a patient who has become sensitive to one of them.

Cephalosporins and Cephamycins

The semi-synthetic derivatives of cephalosporin C (a product of the mould *Cephalosporium acremonium*) resemble the penicillins in general structure, including possession of a β-lactam ring (see p 334), and in their mode of action. In general their antibacterial ranges are those of the ampicillin group, with the additional advantage of being in varying degree resistant to the penicillinases of *Staph. aureus* and of some enterobacterial strains. They do not as a rule provoke hypersensitivity reactions in patients sensitized to the penicillins. *Cephaloridine*, which must be given by injection, is the most active against Gram-positive cocci, but it is potentially nephrotoxic, particularly when it is given to patients who already have low glomerular filtration rates and in whose blood it consequently accumulates, or when given with certain other drugs (see p 330). *Cephalothin* has to be given intravenously (or by painful intramuscular injection), but its renal excretion is tubular and it is rapidly metabolized by the liver, so it can be given in circumstances in which cephaloridine would be dangerous. *Cephradine* resembles ampicillin in that it can be given by mouth or parenterally, but intramuscular injection gives rather poor blood levels. It is highly resistant to staphylococcal penicillinase, but less effective than other cephalosporins or the ampicillin group against faecal streptococci and *H. influenzae*–a disadvantage for an oral drug which might otherwise be valuable in two of the commonest conditions that need oral treatment, urinary tract infection and chronic bronchitis. *Cephalexin* closely resembles cephradine but is not available for parenteral use. *Cefazolin*, which must be injected, has a promising range of activity *in vitro* and gives good blood levels, but it seems that its high degree of protein binding may limit its value. Of the most recent cephalosporins, *cefamandole* and *cefuroxime* have promisingly high levels of activity against *N. gonorrhoeae* and *H. influenzae*.

The cephamycins are closely related to the cephalosporins but derived from a different natural antibiotic, cephamycin C. They have the advantage of high levels of resistance to certain enterobacterial β-lactamases that destroy penicillins and cephalosporins. *Cefoxitin* is the first of this series to be widely available.

Fucidin

This sodium salt of fusidic acid derived from the fungus *Fusidium coccineum* is unusual among antibiotics in having a steroid molecular structure. It is well absorbed when given by mouth, is apparently free from serious toxic effects, and is highly effective against most strains of *Staph. aureus*, including penicillinase-producers. Claims have been made that it is particularly good at eradicating staphylococcal infections of bones and joints. Resistance to it develops readily among staphylococci in culture, and sometimes occurs during treatment also. In order to preserve its value, it seems best to use it against staphylococci only, and always in conjunction with another antibiotic so as to reduce the risk of developing resistance (see p 334).

Aminoglycosides

With one exception the members of this group (like nearly all of the remaining antibiotics to be considered in this chapter) are derived from *Streptomyces* species (see p 151); the exception, derived from the somewhat similar *Micromonospora purpurea*, is named 'gentamicin', not 'gentamycin', to mark this distinction. All members of the group are bactericidal to a wide range of bacteria, including many strains of *Staph. aureus* and of enterobacteria, but they do not have useful levels of activity against *Clostridium* or *Bacteroides* species or against streptococci (except when acting synergically with a penicillin–see pp 328 and 353). All are toxic to the 8th nerve unless given in carefully controlled dosage and with due regard to any impairment of renal excretion; but some affect mainly the vestibular and some mainly the auditory branch of the nerve. All may provoke hypersensitivity reactions.

Streptomycin, introduced in 1944 by Waksman and his colleagues, was the first antibiotic with useful activity against enterobacteria and for many years the only one that was of value in treatment of tuberculosis. When given by mouth it is not absorbed and so, like later members of the group, it has been used for suppression of bowel flora. It is usually given intramuscularly or intravenously (or intrathecally in treatment of tuberculous meningitis). Bacterial strains frequently become resistant to it during treatment, but are not then necessarily resistant to other aminoglycosides (whereas strains resistant to the others are usually streptomycin-resistant). For this reason, and because of greater activity against some *Proteus* and other strains and less serious toxicity, *kanamycin* has been more generally used than streptomycin as a broad-spectrum bactericidal antibiotic, especially by paediatricians; but its role has now been taken over by *gentamicin*, which has a higher level of activity against many bacteria, but in particular is one of the few antibacterial drugs that are effective against *Pseudomonas aeruginosa*. Gentamicin is thus a most useful drug for treatment of proven or suspected septicaemia due to organisms presumably originating from the alimentary or urinary tracts–after surgery or as a complication of a malignant growth, for example; but for such purposes it needs the assistance of metronidazole or some other drug capable of dealing with *Clostridium* and *Bacteroides* species, and possibly also of a penicillin to deal with streptococci. We have mentioned earlier the importance of monitoring levels of gentamicin (pp 333 and 339) and that it must not be given with cephaloridine (p 330).

(Whether other cephalosporins should be avoided is less clear.) *Tobramycin* is less active than gentamicin against many species but rather more active against many *Pseudomonas* strains, and since attainable blood levels and toxic levels are much the same as for gentamicin, full advantage can be taken of this difference. Unfortunately, however, there has been a marked increase in the frequency of *Ps. aeruginosa* strains that are resistant to gentamicin by means of enzymes that also destroy tobramycin. Such enzymes are not usually effective against *amikacin*, a derivative of kanamycin which is also effective against *Ps. aeruginosa* but of which clinical experience is still limited.

Neomycin and *framycetin* are kanamycin-like drugs too toxic for systemic use. Neomycin is sometimes given by mouth as a means of attack on intestinal pathogens, but may do more harm than good (see p 130). Either can be applied topically in the form of powder, cream, ointment, eye or ear drops, etc., though prolonged and heavy topical application can lead to absorption of toxic amounts. Gentamicin has also been extensively used in such topical forms, but this practice seems to have been responsible for the increasing frequency of gentamicin-resistant strains of *Ps. aeruginosa* and other species.

Chloramphenicol

Originally derived from *Streptomyces venezuelae* in 1947, chloramphenicol is now made synthetically. It is well absorbed when given by mouth, and passes from the blood stream into the cerebrospinal fluid more readily than any other antibiotic. It can also be given parenterally, but the intravenous route should be used, as absorption after intramuscular injection is slow and gives relatively poor blood levels. It is effective against a wide range of bacteria, and also against rickettsiae and chlamydiae. It is bactericidal to *H. influenzae*, and a most valuable drug for treatment of the life-threatening infections of children caused by type b strains of this species (see p 137). Against other genera it is bacteriostatic only. This may explain its failure to eradicate *S. typhi* infections (see p 129), even though it is highly effective – until recently the only drug that was effective – in controlling the acute illness of typhoid (except when this is due to a chloramphenicol-resistant strain). When it was introduced it seemed to have many features of the ideal antibiotic. However, after it had been used enthusiastically and on a large scale for a few years, reports began to appear of fatal bone marrow depression following its use. Since then there has been a general tendency to regard it as highly dangerous and to reserve it for the treatment of typhoid and paratyphoid (for which it now seems that amoxycillin may be equally effective and safer – see p 345) and of severe infections due to *H. influenzae* or to bacteria resistant to all of the antibiotics that are reputedly safer. On the available evidence it is impossible to be sure how dangerous chloramphenicol is, or indeed whether all batches are equally dangerous. Possibly because it has been 'in disgrace', it is sometimes a valuable drug in an emergency because most strains of staphylococci and of other troublesome bacteria are still sensitive to it. Caution is necessary when giving it to new-born infants, since they inactivate and excrete it very slowly and therefore high dosage may lead to excessive blood levels, collapse and death ('the grey syndrome'). It is of little value in urinary tract infection because the kidneys excrete it mainly in a form that is not active against bacteria.

Tetracyclines

Chlortetracycline (first isolated in 1948), *oxytetracycline* and *tetracycline* can all be derived from *Streptomyces* species, or tetracycline can be derived chemically from chlortetracycline. They are closely similar in their properties. Like chloramphenicol, they are effective when given by mouth, though absorption is inefficient and somewhat irregular. They are purely bacteriostatic. They have much the same antimicrobial range as chloramphenicol, including the rickettsiae and chlamydiae. Bacterial resistance develops rather readily, and has become increasingly common even in species such as *Str. pyogenes* and *Str. pneumoniae* which do not readily become resistant to drugs of most other groups. Administration of a tetracycline may cause nausea and vomiting, and diarrhoea is a common complication, probably as a result of derangement of the normal bowel flora by the unabsorbed part of the drug. In the extreme form this derangement may lead to intestinal moniliasis, or rarely to staphylococcal enteritis (see p 95). Tetracycline is claimed to cause less alimentary disturbance than the other two. Permanent yellow staining of teeth may follow administration of tetracyclines to children during the early years of life or to their mothers during the later months of pregnancy. Other reasons for avoiding these drugs during pregnancy are reports of severe liver damage in pregnant women following high dosage and unconfirmed allegations of teratogenic effects on foetuses.

In attempts to avoid alimentary side-effects a number of new tetracyclines have been developed which are better absorbed from the intestine or for one reason or another are effective when given in smaller doses than those necessary with the established members of the group. *Demethylchlortetracycline* (DMCT) is comparatively well absorbed and rather slowly excreted. Excretion of *doxycycline* is so slow that a daily dose is sufficient, as against 6-hourly doses for the older tetracyclines. *Minocycline* is very well absorbed and slowly excreted, so that it too can be given as a daily dose, and it has the additional valuable and interesting property of being effective against many staphylococcal and other strains that are resistant to other tetracyclines; but unfortunately it makes many patients giddy.

Macrolides

Erythromycin, isolated from *Streptomyces erythreus*, has an antibacterial range similar to that of benzyl penicillin. In high concentrations *in vitro* it is bactericidal to susceptible organisms, but this probably has only limited relevance to its action in the body. Taken by mouth in the form of the base it is rather poorly absorbed from the intestine but has negligible toxicity, whereas *erythromycin estolate*, the lauryl sulphate of the propinyl ester, is efficiently absorbed but sometimes causes cholestatic jaundice. Intramuscular injection is painful, and intravenous administration, though possible, is seldom convenient. Staphylococci in particular readily become resistant to erythromycin but this can be discouraged by giving another antibiotic at the same time (see p 334).

Oleandomycin, *spiramycin* and other antibiotics of this group are similar to erythromycin in their range of activity but less potent, and therefore of little value.

Clindamycin

This is a synthetic derivative of another streptomyces antibiotic, *lincomycin*. It closely resembles the macrolide antibiotics in most of its properties, in spite of having a markedly different molecular structure. It is well absorbed when taken orally, and penetrates into bone better than most antibiotics; it is therefore a useful weapon for dealing with osteomyelitis. It is an effective alternative to penicillin for use against *Str. pyogenes*, and is also valuable for dealing with *Bacteroides* infections. Being better absorbed from the alimentary tract than lincomycin, it does not cause the immediate gastro-intestinal upsets commonly associated with use of that drug. Pseudomembranous colitis, a severe and sometimes fatal condition that occasionally follows antibiotic treatment and is perhaps more often induced by one of these two drugs than by any other, is due to proliferation of a toxin-producing clostridium in the patient's intestine.

Vancomycin

This is another streptomyces antibiotic. Despite its toxicity and the necessity of giving it intravenously, it occasionally has a place in the treatment of a severe staphylococcal or streptococcal infection for which less toxic drugs are contraindicated by resistance of the organism or hypersensitivity of the patient.

Rifamycins

Although the members of this group of antibiotics derived from

Streptomyces mediterranei have promising antibacterial activities *in vitro*, their clinical usefulness is impaired by their rapid excretion in the bile and the consequent impossibility of maintaining adequate blood levels. *Rifampicin*, a synthetic derivative of one of them, is less rapidly excreted, is well absorbed when given by mouth, and is bactericidal to staphylococci and non-faecal streptococci (at remarkably low concentrations), to *Myco. tuberculosis* and to many other bacteria. However, its most serious limitation is the speed with which resistant mutants emerge, and because of this it should probably never be used alone. Its considerable value as an anti-tuberculous agent is likely to be best preserved by using it only in exceptional circumstances for non-tuberculous infections (e.g. in treatment of endocarditis due to a staphylococcus resistant to most other drugs). It has been used for treatment of meningococcal carriers, and this has resulted in the emergence of resistant meningococci, but if any of the carriers had undiagnosed tuberculosis it could at the same time have selected out resistant tubercle bacilli. When given in low dosage it is mostly excreted in the bile, but higher dosage saturates this excretory mechanism and it then appears in useful concentrations in the urine, which it colours red (as it may also do to the tears).

Spectinomycin
This, the last streptomyces antibiotic that we shall describe, has a wide antibacterial range but its value as a therapeutic agent has not been fully assessed. Currently its one clinical use is as a 'single shot' intramuscular injection for gonorrhoea (see pp 109 and 333).

Polymyxins
These are polypeptides derived from bacteria of the genus *Bacillus* and first reported in 1947. *Colistin*, discovered in 1950 and at first thought to be a new antibiotic, is identical with polymyxin E. All are nephrotoxic but the toxicity of polymyxins B and E is not sufficient to preclude their systemic use when necessary. For this purpose they are administered intramuscularly (and intrathecally for treatment of meningitis). They are also used in the form of powders and ointments for the treatment of wounds and burns, and given by mouth for treatment of alimentary infections. They are not absorbed from the intestine. They are administered either as sulphates or as sulphomethyl derivatives (methane sulphonates), and the latter are preferred by some for parenteral use because they give less pain when injected and are less toxic. However, they are also less potent and more rapidly excreted by the kidneys–an advantage, perhaps, when treating urinary tract infections but not when sustained blood levels are needed. The polymyxins are bactericidal and are effective against *Ps. aeruginosa* and against Gram-negative bacilli of

most other genera except *Proteus*, but unfortunately their efficacy against *Ps. aeruginosa* is markedly reduced in the presence of calcium ions in concentrations found in blood and other body fluids.

Bacitracin
This is another polypeptide antibiotic. It has a bactericidal range similar to that of benzyl penicillin. Nephrotoxicity makes it unsuitable for systemic use, but it is commonly used in powders or ointments for topical application.

SOME SPECIAL PROBLEMS
Staphylococcus aureus Infections
This most adaptable species has continued to be a special problem throughout the antibiotic era. Apart from the strains mentioned in the next paragraph, *Staph. aureus* strains are all *intrinsically* penicillin sensitive, but many protect themselves against the action of most penicillins by producing penicillinases. For those which do not do so benzyl penicillin is still the most effective antibiotic. For dealing with penicillinase-producers (usually reported as 'penicillin resistant'), or with strains that are inaccessible for testing (e.g. because they are in deeply placed lesions) or that require urgent treatment before results of tests are available, the cloxacillins (penicillinase-resistant penicillins – see p 345) are currently the first choice – with the cephalosporins as perhaps the best alternatives when there is a possibility that the patient is hypersensitive to penicillins. Other antibiotics that can be used against *Staph. aureus* (in combination with one another or with some other effective drugs, to prevent rapid emergence of resistant variants) are erythromycin, fucidin, clindamycin and the aminoglycosides, with the more toxic vancomycin in reserve for special problems.

There are some *Staph. aureus* strains, once very rare but encountered with increasing frequency in hospitals as penicillin consumption has increased, which show genuine penicillin resistance – as distinct from the ability to destroy penicillins. Their resistance includes all penicillins, and usually the cephalosporins as well. It depends on unusual cell-wall composition, and is as a rule shown by only a very small proportion of any given population of such a *Staph. aureus* strain when incubated at 37°C, but this proportion is greatly increased at lower incubation temperatures (e.g. 30°C). Perhaps because of this, such strains (in our experience at least) occur mainly in surface wounds and ulcers and seldom cause serious systemic disease. There are reports that when they do cause major infections they respond poorly to treatment with any of the penicillins.

Subacute Bacterial Endocarditis

The paradox of antibacterial treatment for this condition, and the need for it to be bactericidal, have been discussed on p 328. It seems probable that in order to attain bactericidal drug levels inside the vegetations it is best to have persistent high blood levels. High penicillin dosage, accompanied if necessary by use of probenicid to block renal excretion of the penicillin, is usually effective against highly or even moderately penicillin-sensitive organisms, such as the viridans streptococci that are the commonest cause of this disease. However, there is evidence that even these are eliminated more rapidly and more surely if in addition to the penicillin the patient receives an aminoglycoside (even in quite low dosage, which minimizes the risk of toxicity). When the causative organism is an enterococcus (see p 105) or other streptococcus which on routine bacteriostatic sensitivity testing is resistant both to penicillin and to the aminoglycosides, bactericidal penicillin-aminoglycoside synergy can often still be demonstrated in the laboratory. In such circumstances combined use of such drugs in high dosage is likely to be successful. For other organisms, however, it is necessary to test various antibiotic combinations for *in vitro* synergy in an attempt to find a form of treatment that might succeed.

A special form of heart-valve infection is that which follows open-heart surgery and installation of a prosthetic heart valve. The organisms are commonly 'non-pathogenic' bacteria, such as coagulase-negative staphylococci, but *Candida* species or other fungi are sometimes involved. Even when backed by laboratory tests to find synergic antibiotic combinations, treatment seldom eradicates the infection and the valve usually has to be replaced. (A closely similar problem often arises with Spitz-Holter valves and other prostheses used in treatment of hydrocephalus.)

Meningitis

This disease illustrates clearly the point, made on p 331 and elsewhere, that a drug with *in vitro* activity against a pathogen cannot be useful in treatment unless it can reach the appropriate site. Presumably in meningitis one such site is in the meninges themselves, but drug levels in the cerebrospinal fluid are much easier to determine and are also important–probably because of the massive bacterial 'reinforcements' that can accumulate there. Some information about drug penetration into the cerebrospinal fluid is given on pp 331–2.

The common causes of bacterial meningitis–the meningococcus, *H. influenzae* type b and the pneumococcus–can often be detected and firmly identified very soon after the cerebrospinal fluid specimen reaches the laboratory (see p 254). Such rapid identification of the pathogen simplifies the choice of treatment. For meningococcal meningitis the first choice was for many years a sulphonamide that penetrates rapidly into cerebrospinal fluid, usually sulphadiazine; but in many parts of the world the frequency of sulphonamide-resistant meningococcal strains now makes such treatment unreliable, and penicillin has to be given as well (or instead). Penicillin itself, which is also the first choice for pneumococcal meningitis, can be made to achieve adequate cerebrospinal levels via inflamed meninges by ensuring a high blood level, and there is probably nothing to be gained by giving it also intrathecally–apart from the small gain in time that is made by giving it by that route at the time of the diagnostic lumbar puncture if turbid fluid is withdrawn. Unfortunately penicillin is never a suitable antibiotic for treatment of haemophilus meningitis, and ampicillin–which was for some years regarded by some authorities as a suitable first choice for dealing with any of these 3 organisms–is ineffective against the increasingly common penicillinase-producing strains of *H. influenzae*. Chloramphenicol is, for this and other reasons, the best drug for treating haemophilus meningitis, but hae-mophilus strains resistant to it are not unknown and may increase in frequency. To treat a case of acute meningitis with a drug that might not be effective against the pathogen is to take a serious risk, as the infection can rapidly cause irreversible damage. Therefore if there is doubt as to the pathogenic species, or as to the reliability of the sensitivity of local strains of that species to a particular drug, a combination of drugs is indicated. The example of penicillin-tetracycline antagonism quoted on p 328 is a warning about the risks of such a bactericidal + bacteriostatic mixture, but there has as yet been no evidence of significant penicillin-chloramphenicol or ampicillin-chloramphenicol antagonism in connection with meningitis, or that sulphadiazine should not be given with any of these. However, the drug combination to be used on any occasion has to be chosen in the light of local circumstances and experience–there is at present no simple and generally applicable answer to the problem. Neonatal meningitis is likely to be enterobacterial, and gentamicin is usually a good choice of drug, though in view of its very poor penetration from blood into cerebrospinal fluid there is a case for giving it intrathecally as well as intramuscularly or intravenously. Treatment of tuberculous meningitis is mentioned below.

Chronic Bronchitis

A large proportion of Britain's drug bill is spent on antibiotics for patients with chronic bronchitis. This disease is not caused by bacteria, but bronchi affected by it lose their ability to keep themselves sterile, and are liable to recurrent or persistent bacterial infection. The commonest offending bacteria are *H. influenzae* and pneumococci. Some patients

harbour these in their bronchi without any significant trouble. Others
have episodes of increased respiratory difficulty and purulent sputum,
with these organisms in profusion in the sputum. Such exacerbations are
often precipitated by colds or other virus infections, and indeed can in
many cases be aborted by a few days of treatment, from the onset of such a
virus infection, with one of the drugs to be mentioned below. This is in
fact probably prophylaxis on some occasions and early treatment on
others. Some patients get over their exacerbations quite rapidly with the
help of bacteriostatic treatment with a tetracycline or co-trimoxazole. In
others the trouble is more persistent, but it may be possible to give them
quite long remissions by means of bactericidal treatment to eradicate the
pathogens from their bronchi. High doses of ampicillin sometimes
achieve this, but penetration of this drug into the sputum falls off sharply
as the bronchial suppuration subsides (see p 332), and it may find itself
shut out from the scene of action before it has completed the job.
Amoxycillin gives good sputum levels much less affected by the state of
the bronchi, and it is therefore preferable to ampicillin for this purpose.
Many advanced bronchitics have such poor bronchial defences that they
have trouble with bacterial infections throughout each winter, or even
throughout the year. For these it may be impossible to achieve true
remissions, but they may be helped by long-term bacteriostatic treatment
which reduces the severity of their bronchial infections.

Urinary Tract Infections

Acute urinary tract infection is another condition that is responsible,
in all parts of the world, for a vast consumption of antibacterials—
sulphonamides (alone or with trimethoprim), ampicillin, amoxycillin,
cephalosporins, tetracyclines, nitrofurantoin, nalidixic acid and others.
These drugs are used because they are excreted in high concentrations
in the urine, and it is these urinary levels, rather than those in
the blood, that are generally used as the basis for laboratory sensitivity
tests—some organisms therefore being reported as sensitive which
would be resistant to the levels attainable in the blood. This is reasonable
if the object of treatment is to deal with organisms that are in the urine
itself, which appears to be all that is necessary for the majority of acute
urinary tract infections. However, for treatment of more chronic
infections involving the renal parenchyma blood levels are probably more
relevant.

Most isolated episodes of acute urinary tract infections in otherwise
healthy people are due to strains of *Esch. coli* or other bacteria that are
sensitive to most or all of the commonly used drugs. Furthermore such
episodes are likely to resolve spontaneously within a few days, and the
main function of antibacterial treatment is merely to shorten the period of

discomfort. In such circumstances it is sufficient to choose a drug which is cheap, relatively harmless and known to be effective against the great majority of prevailing strains, though it is a good idea to send to the laboratory a pre-treatment urine specimen in case all does not go well and a follow-up specimen to ensure that the infection has been eradicated. Relapses, recurrent infections and infections acquired in hospital following catheterization or operation are likely to be due to more sophisticated strains, which need to have their sensitivities determined as a basis for treatment. (Recurrent infections also require thorough investigation of possible anatomical or pathological causes.) Patients with indwelling catheters because of neurological or other long-standing problems are liable to repeated bouts of infection due to organisms which, as a result of antibacterial treatment, are progressively more resistant to the drugs used; they commonly reach a stage of intractable infection with highly resistant klebsiellae or pseudomonads.

Tuberculosis

Antibacterial treatment of tuberculosis has three unusual features: the need for combinations of drugs at all times, to avoid the emergence of resistance; the need for prolonged treatment, related to the very slow metabolism and multiplication rate of the tubercle bacillus; and the nature of the drugs used. *Streptomycin* (see p 347) and the oral chemotherapeutic drugs *isoniazid* and *p-aminosalicyclic acid* (PAS) were the first and for many years the only 3 drugs available for this purpose. All 3 were commonly given together to a newly-diagnosed patient, in 'standard triple therapy'. This meant that even if the patient's organism was resistant to one of them (a point which may take 2 months or more to establish in the laboratory), he was still receiving 2 effective drugs. Such treatment has to be continued for 18 months or more, though one drug can be dropped when tests have shown the patient's organism to be sensitive to the other two. Streptomycin has the disadvantage of having to be injected. Isoniazid is cheap, orally administered and highly effective, and remains a valuable drug. PAS, itself relatively ineffective against the tubercle bacillus, has been used merely to discourage development of resistance to the others, and is unpleasant to take because it causes gastrointestinal disturbances; it has now been superseded, except where low cost is an important consideration. The oral antibiotic *rifampicin* (see p 340) is an excellent antituberculous drug in all respects except its high cost, which limits its availability in many of the countries that still have high incidences of tuberculosis. Rifampicin and isoniazid together have a synergic bactericidal action on the tubercle bacillus, and this fact has been the basis for some encouraging trials of relatively short courses of treatment–6 months or less–using these 2 drugs, initially accompanied by either streptomycin or the oral chemotherapeutic agent *ethambutol*. The 4 drugs mentioned in the last sentence are our principal anti-tuberculous agents at present, used in combinations and regimens that have to be adapted to the economic circumstances of the country and the particular needs of the patient. As an example of the latter, weekly or twice weekly supervised administration of high doses may be more effective for some types of patient than daily (and erratically) self-administered standard doses. Reserve drugs, available for patients whose bacilli are resistant to two or more of the 4 in general use or who have other special problems, include *ethionamide*, *pyrazinamide*, *cycloserine* and *thiacetazone*.

Patients with Impaired Renal Function

If a patient who needs antimicrobial therapy also has impaired renal function, additional factors must be borne in mind when selecting appropriate drugs and dosage schedules. The renal excretion rate is a major factor in determining the blood and tissue levels of many antimicrobial drugs. The aminoglycosides and the polymyxins are examples of drugs which are normally excreted mainly by the kidneys and which have serious toxic effects at blood levels not far above those required for therapy; impairment of their renal excretion calls for carefully calculated dose-reduction and close attention to the levels actually achieved. On the other hand, the penicillins and clindamycin are also mainly excreted by the kidneys, but their lack of toxicity at much higher levels than those usually required means that they can safely be given to patients with impaired renal function, though it is usually wise to keep down to modest dosage. Drugs that are themselves potentially nephrotoxic clearly need special care—e.g. cephaloridine, see p 346. Blood levels of chloramphenicol, as determined by bio-assay, are little affected by renal failure, as the main mechanism of removal of this drug from the blood is conjugation by the liver to an inactive form. Therefore if the drug is to be used in the presence of renal failure it should be given in normal dosage, but it is best to avoid it if possible, as in the absence of renal excretion the conjugates accumulate in the blood and they are not free from suspicion of toxicity. The tetracyclines too should be avoided in such circumstances, as they are liable to precipitate severe and sometimes fatal uraemia—by direct action on the kidneys and also by an anti-anabolic effect which increases the amount of urea needing to be cleared from the blood. Fucidin and the rifamycins are among the few antimicrobial drugs that are excreted almost entirely by non-renal mechanisms.

Suggestions for Further Reading

Antibiotic and Chemotherapy by L. P. Garrod, H. P. Lambert and F. O'Grady, 4th edn. (Churchill Livingstone, Edinburgh and London, 1973).

Antibiotics in Clinical Practice by Hillas Smith, 3rd edn. (Pitman Medical, Tunbridge Wells, 1977).

A Clinician's Guide to Antibiotic Therapy by Paul Noone (Blackwell, Oxford, 1977)–a short book of tabulated advice in a format that allows little room for reasons and none for distinction between the author's preference and generally accepted practice.

TABLE VIII

Summary of Factors Determining the Clinical Value of some Antimicrobial Drugs

Usefulness in treatment of

	Staph. aureus	Str. pyogenes	Str. pneumoniae	Neisseriae	Clostridia	Enterobacteria	Ps. aeruginosa	H. influenzae	Bact. fragilis	Rickettsiae and Chlamydiae	Bactericidal in vivo	Systemic effect when given by mouth	Toxicity
Sulphonamides*	o	v	v	.	v	v	.	.	.	v	No	Yes	+
Metronidazole	.	.	.	.	X	.	.	.	X	.	No	Yes	−
Penicillins (other than those below)	v	X	X	X	.	.	.	.	.	.	Yes	SM	−
Cloxacillins	X	x	.	.	.	.	.	.	.	.	Yes	Yes	−
Ampicillin	v	x	X	X	.	v	.	X	.	.	Yes	Yes	−
Amoxycillin	v	x	X	X	.	v	.	X	.	.	Yes	Yes	−
Carbenicillin	.	.	.	.	.	v	v	x	.	.	Yes	No	−
Cephalosporins	X	X	o	.	.	v	o	.	.	.	Yes	SM	−
Fucidin	o	.	.	.	.	.	.	.	.	.	Yes	Yes	−
Gentamicin	X	.	.	.	v	v	.	.	.	.	Yes	No	+ +
Tobramicin	.	.	.	.	.	v	.	.	.	.	Yes	No	+ +
Amikacin	.	.	.	.	v	o	.	.	.	.	Yes	No	+ +
Chloramphenicol	x	.	.	.	.	v	.	X	x	X	No	Yes	+ +
Tetracyclines	v	v	o	.	.	v	.	X	x	X	No	Yes	+
Erythromycin	v	X	.	.	.	.	.	.	.	.	(Yes)	Yes	−
Clindamycin	v	X	.	.	.	.	.	.	X	.	No	Yes	+
Vancomycin	o	.	.	.	.	.	.	.	.	.	Yes	No	+ +
Polymyxins	.	.	.	.	v	o	.	.	.	.	Yes	No	+ +

Usefulness: (Many of these entries greatly oversimplify complicated situations.)

X = most or all strains sensitive, commonly useful.
x = most or all strains sensitive, but unlikely to be be chosen primarily for treating these organisms.
v = usefulness limited by variations in sensitivity.
o = occasionally useful.
. = ineffective *or* more suitable drugs available.

Systemic effect: SM = some members of the group can be given by mouth for this purpose.

Toxicity:
− = seldom serious (excluding hypersensitivity reactions).
+ = sometimes serious.
+ + = sufficiently common or serious to require special caution.

* Sulphonamides are often more effective when given with trimethoprim (see p 342).

APPENDICES

A
Glossary of Technical Terms

For the reader's convenience definitions of some terms in common use in medical microbiology are brought together here. Definitions, or at least indications of the meanings, of many of them are also given in the main text on the pages cited. The meanings of many other terms not quoted here can be found by reference to the Index.

Acid-fast (acid-alcohol-fast): Resistant to decolorization by acid (or by acid and by alcohol) after staining with hot carbol fuchsin, and so retaining a red colour when stained by the Ziehl–Neelsen method–*page* 145.

Active (immunity, immunization): Dependent upon stimulation of the subject's own immunological mechanisms–*page* 56. (Cf. *passive*.)

Adjuvant: A substance which, by delaying absorption of an antigen or by other means, enhances its antigenic efficiency–*page* 65.

Aerobe: An organism which can live and multiply in the presence of atmospheric oxygen–*page* 27.

Agglutination: Clumping together, e.g. of red blood cells or micro-organisms, on exposure to an appropriate antiserum–*page* 69.

Anaerobe: An organism which can live and multiply in the absence (*facultative* anaerobe) or *only* in the absence (*strict* anaerobe) of free oxygen–*page* 27.

Anamnestic reaction: A rise of an existing antibody level in response to an irrelevant stimulus, such as an infection with an organism unrelated to that against which the antibody was originally formed–*page* 259.

Antagonism (between antimicrobial drugs): Impairment of the efficacy of one or of each drug in the presence of the other–*page* 328. (Cf. *synergy*.)

Antibiotic: A product of micro-organisms which, even when much diluted, is lethal or inhibitory to other micro-organisms–*page* 40.

Antibody: A globulin which is formed by the human or animal body in response to contact with some foreign substance and which reacts in special ways with that substance—*page* 60.

Antigen: A substance which provokes formation of antibodies—*page* 59.

Antiseptic: Roughly synonymous with *disinfectant* (q.v.)—*page* 285.

Antiserum: A serum containing antibodies for a given organism or toxin—*page* 307.

Antitoxin: An antibody for a given toxin—*page* 307.

Asepsis: Avoidance of infection—*page* 10.

Attack rate: The proportion of a population at risk which develops clinical illness as a result of a given infection.

Attenuated (organism): Reduced in virulence for a given host (but often retaining useful antigenicity for that host)—*page* 51.

Bacillus: A 'little stick', a rod-shaped bacterium—*page* 18.

Bacteraemia: Presence of bacteria in the blood-stream with or without resulting illness—*page* 55. (Cf. *septicaemia.*)

Bactericidal: Lethal to bacteria—*page* 38.

Bacteriostatic (bacteristatic): Preventing multiplication of bacteria—*page* 38.

Bacteriuria (bacilluria): Presence of bacteria (bacilli) in freshly voided non-purulent urine—*page* 250.

Brownian movement: Passive to-an-fro movement of small particles such as bacteria when suspended in a fluid medium, due to irregular bombardment by molecules of the fluid or its solutes—*page* 20.

Candling: Inspection of an unbroken egg by holding it in front of a bright light-source and using the transmitted light to determine whether the embryo is alive—*page* 173.

Capsid: The protein coat surrounding the genome (q.v.) of a virus—*page* 19.

Capsomere: One of the units of which a virus capsid is composed—*page* 170.

Capsule: A coating, commonly of polysaccharide, outside the cell walls of some bacteria and fungi—*page* 86.

Carrier: One who is harbouring but not currently suffering any ill-effects from a pathogenic organism—*page* 46.

Cell line: An *in vitro* culture of mammalian cells of known origin, suitable for propagation of viruses—*page* 173. (The word 'mammalian' in this definition is of course appropriate only in connection with the study of viruses that are parasites of mammals.)

Chemotherapeutic agent: A synthetic chemical suitable for systemic administration and effective in the treatment of microbial infections—*pages* 39 and 341–3.

Clone: A 'race' of cells derived from a single ancestral cell and sharing a single function, e.g. of producing a particular antibody—*page* 62.

Coccus: A spherical or ovoid bacterium—*page* 18.

Coliform bacillus: Not, as the name ought to mean, one that is shaped like a colon but one that resembles *Esch. coli.*—*page* 122. Authorities differ, however, on the closeness of the resemblance which is required for use of this term.

Colony: A visible pile or mass of micro-organisms on the surface of a solid culture medium, resulting in most cases from the multiplication of a single organism or a very small number—*page* 88.

Commensal: Deriving nourishment from a host without being either beneficial or harmful to him—*page* 23. (Cf. *pathogenic, symbiotic.*)

Complement: A heat-labile system with many components, present in the serum of man and of animals and necessary for the completion of some processes that result from antigen-antibody interactions—*page* 65.

Conjugation (bacterial): Exchange of genetic material between bacteria, a primitive form of sexual reproduction—*page* 34.

Constitutive (enzyme): Produced under nearly all circumstances, not dependent upon the presence of appropriate substrate—*page* 27. (Cf. *inducible.*)

Cytopathic effect: Degenerative changes occurring in tissue-culture cells as a result of virus infection, the nature of the changes sometimes indicating the identity of the virus—*page* 174.

Disinfectant: A substance, not an antibiotic, which has useful anti-microbial activity but is too toxic for systemic administration—*page* 38.

Elementary bodies: Single virus particles of some of the larger viruses, visible by ordinary light microscopy after appropriate staining—*page* 169.

Endemic (disease): Persistently present in a given community—*page* 46.

Endogenous (infection or disease): Originated by organisms or factors already present in the patient's body before onset of the condition—*page* 51. (Cf. *exogenous.*)

Endotoxin: A toxic component of a micro-organism, largely dependent for its release on the death and disruption of the organism. In particular, complex material derived from the cell walls of Gram-negative bacteria—*page* 29. (Cf. *exotoxin.*)

Enrichment medium: A medium used to encourage preliminary growth of an organism so as to enhance the chances of growing it on subsequent plate cultures—*page* 128. (Cf. *selective medium.*)

Epidemic (noun or adjective): A disease that temporarily has a high frequency in a given community—*page* 46.

Exogenous (infection or disease): Originated by organisms or factors from outside the patient's body. (Cf. *endogenous*.)

Exotoxin: A toxin released by living micro-organisms into the surrounding medium or tissues–*page* 29.

Facultative: Able to behave in a specified way, with the implication that this is not however the usual behaviour–e.g. facultative *anaerobe* (q.v.)–*page* 27.

Fimbria (plural *fimbriae*): Hair-like protrusions from bacterial cells, shorter than a *flagellum* (q.v.). Synonym *pilus*–*page* 18.

Flagellum (plural *flagella*): Whip-like organ of motion possessed by some bacteria and protozoa–*pages* 18, 86, 225.

Formites (Latin, 3 syllables): Literally 'kindling wood', hence personal properties liable to convey agents that initiate diseases–*pages* 7 and 48.

Genome: The total genetic material of an organism; the nucleic acid core of a virus–*page* 19.

Genotype: Genetic composition, whether manifest or not–*page* 32. (Cf. *phenotype*.)

Gram-negative: Staining red by Gram's method, through losing the primary stain during decolorization and taking up the counter-stain–*page* 91.

Gram-positive: Staining violet or blue by Gram's method, through retention of the primary stain–*page* 91.

Growth factor: An ingredient of which at least a small amount must be present in a culture medium in order that it may support the growth of a given organism or group of organisms–*page* 28.

Haemolysis: Disruption of red blood cells. In connection with growth of streptococci on blood agar, destruction of all red cells around a colony and decolorization of the medium is called β-haemolysis, whereas destruction of most of the red cells and production of a green pigment is called α-haemolysis–*page* 99.

Hapten: A substance which acts as an antigenic stimulus only when combined with a protein, but which, even in the uncombined state, can react with the resultant antibody in the manner of a true antigen–*page* 60.

Heterologous: Related to a different kind of organism, a different disease, etc.–e.g. an *anamnestic reaction* (q.v.) is due to a heterologous stimulus.

Homologous: Related to the same kind of organism, the same disease, etc.–e.g. diphtheria requires treatment with homologous serum, serum containing diphtheria antitoxin.

In vitro: 'In glass', hence in laboratory apparatus.

In vivo: In a living animal or human being.

Inclusion bodies: Aggregates of virus particles, visible by light microscopy after appropriate staining, within the nuclei or the cytoplasm of infected cells–*pages* 169 and 177.

Inducible (enzyme): Produced only in the presence of an appropriate substrate–*page* 27. (Cf. *constitutive*.)

Infection: The arrival or presence of potentially pathogenic organisms on the surface or in the tissues of an appropriate host–*page* 45.

Inoculation: (1) of man or animals: Introduction of material containing micro-organisms or their products into the tissues–usually for prophylactic purposes in the case of man.

(2) of culture media: Introduction into a fluid medium, or application to the surface of a solid medium, of material known or suspected of containing living organisms–e.g. Fig. 2–*page* 89.

Inoculum: The particular portion of material used for a single inoculation.

Interference (by viruses): Modification of host cells infected with one type of virus so that other viruses are unable to multiply in them–*page* 176.

L-form: Cell-wall deficient mutant bacterium–*page* 87. (Cf. *protoplast*, *spheroplast*.)

Lyophilization: Combined freezing and desiccation (freeze-drying), a means of long-term preservation of micro-organisms–*page* 37.

Lysis: Disruption (literally 'dissolving') of a microbial or other cell–*page* 65.

Lysogenic conversion: Alteration of the properties of a bacterium as a result of *lysogeny* (q.v.)–*page* 212.

Lysogeny: A temporary stable relationship between a bacteriophage and its bacterial host, in which the phage is reproduced in step with the bacterium and thus handed on to succeeding generations of bacteria –*page* 212.

Micro-aerophile: An organism which grows best in sub-atmospheric concentrations of oxygen–*page* 27.

Monolayer: A sheet of tissue-culture cells one cell thick–*page* 174.

Mutation: An alteration in genetic material–*page* 32.

Nucleoid (virus): Former synonym of *genome* (q.v.).

Nucleocapsid: The genome and *capsid* (q.v.) of a virus–*page* 170.

Pandemic (noun or adjective): World-wide *epidemic* (q.v.)–*page* 46.

Passage (French): Administration of a micro-organism to a host and its subsequent recovery from the host, usually carried out with a view to modifying the pathogenicity of the organism–*page* 179.

Passive (immunity, immunization): Dependent upon injection of ready-made antibodies and not upon the subject's own immunological mechanisms–*page* 56. (Cf. *active*.)

Pathogenic: Actually producing or capable of producing disease–*page* 24. (*Cf. commensal, symbiotic.*)

Petri dish: A shallow circular flat-bottomed glass or plastic dish used as a container for solid media–*page* 88.

Phage-type: The identity of a bacterial strain as indicated by its sensitivity or resistance to the lytic action of the members of a standard panel of bacteriophages (its 'phage-pattern'); *or* a group of strains having identical or closely similar phage-patterns–*pages* 97 and 211.

Phenotype: That part of the *genotype* (q.v.) of an organism which is expressed in a given situation–*page* 34.

Pilus (plural *pili*): Synonym of *fimbria* (q.v.).

Plaque: A small roughly circular deficiency in the growth of a bacterial culture on a solid medium, resulting from local destruction of bacteria by bacteriophages–*page* 211.

Plasmid: An extrachromosomal portion of genetic material (DNA)–*page* 34.

Prophage: Bacteriophage in a lysogenic relationship with its host–*page* 212. (See *lysogeny*.)

Protoplast: A bacterium deprived of its cell wall and thus highly susceptible to osmotic distension and rupture–*page* 17. (Cf. *L-form, spheroplast*.)

Prozone: See *zoning*.

Reagin(s): *Either* the serum component responsible for the Wassermann and related reactions–*page* 262; *or* the antibodies associated with certain types of hypersensitivity reactions–*pages* 61 and 74.

Replication: Virus reproduction, so called to emphasize that a virus does not reproduce *itself* but causes the host cell to make replicas of it–*pages* 19 and 172.

Saprophytic: Living on dead organic matter–*page* 23.

Satellitism: Enhancement of bacterial growth on a solid medium around a source of a growth factor–*page* 138.

Selective medium: A solid culture medium on which all but the desired microbial species are wholly or largely inhibited–*page* 128. A *selective enrichment medium* is a fluid medium in which the desired species can multiply more rapidly than others likely to be present, so that a sample subsequently taken from it for inoculation of plate cultures is 'richer' than the original material in organisms of the desired species–*page* 128. (Cf. *enrichment medium*.)

Septicaemia: Presence and multiplication of pathogenic bacteria in the blood stream, with consequent and often severe illness–*page* 55. (Cf. *bacteraemia*.)

Serology: Study of the antibody content of sera–*page* 257–and also use of antisera in the antigenic analysis of micro-organisms and their products.

Serotype: The identity of a bacterial strain as indicated by antigenic analysis: *or* a group of strains shown by serological tests to be antigenically identical or closely similar–*page* 126. (Synonyms: antigenic type, serological type.)

Specific: (1) relating to a species.

(2) relating particularly to some other unit–e.g. type-specific. Hence commonly used in much the same sense as *homologous* (q.v.).

Spheroplast: A bacterium similar to a *protoplast* (q.v.) except that the cell-wall damage is partial and reversible–*page* 87. (Cf. *L-form.*)

Spirochaete: A member of one of a group of genera of spiral bacteria–*page* 153.

Sterilization: The process of making sterile, i.e. free from all living micro-organisms–*page* 36.

Strain (of an organism): A culture all members of which are believed to be the progeny of a single organism–*page* 84. (This is not an entirely satisfactory definition, and indeed the variations which inevitably accompany bacterial reproduction make the whole concept of a 'pure' strain fallacious.)

Symbiotic: Living in a mutually beneficial relationship with the host –*page* 23. (Cf. *commensal, pathogenic.*)

Synergy (between antimicrobial drugs): Action of a combination of drugs which exceeds the sum of the actions of the drugs used singly–*page* 328.

Temperate phage: A phage capable of a lysogenic relationship with its bacterial host–*page* 212. (See *lysogeny, prophage.*)

Titre: The highest dilution of a serum or an antigen preparation which gives a positive reaction under defined conditions–*page* 258.

Toxoid: Toxin rendered harmless but still effective as an antigen–*page* 309.

Transduction: Conveyance of genetic characters from one bacterial strain to another by means of a transfer of bacteriophage–*page* 33.

Transformation: Acquisition of genetic characters of one bacterial strain by a related strain grown in the presence of DNA from the first strain–*page* 33.

Transport medium: A medium which increases the chances of survival of a micro-organism during transit from the patient to the laboratory –*page* 236.

Vaccination: Originally, the use of cowpox material or of vaccinia virus in active immunization against smallpox; then all forms of active immunization using live organisms; now all forms of active immunization–*page* 308.

Vaccine: Material used in vaccination; therefore this term also has an expanding meaning–*page* 308.

Viraemia: Presence of viruses in the blood-stream–*page* 177.

Virion: A virus particle, the virus unit corresponding to a single cell of a larger organism–*page* 19.

Zoning: The occurrence of an antigen-antibody reaction when a serum is adequately diluted but not when it is used at higher concentrations –*page* 69. (Synonym: the *prozone* phenomenon.)

B

Meanings of Some Abbreviations

Convenient though abbreviations may be, they are liable to cause confusion by meaning different things to specialists in different fields. The meanings given below are those which the appropriate abbreviations customarily have when they are encountered in the field of medical microbiology. The use of capital letters without intervening stops–e.g. DNA–has become conventional for abbreviations of chemical names and is extending into other fields. The terms are further explained on the pages cited.

A.A.F.B.   acid-alcohol-fast bacilli–*page* 145 and Appendix A.
A.F.B.   acid-fast bacilli–*page* 145 and Appendix A.
A.H.G.   anti-human globulin (antibodies, serum)–*page* 71.
A.P.M.   anterior poliomyelitis–*page* 186.
A.P.T.   alum precipitated toxoid–*page* 313.
A.R.T.   automated reaginic test–*page* 263.
A.S.O.   antistreptolysin O–*page* 100.
A.T.S.   anti-tetanus serum–*page* 314.
B.C.G.   Bacille Calmette Guerin–*page* 310.
C.F.T.   complement-fixation test–*page* 70.
C.I.E.   countercurrent immunoelectrophoresis–*page* 5.
C.P.E.   cytopathic effect–*page* 174 and Appendix A.
C.S.F.   cerebrospinal fluid – *page* 253.
C.S.U.   catheter specimen of urine–*page* 250.
D.C.A.   deoxycholate citrate agar–*page* 128.
DMCT   demethylchlortetracycline–*page* 349.
DNA   deoxyribonucleic acid–*page* 18.
E.B.   Epstein-Barr (virus)–*page* 204.
ECHO   enteric cytopathic human orphan (viruses)–*page* 188.

ELISA	enzyme-linked immunosorbent assay–*page* 72.
E.M.U.(E.M.S.U.)	early morning (specimen of) urine–*page* 250.
F.T.	formol toxoid–*page* 312.
F.T.A.T.	fluorescent treponemal antibody test–*page* 263.
G.C.	gonococcus–*page* 108.
G.C.F.T.	gonococcal complement-fixation test–*page* 109.
G.L.C.	gas-liquid chromatography–*page* 5.
H	flagellar (antigens, antibodies)–from German *Hauch*, see *page* 124.
HBcAg etc.	antigenic components of hepatitis B virus–*page* 209.
H.V.S	high vaginal swab–*page* 252.
IDU	idoxuridine–*page* 180.
IgA, IgE, etc.	immunoglobulins of classes A, E, etc.–*page* 61.
INAH	isonicotinic acid hydrazide = isoniazid–*page* 356.
K	capsular or envelope (antigens, antibodies)–*page* 124.
LD 50	dose lethal to 50% of a group of experimental animals–*page* 50.
L.F.	lactose-fermenter–*page* 123
LGV	lymphogranuloma venereum–*page* 167.
M.B.C.	minimal bactericidal concentration–*page* 338.
M.I.C.	minimal inhibitory concentration–*page* 338.
M.L.D.	minimum lethal dose (of a drug or microbial preparation).
mRNA	messenger ribonucleic acid–*page* 41.
M.S.U.(M.S.S.U.)	mid-stream (specimen of) urine–*page* 249.
N.G.U.	non-gonococcal urethritis–*page* 168.
N.L.F.	non-lactose-fermenter–*page* 123.
N.S.U.	non-specific urethritis–*page* 168.
O	somatic (antigens, antibodies)–from German *ohne Hauch*, see *page* 124.
O.T.	old tuberculin–*page* 266.
PABA	*p*-aminobenzoic acid–*page* 40.
PAS	*p*-aminosalicylic acid–*page* 356.
P.P.D.	purified protein derivative (of old tuberculin)–*page* 266.
PPLO	pleuropneumonia-like organisms–*page* 158.
P.T.A.H.	purified toxoid, aluminium hydroxide–*page* 313.
P.T.A.P.	purified toxoid, aluminium phosphate–*page* 313.
P.U.O.	pyrexia of unknown origin–*page* 262.
R.D.E.	receptor-destroying enzyme (= neuraminidase)–*page* 193.

REO	respiratory enteric orphan (viruses)–*page* 189.
RNA	ribonucleic acid–*page* 18.
R.P.C.F.T.	Reiter protein complement-fixation test–*page* 263.
R.P.R.	rapid plasma reagin (test)–*page* 262.
R.S.(R.S.V.)	respiratory syncytial (virus)–*page* 196.
R.T.D.	routine test dilution (of bacteriophage)–*page* 97.
S (as in 7S, etc.)	Svedberg units–*page* 61.
T.A.B. (T.A.B.C.)	typhoid + paratyphoids A and B (and C) vaccine–*page* 312.
T.A.F.	toxoid-antitoxin floccules–*page* 313.
T.B.	tubercle bacilli–*page* 144–and hence loosely used to denote tuberculosis.
T.C.B.S.	thiosulphate citrate bile salts sucrose (agar)–*page* 136.
T.P.H.A.	*Treponema pallidum* haemagglutination (test)–*page* 264.
T.P.I.	*Treponema pallidum* immobilization (test)–*page* 263.
TRIC	trachoma and inclusion conjunctivitis agents–*page* 167.
T.T.	(1) tetanus toxoid–*page* 313.
	(2) tuberculin tested (cattle)–*page* 267.
U.H.T.	Ultra heat treated (milk)–*page* 299.
U.V.	ultra-violet (light).
Vi	virulence (antigen of *S. typhi*, etc.)–*page* 129.
V.D.R.L.	Venereal Disease Research Laboratory (test)–*page* 262.
V.Z.	varicella-zoster (virus)–*page* 202.
W.R.	Wassermann reaction–*page* 262.
Z.N.	Ziehl-Neelsen (staining method)–*page* 145.

Index